Sport Modalities, Performance and Health

Sport Modalities, Performance and Health

Editors

**José Alberto Frade Martins Parraca
Diego Muñoz Marín
Bernardino Javier Sánchez-Alcaraz Martínez**

MDPI • Basel • Beijing • Wuhan • Barcelona • Belgrade • Manchester • Tokyo • Cluj • Tianjin

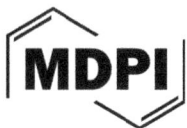

Editors

José Alberto Frade Martins
Parraca
Departamento de Desporto e
Saúde
Universidade de Évora
Évora
Portugal

Diego Muñoz Marín
Faculty of Sport Sciences
University of Extremadura
Caceres
Spain

Bernardino Javier
Sánchez-Alcaraz Martínez
Faculty of Sport Sciences,
University of Murcia
University of Murcia
Murcia
Spain

Editorial Office
MDPI
St. Alban-Anlage 66
4052 Basel, Switzerland

This is a reprint of articles from the Special Issue published online in the open access journal *International Journal of Environmental Research and Public Health* (ISSN 1660-4601) (available at: www.mdpi.com/journal/ijerph/special_issues/sport_modalities).

For citation purposes, cite each article independently as indicated on the article page online and as indicated below:

LastName, A.A.; LastName, B.B.; LastName, C.C. Article Title. *Journal Name* **Year**, *Volume Number*, Page Range.

ISBN 978-3-0365-3342-1 (Hbk)
ISBN 978-3-0365-3341-4 (PDF)

© 2022 by the authors. Articles in this book are Open Access and distributed under the Creative Commons Attribution (CC BY) license, which allows users to download, copy and build upon published articles, as long as the author and publisher are properly credited, which ensures maximum dissemination and a wider impact of our publications.

The book as a whole is distributed by MDPI under the terms and conditions of the Creative Commons license CC BY-NC-ND.

Contents

About the Editors vii

Aldo Seffrin, Beat Knechtle, Rodrigo Luiz Vancini, Douglas de Assis Teles Santos, Claudio Andre Barbosa de Lira and Lee Hill et al.
Origin of the Fastest 5 km, 10 km and 25 km Open-Water Swimmers—An Analysis from 20 Years and 9819 Swimmers
Reprinted from: *Int. J. Environ. Res. Public Health* **2021**, *18*, 11369, doi:10.3390/ijerph182111369 . 1

Adrien Mater, Pierre Clos and Romuald Lepers
Effect of Cycling Cadence on Neuromuscular Function: A Systematic Review of Acute and Chronic Alterations
Reprinted from: *Int. J. Environ. Res. Public Health* **2021**, *18*, 7912, doi:10.3390/ijerph18157912 . . . 13

Joana Barreto, Filipe Casanova, César Peixoto, Bradley Fawver and Andrew Mark Williams
How Task Constraints Influence the Gaze and Motor Behaviours of Elite-Level Gymnasts
Reprinted from: *Int. J. Environ. Res. Public Health* **2021**, *18*, 6941, doi:10.3390/ijerph18136941 . . . 27

Mabliny Thuany, Beat Knechtle, Thomas Rosemann, Marcos B. Almeida and Thayse Natacha Gomes
Running around the Country: An Analysis of the Running Phenomenon among Brazilian Runners
Reprinted from: *Int. J. Environ. Res. Public Health* **2021**, *18*, 6610, doi:10.3390/ijerph18126610 . . . 39

Henrique Nascimento, Clara Martinez-Perez, Cristina Alvarez-Peregrina and Miguel Ángel Sánchez-Tena
Reply to Laby, D.M.; Appelbaum, L.G. Comment on "Nascimento et al. Citations Network Analysis of Vision and Sport. *Int. J. Environ. Res. Public Health* 2020, *17*, 7574"
Reprinted from: *Int. J. Environ. Res. Public Health* **2021**, *18*, 6521, doi:10.3390/ijerph18126521 . . . 49

Daniel M. Laby and Lawrence G. Appelbaum
Comment on Nascimento et al. Citations Network Analysis of Vision and Sport. *Int. J. Environ. Res. Public Health* 2020, *17*, 7574
Reprinted from: *Int. J. Environ. Res. Public Health* **2021**, *18*, 6488, doi:10.3390/ijerph18126488 . . . 51

Francisco Pradas, María Pía Cádiz, María Teresa Nestares, Inmaculada C. Martínez-Díaz and Luis Carrasco
Effects of Padel Competition on Brain Health-Related Myokines
Reprinted from: *Int. J. Environ. Res. Public Health* **2021**, *18*, 6042, doi:10.3390/ijerph18116042 . . . 53

Henrique Nascimento, Clara Martinez-Perez, Cristina Alvarez-Peregrina and Miguel Ángel Sánchez-Tena
The Role of Social Media in Sports Vision
Reprinted from: *Int. J. Environ. Res. Public Health* **2021**, *18*, 5354, doi:10.3390/ijerph18105354 . . . 65

Francisco Pradas, David Falcón, Carlos Peñarrubia-Lozano, Víctor Toro-Román, Luis Carrasco and Carlos Castellar
Effects of Ultratrail Running on Neuromuscular Function, Muscle Damage and Hydration Status. Differences According to Training Level
Reprinted from: *Int. J. Environ. Res. Public Health* **2021**, *18*, 5119, doi:10.3390/ijerph18105119 . . . 75

Adrián Escudero-Tena, Bernardino Javier Sánchez-Alcaraz, Javier García-Rubio and Sergio J. Ibáñez
Analysis of Game Performance Indicators during 2015–2019 World Padel Tour Seasons and Their Influence on Match Outcome
Reprinted from: *Int. J. Environ. Res. Public Health* **2021**, *18*, 4904, doi:10.3390/ijerph18094904 . . . 89

Elena Pardos-Mainer, Chris Bishop, Oliver Gonzalo-Skok, Hadi Nobari, Jorge Pérez-Gómez and Demetrio Lozano
Associations between Inter-Limb Asymmetries in Jump and Change of Direction Speed Tests and Physical Performance in Adolescent Female Soccer Players
Reprinted from: *Int. J. Environ. Res. Public Health* **2021**, *18*, 3474, doi:10.3390/ijerph18073474 . . . 97

Aldo A. Vasquez-Bonilla, Alba Camacho-Cardeñosa, Rafael Timón, Ismael Martínez-Guardado, Marta Camacho-Cardeñosa and Guillermo Olcina
Muscle Oxygen Desaturation and Re-Saturation Capacity Limits in Repeated Sprint Ability Performance in Women Soccer Players: A New Physiological Interpretation
Reprinted from: *Int. J. Environ. Res. Public Health* **2021**, *18*, 3484, doi:10.3390/ijerph18073484 . . . 111

Andreas Konrad, Richard Močnik, Sylvia Titze, Masatoshi Nakamura and Markus Tilp
The Influence of Stretching the Hip Flexor Muscles on Performance Parameters. A Systematic Review with Meta-Analysis
Reprinted from: *Int. J. Environ. Res. Public Health* **2021**, *18*, 1936, doi:10.3390/ijerph18041936 . . . 125

Alejandro Sánchez-Pay, Rafael Martínez-Gallego, Miguel Crespo and David Sanz-Rivas
Key Physical Factors in the Serve Velocity of Male Professional Wheelchair Tennis Players
Reprinted from: *Int. J. Environ. Res. Public Health* **2021**, *18*, 1944, doi:10.3390/ijerph18041944 . . . 145

Hanming Li, Xingquan Chen and Yiwei Fang
The Development Strategy of Home-Based Exercise in China Based on the SWOT-AHP Model
Reprinted from: *Int. J. Environ. Res. Public Health* **2021**, *18*, 1224, doi:10.3390/ijerph18031224 . . . 155

Bernardino Javier Sánchez-Alcaraz, Rafael Martínez-Gallego, Salvador Llana, Goran Vučković, Diego Muñoz and Javier Courel-Ibáñez et al.
Ball Impact Position in Recreational Male Padel Players: Implications for Training and Injury Management
Reprinted from: *Int. J. Environ. Res. Public Health* **2021**, *18*, 435, doi:10.3390/ijerph18020435 . . . 167

Javier Alves, Gema Barrientos, Víctor Toro, Francisco Javier Grijota, Diego Muñoz and Marcos Maynar
Correlations between Basal Trace Minerals and Hormones in Middle and Long-Distance High-Level Male Runners
Reprinted from: *Int. J. Environ. Res. Public Health* **2020**, *17*, 9473, doi:10.3390/ijerph17249473 . . . 177

Jesús Ramón-Llin, José Guzmán, Rafael Martínez-Gallego, Diego Muñoz, Alejandro Sánchez-Pay and Bernardino J. Sánchez-Alcaraz
Stroke Analysis in Padel According to Match Outcome and Game Side on Court
Reprinted from: *Int. J. Environ. Res. Public Health* **2020**, *17*, 7838, doi:10.3390/ijerph17217838 . . . 189

Henrique Nascimento, Clara Martinez-Perez, Cristina Alvarez-Peregrina and Miguel Ángel Sánchez-Tena
Citations Network Analysis of Vision and Sport
Reprinted from: *Int. J. Environ. Res. Public Health* **2020**, *17*, 7574, doi:10.3390/ijerph17207574 . . . 199

Bernardino J. Sánchez-Alcaraz, Daniel T. Perez-Puche, Francisco Pradas, Jesús Ramón-Llín, Alejandro Sánchez-Pay and Diego Muñoz
Analysis of Performance Parameters of the Smash in Male and Female Professional Padel
Reprinted from: *Int. J. Environ. Res. Public Health* **2020**, *17*, 7027, doi:10.3390/ijerph17197027 . . . **221**

Víctor Toro, Jesús Siquier-Coll, Ignacio Bartolomé, María C. Robles-Gil, Javier Rodrigo and Marcos Maynar-Mariño
Effects of *Tetraselmis chuii* Microalgae Supplementation on Ergospirometric, Haematological and Biochemical Parameters in Amateur Soccer Players
Reprinted from: *Int. J. Environ. Res. Public Health* **2020**, *17*, 6885, doi:10.3390/ijerph17186885 . . . **231**

Hae Joo Nam, Joon-Hee Lee, Dae-Seok Hong and Hyun Chul Jung
The Effect of Wearing a Customized Mouthguard on Body Alignment and Balance Performance in Professional Basketball Players
Reprinted from: *Int. J. Environ. Res. Public Health* **2020**, *17*, 6431, doi:10.3390/ijerph17176431 . . . **243**

Javier Alves, Víctor Toro, Gema Barrientos, Ignacio Bartolomé, Diego Muñoz and Marcos Maynar
Hormonal Changes in High-Level Aerobic Male Athletes during a Sports Season
Reprinted from: *Int. J. Environ. Res. Public Health* **2020**, *17*, 5833, doi:10.3390/ijerph17165833 . . . **253**

About the Editors

José Alberto Frade Martins Parraca

José Alberto Frade Martins Parraça completed a Degree in Sports Science (2006/06/23) at the University of Évora, a PhD in Physiology (2012/05/05) at the "Universidad de Extremadura"and Master's Degree in "Ejercicio e Salud"in (2010/05/16) at the "Universidad Internacional de Andalucía". He is an Assistant Professor at the University of Évoran and has published numerous articles in specialized journals. He also participates and/or has participated as a researcher in several projects, being the principal investigator in several of them.

Diego Muñoz Marín

Diego Munoz Mariño, born in Lorca (Murcia), is currently a full professor at the University of Extremadura's Faculty of Sports Sciences.

He graduated in Sciences of Physical Activity and Sports in the year 2000. He studied for a doctorate in the Department of Physiology of the University of Extremadura, obtaining a degree of Doctor in the year 2007.

He was an assistant professor at the Faculty of Sports Sciences starting from 2007, being promoted to Professor Contracted Doctor in 2010. His main lines of research are related to the physiology of exercise, health, and training, with particular focus on the sport of paddle tennis. He has been published in numerous national and international scientific publications, and is currently being recognized for two six-year research periods by the National Agency for Quality Assessment and Accreditation (ANECA).

Bernardino Javier Sánchez-Alcaraz Martínez

Bernardino Javier Sánchez-Alcaraz Martínez obtained a degree in Physical Activity and Sports Sciences from the Catholic University of San Antonio, starting in 2009, and Diploma in Physical Education Teaching from the Camilo Jose Cela University, from 2012. In addition, he passed the Training Master of the Teacher of Compulsory Secondary Education from the University of Murcia in 2010 and the Official Master of Management and Administration of Sports Entities in 2011. He has been a Doctor in Physical Activity and Sports Sciences, having attended the University of Murcia, since the year 2014. Currently, he is a professor of the subject of Methodological Aspects of Physical Activity and Sport at the Faculty of Sports Sciences of the University of Murcia.

He highlights as main lines of research the analysis of the aspects that influence the teaching of Physical Education and Sports, as well as the performance of racket sports.

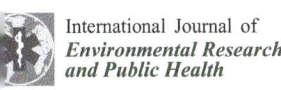

Origin of the Fastest 5 km, 10 km and 25 km Open-Water Swimmers—An Analysis from 20 Years and 9819 Swimmers

Aldo Seffrin [1], Beat Knechtle [2,3,*], Rodrigo Luiz Vancini [4], Douglas de Assis Teles Santos [5], Claudio Andre Barbosa de Lira [6], Lee Hill [7], Thomas Rosemann [3] and Marilia Santos Andrade [1]

1. Department of Physiology, Federal University of São Paulo, São Paulo 04021-001, Brazil; netoseffrin@gmail.com (A.S.); marilia1707@gmail.com (M.S.A.)
2. Medbase St. Gallen Am Vadianplatz, 9000 St. Gallen, Switzerland
3. Institute of Primary Care, University of Zurich, 8006 Zurich, Switzerland; thomas.rosemann@usz.ch
4. Center for Physical Education and Sports, Federal University of Espírito Santo, Vitória 29075-910, Brazil; rodrigo.luiz.vancini@gmail.com
5. Faculty of Physical Education, State University of Bahia, Teixeira de Freitas 45992-255, Brazil; datsantos@uneb.br
6. Human and Exercise Physiology Division, Faculty of Physical Education and Dance, Federal University of Goiás, Goiânia 74690-900, Brazil; andre.claudio@gmail.com
7. Department of Pediatrics, McMaster University, Hamilton, ON L8S 4L8, Canada; hilll14@mcmaster.ca
* Correspondence: beat.knechtle@hispeed.ch; Tel.: +41-(0)-71-226-93-00; Fax: +41-(0)-71-226-93-01

Abstract: In elite pool swimmers competing at world class level, mainly athletes from the United States of America and Australia are dominating. Little is known, however, for the nationality of dominating swimmers in elite open-water long-distance swimming races such as the official FINA races over 5 km, 10 km and 25 km—held since 2000. The aim of this study was to investigate the participation and performance trends by nationality of these elite open-water swimmers. Race results from all female and male swimmers competing in 5 km, 10 km and 25 km FINA races between 2000 and 2020 were analyzed. A total of 9819 swimmers competed between 2000 and 2020 in these races. The five countries that figure most times among the top ten in 5 km, 10 km and 25 km races over the years were Italy, Germany, Russia, Brazil and the Netherlands. In 10 km races, considering the all the athletes from each country, male athletes from Germany, Italy, and France presented faster race times than the other countries. In 10 km, female athletes presented no significant difference among the countries. In 5 and 25 km races, there were no differences between countries, for male and female athletes. Moreover, comparing only the 10 best results (top 10) from each country, there were no differences between countries in 5 km, 10 km and 25 km, for male and female athletes. Men were faster than women for all three distances. In summary, male swimmers from Europe (i.e., Germany, Italy, France) are dominating the 10 km FINA races. In the 5 km and 25 km FINA races, there is no dominating nationality, but among the top five countries in the top 10 over the years, three are European countries.

Keywords: water sport; endurance; origin; nationality

1. Introduction

Competitive open-water swimming (OWS) is a relatively young sports discipline to the Olympic program, but has been a feature of the Fédération Internationale de Natation (FINA) World Championships since 1991 [1]. As the popularity of OWS increased over the years, the 10 km marathon swim race made its debut at the 2008 Olympic Games in Beijing [2]. Although the current Olympic program only offers the 10 km event, the FINA World Championships Ligue Européenne de Natation (LEN) European Championships have an expanded programs including the 5 km, 10 km and 25 km distances, and a recently introduced mixed team relay event [3,4].

The increased number of competitions have stimulated the interest in OWS worldwide and as a result, the number of participants has substantially increased in the last years [5]. Secondly, it is interesting to note that there has been an exponential growth in women participating [5], including a trend towards an over overall higher competitive level of women than of men [5–7]. It has been shown that women were faster than men in the 'Triple Crown of Open Water Swimming' with 'Catalina Channel Swim', 'English Channel Swim' and 'Manhattan Island Marathon Swim' [8]. However, in the 5 km, 10 km and 25 km FINA races, men were faster than women in all race distances [9,10] although women improved their performance in the 10 km race distance, but not for the other distances [10,11]. Interestingly, in the 3000 m FINA World Championships between 1992 and 2014, women were not able to reduce the sex difference in performance to men across years [12].

Regarding to the origin of elite pool swimmers at world class level [13,14], mainly athletes from the United States of America (USA) and Australia (AUS) were more likely to finish in the Top 10 or medal positions [15,16]. However, regarding the relationship between the origin of open-water long-distance swimmers and their performance little is known, and the few published data are not from World Championships [8,17–19]. In the 'English Channel Crossing' between 1875 and 2013, most swimmers were from Great Britain (GB), the USA, AUS and Ireland. Secondly, the fastest swim times were achieved by athletes from the USA, AUS and GB [18] and in the 'Strait of Gibraltar', local Spanish swimmers were the fastest [19]. In long-distance open-water events in the 'Triple Crown of Open Water Swimming' from 1875 to 2017 ('Catalina Channel Swim', 'English Channel Swim' and 'Manhattan Island Marathon Swim') the fastest swimmers were from AUS, USA, GB and Canada [8] were recorded the fastest performances. Therefore, there is little knowledge from where the swimmers competing in world championships originate from [9].

Therefore, the aim of the study was to investigate the participation and performance trends of elite open-water swimmers competing 5 km, 10 km and 25 km races held since 2000. Based upon existing findings for pool and open-water swimmers we hypothesized that the fastest swimmers competing in that discipline would also originate from the USA and AUS.

2. Methods

2.1. Ethical Approval

This study was approved by the Institutional Review Board of Kanton St. Gallen, Switzerland, with a waiver of the requirement for informed consent of the participant as the study involved the analysis of publicly available data (EKSG 01-06-2010).

2.2. Data

Race results from all female and male swimmers competing in 5 km, 10 km and 25 km FINA races between 2000 and 2020 were obtained from the FINA website [4]. From the entire FINA website database of the competitions of 5, 10 and 25 km races, the following data were selected to tabulation and subsequent analysis: nationality, sex, race time, race distance (5, 10 or 25 km), competition date and local.

2.3. Statistical Analysis

Descriptive data were presented by mean, standard deviation, maximum and minimum values. In order to compare race time between sexes, Student-t test for independent samples was used. The mean values of the entire sample and top 10 results of each country and sex were selected for analysis. Data did not follow a normal distribution nor had homogeneous variances according to Shapiro–Wilk and Levene's test, respectively. A generalized linear model (GLM) with a gamma or tweedie probability distribution and identity or log link function was used to assess the effect of nationality of the athlete and the advancement of the years on race time for the entire sample and for top 10 sample the method of choosing the distribution of the dependent variable and the link function was the Akaike information criterion (AIC), using its lowest value. For this analysis, the nationalities were grouped into six groups, the five nationalities that were most present in the top 10 times in each event and one group with the other nationalities by sex. Differences found were investigated with posthoc Bonferroni test. The level of significance was set at 0.05. SPSS version 26.0 (SPSS, Inc., Chicago, IL, USA) was used for all statistical analyses.

3. Results

In order to compare the performance of the countries that participated in the 5, 10 or 25 km swim events, the 5 countries that were most often among the top 10 were first selected (Table 1). The other countries were grouped into a single group called "Others" (Table 1). First, the mean value of each swim distance of all participants from each country (divided by sex) was compared. After this initial analysis, the mean values of each swim distance of the top 10 swimmers of each country were compared. The results section was divided in these two parts. First, data from the entire sample are presented, and, secondly, data from the top 10 comparison are presented.

Table 1. Sum of nationality that figure in the top 10 times in each event by sex.

Distance	Female Nationality	Female (n)	Male Nationality	Male (n)
5 km	Italy	31	Italy	35
	Germany	19	Germany	26
	Russia	19	Russia	25
	USA	17	France	19
	Spain	12	Spain	14
	Others	82	Others	61
10 km	Germany	29	Germany	33
	Italy	25	Italy	28
	Brazil	22	Russia	17
	Russia	14	France	14
	USA	13	Brazil	13
	Others	87	Others	85
25 km	Russia	28	Italy	30
	Italy	27	France	26
	Germany	21	Russia	24
	Spain	14	Germany	12
	USA	11	Czech R.	9
	Others	68	Others	68

3.1. Comparison among All Athletes from Each Country

A total of 9819 swimmers competed between 2000 and 2020 in 5, 10 and 25 km races. Most of the swimmers (76.1%) competed in the 10 km (n = 7476, 3227 women and 4249 men), followed by 5 km (16%, n = 1575, 740 women and 835 men) and 25 km (7.9%, n = 768, 323 women and 445 men).

The 5 km event (n = 1575) had a total mean time of 01:00:15 ± 05:12 (minimum 00:51:17/maximum 01:47:37) h:min:s, the 10 km event (n = 7476) had a mean time of 02:02:21 ± 11:43 (minimum 01:29:51/maximum 03:01:00) h:min:s, while the 25 km (n = 768) had a mean time of 05:23:07 ± 27:30 (minimum 04:10:41/maximum 07:02:38) h:min:s for the entire sample. The time spend in each distance by each sex were presented in Table 2.

Table 2. Race time in each event by sex.

		Female		Male		
Event	n (%)	Time	n (%)	Time		p Value *
5 km	740 (47)	01:02:40 ± 04:29 (00:55:40/01:31:43)	835 (53)	00:58:07 ± 04:50 (00:51:17/01:47:37)		<0.001
10 km	3227 (43.2)	02:07:29 ± 11:20 (01:37:29/03:01:00)	4249 (56.8)	01:58:27 ± 10:27 (01:29:51/02:46:56)		<0.001
25 km	323 (42.1)	05:37:36 ± 24:35 (04:18:28/07:02:38)	445 (59.1)	05:12:36 ± 24:34 (04:10:41/06:39:33)		<0.001

n = sample size; % = percentage values; * $p < 0.05$ (race time for male group was significantly lower than for female group).

Regarding nationality, there were observed no significant differences on the mean time in the 5 km events for females [x^2 (5) = 3.608, p = 0.607, AIC = 10,297.59] (Figure 1a) and males (Figure 1b) [x^2 (5) = 9.706, p = 0.084, AIC = 11,669.47]. In addition, there was a significant effect of the advancement of the years on the mean time in the 5 km events for males [x^2 (1) = 27.880, p < 0.001], a reduction of 11,906 s/year [IC = −16.325/−7.486], but not for females [x^2 (1) = 2.978, p = 0.084] (Figure 2a).

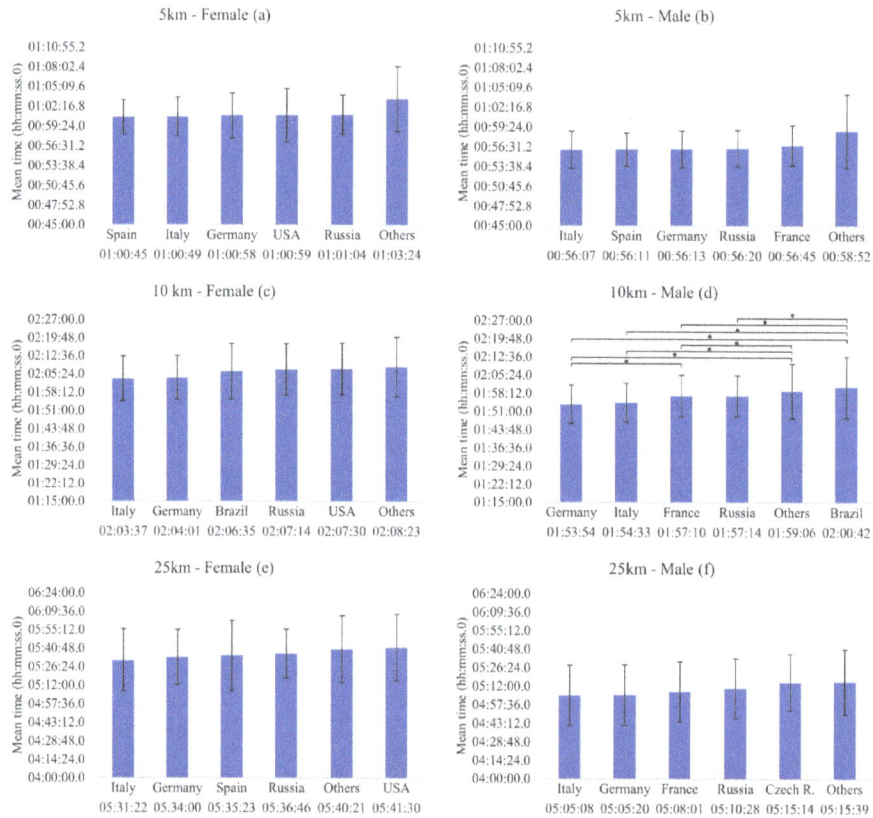

Figure 1. Mean race times and significant differences among nationalities, regarding the entire sample, in the female and male 5, 10 and 25 km events. * $p < 0.005$.

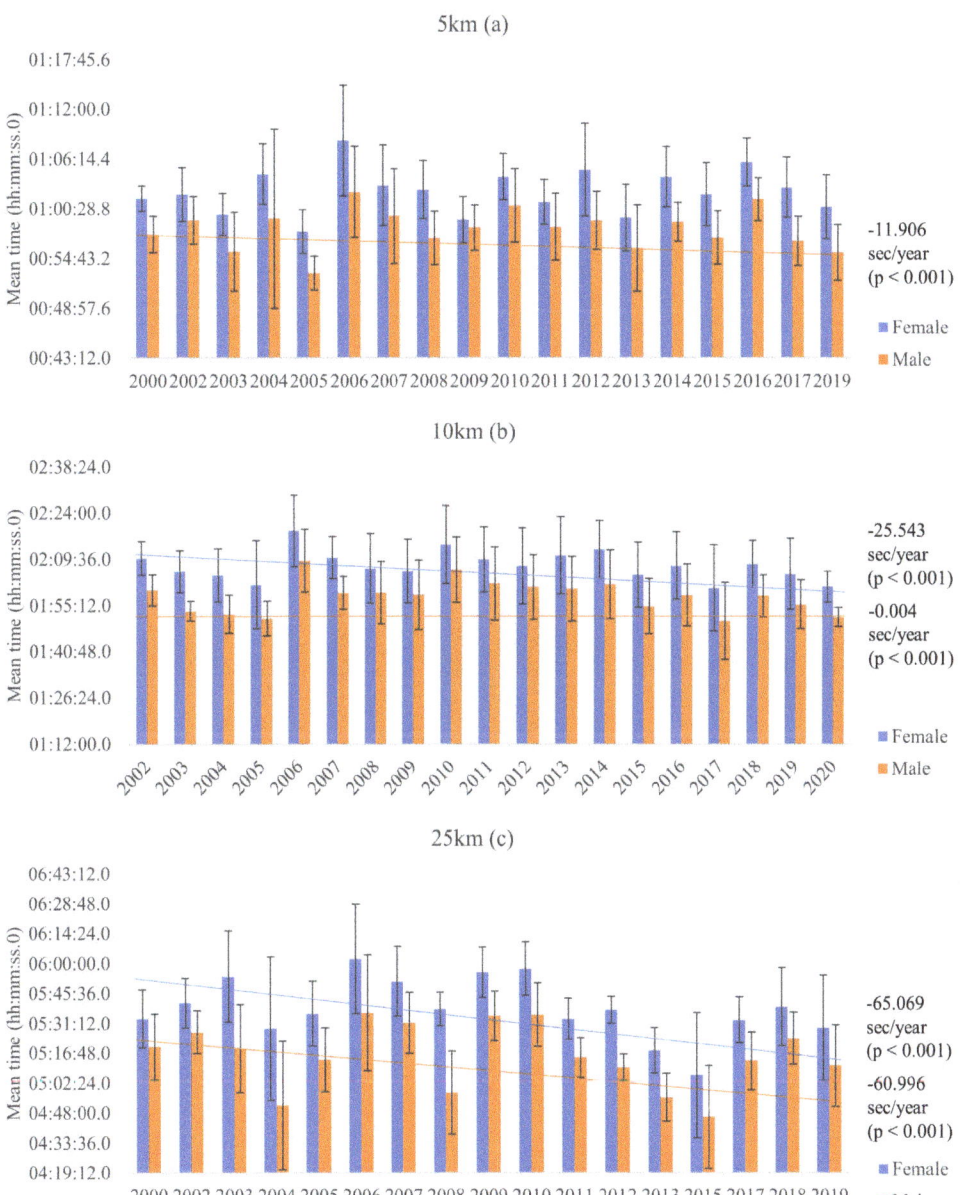

Figure 2. Mean values, of entire sample results, for each race over the years for both sexes in 5, 10 and 25 km events.

For 10 km events, no significant differences on the mean time were found based on the nationality of the athlete for females [x^2 (5) = 6.035, p = 0.303, AIC = 51,047.39] (Figure 1c), but there were significant differences on the mean time in the 10 km events for males [x^2 (5) = 26.388, $p < 0.001$, AIC = 66,358.82], where Germany, Italy and France presented significantly better times than the other countries (Figure 1d). Besides that, there was a significant effect of the advancement of the years on the mean time in the 10km events for females [x^2 (1) = 50.672, $p < 0.001$], a reduction of 25.543 s/year [IC = −32.576/−18.510], and for males [x^2 (1) = 76.638, $p < 0.001$], a reduction of 0.004 s/year [IC = −0.005/−0.004] (Figure 2b).

No significant differences on the mean time of 25 km events were found based on nationality of the athlete for females [x^2 (5) = 9.417, $p = 0.094$, AIC = 5617.71] (Figure 1e) and males [x^2 (5) = 1.384, $p = 0.926$, AIC = 7755.62] (Figure 1f). Moreover, there was a significant effect of the advancement of the years on the mean time in the 25 km events for females [x^2 (1) = 10.683, $p = 0.001$], a reduction of 65.069 s/year [IC = −104.089/−26.049], and for males [x^2 (1) = 12.197, $p < 0.001$], a reduction of 60.996 s/year [IC = −95.227/−26.765] (Figure 2c).

3.2. Comparison between Top 10 Athletes from Each Country

Comparing the race time mean among the top ten athletes from each nationality, there were no significant differences on the mean time in the 5 km events for females [x^2 (5) = 3.903, $p = 0.5.64$, AIC = 2269.27] (Figure 3a) and males (Figure 3b) [x^2 (5) = 2.002, $p = 0.849$, AIC = 2264.16] based on the nationality of the athlete. In addition, there were no significant effect of the advancement of the years on the mean time in the 5 km events for females [x^2 (1) = 0.095, $p = 0.759$] and males [x^2 (1) = 1.330, $p = 0.249$] (Figure 4a).

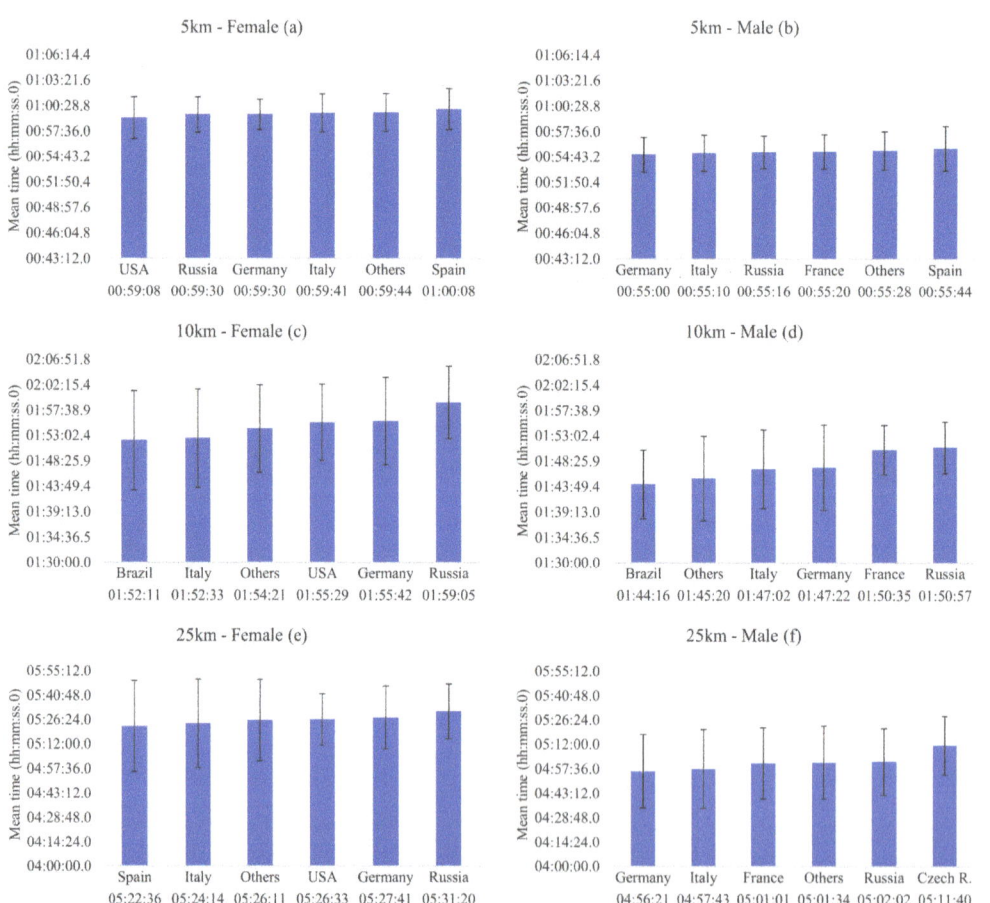

Figure 3. Mean race times for each nationality, regarding the top 10 sample, in the female and male 5, 10 and 25 km events.

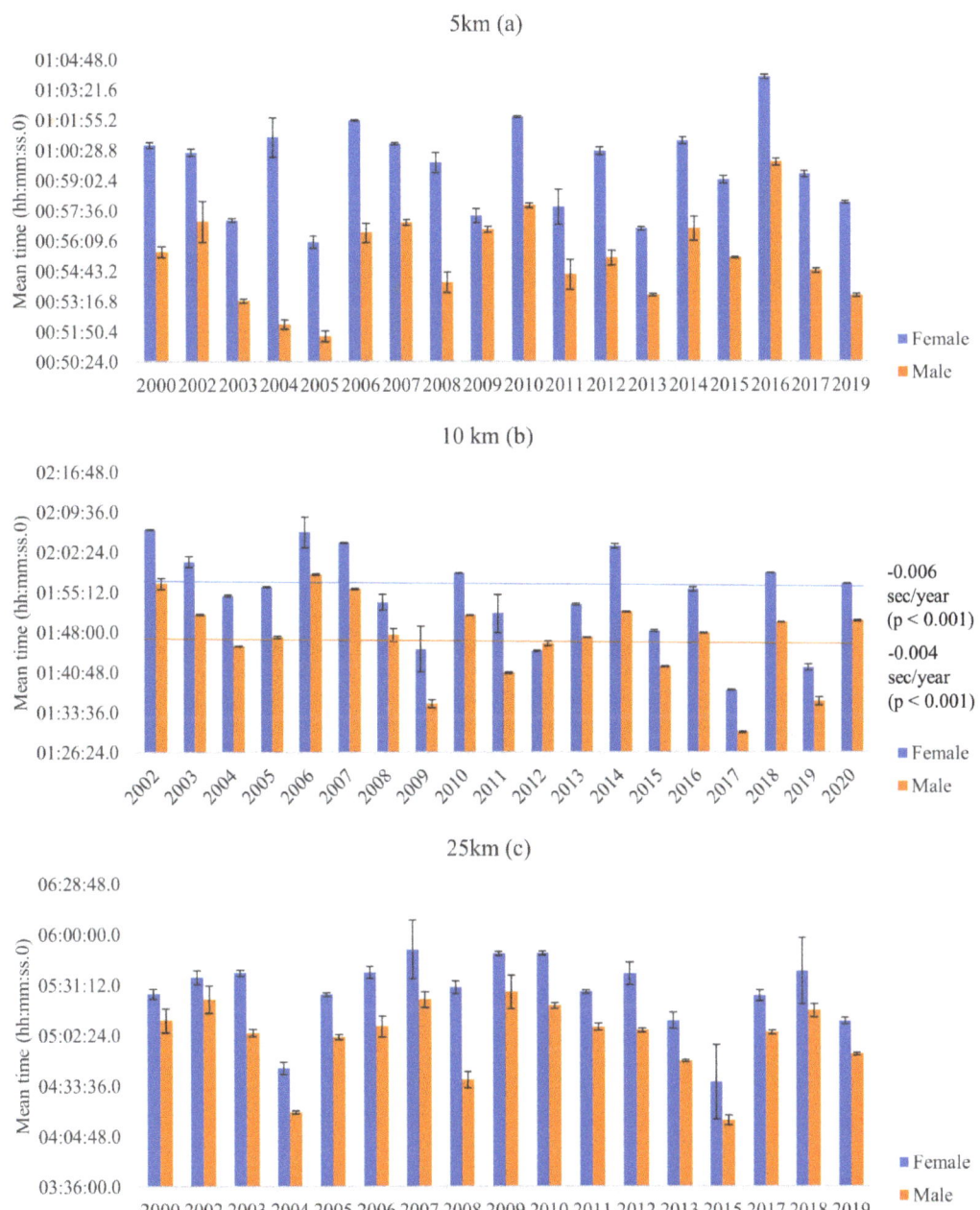

Figure 4. Mean values, of top 10 sample results, for each race over the years for both sexes in 5, 10 and 25 km events.

For 10 km events, no significant differences on the mean time were found based on the nationality of the athlete for females [x^2 (5) = 1.936, p = 0.858, AIC = 2870.49] (Figure 3c), and males [x^2 (5) = 6.852, p = 0.232, AIC = 2825.39] (Figure 3d). Besides that, there was a small but significant effect of the advancement of the years on the mean time in the 10 km events for females [x^2 (1) = 29.530, p < 0.001], a reduction of 0.006 s/year [IC = −0.009/−0.004], and for males [x^2 (1) = 34.709, $p < 0.001$], a reduction of 0.004 s/year [IC = $-0.010/-0.005$] (Figure 4b).

In the same way, no significant differences on the mean time of 25 km events were found based on nationality of the athlete for females [x^2 (5) = 5.415, $p = 0.367$, AIC = 2933.24] (Figure 3e) and males [x^2 (5) = 0.795, $p = 0.977$, AIC = 2934.96] (Figure 3f). Moreover, there were no significant effect of the advancement of the years on the mean time in the 25 km events for females [x^2 (1) = 1.614, $p = 0.204$ and for males [x^2 (1) = 1.359, $p < 0.244$] (Figure 4c).

4. Discussion

This study intended to investigate participation and performance trends by nationality of elite open-water swimmers competing in 5 km, 10 km and 25 km races held between 2000 and 2020. We hypothesized that the fastest swimmers competing in these races would originate from the USA and AUS, similarly to the observations of elite pool swimmers.

The main findings considering the entire sample were, (i) Germany, Italy and France presented significantly better times than the other countries in the 10 km races for males, (ii) there were no differences among the countries in the 10 km races for females, (iii) there were no differences among countries in the 5 km and 25 km races for both sexes, (iv) there were significant decreases among the race times over the last 20 years in 5 km, 10 km and 25 km races for both sexes, except for females in the 5 km event, and (v) male athletes presented better race times in 5 km, 10 km and 25 km races than females. Moreover, considering the top 10 athletes from each country, there were no differences among the countries in the 5 km, 10 km or 25 km races for both males and females.

A first important finding, considering the entire sample, was those male swimmers mainly from Europe were the fastest in 10 km events and the hypothesis that swimmers from the United States of America and Australia would be the fastest could not be confirmed. Regarding female athletes, there were no significant differences in swimming times between nations in the 10 km events, despite athletes from Germany, Italy, Brazil Russia and USA featured more frequently in the top 10 positions. In the 5 km and 25 km events, there was no significant difference in the race times between athletes from different countries for both male and female athletes. Comparing the average time of the 10 best athletes from each country, there were also no significant differences between countries Obviously, the density of high-performance athletes seems to be high in the countries where both all swimmers and the top ten per country were the fastest.

Previous studies investigated the aspect of nationality in long-distance open-water swimming events where non-elite swimmers were performing in a solo event such as the 'English Channel Crossing" [17,18,20], the "Strait of Gibraltar" [19], the "Triple Crown" [8] "Manhattan Island Cross [6], "Maratona del Golfo Capri-Napoli" [7] and the "Robben Island Crossing" [21]. Although some swimmers from the USA and AUS did feature in the solo OWS events could possibly be attributed to non-elite nature of the events. Ultra-long OWS events are often performed on an individual basis by recreational swimmers or swimmers seeking an individual challenge. These events are often self-funded and as a result selects for a very specialized group who wish to complete these challenges, and not necessarily in the fastest time, therefore the characteristics of athletes are very different from those who participate in World Championships.

We found that female swimmers from Italy achieved the best performances and male swimmers from Italy the second-best performances behind Germany although they were not significantly faster than swimmers from other countries. The finding that Italians are among the best in this sport discipline is not accidentally. A very actual study investigating 9247 female and male swimmers competing between 1986 and 2019 in the 3000 m open water swimming Master World Championships found that female and male swimmers from Italy were the fastest during this period of 27 years and 15 editions all over the world [22].

A potential explanation that swimmers from Italy and Germany are the best in the world in this sports discipline could be their national efforts. For example, Italy has its 'Circuito Nuoto in Acque Libere' where open-water swimmers are organized to compete in different formats of open-water swimming [23]. In addition, in Germany, open-water swimming is promoted with information about training, equipment and events [24].

In terms of performance, considering the top 10 results from each country there were no improvement in mean time in the last 20 years, and although a significant decrease in mean times was observed considering the entire sample, sometimes the effect was very small, for example in male 10 km events a reduction of 0.004 s/year was observed. In the 25 km events, there was a slightly greater decrease in time over the years (a reduction of 65.069 s/year for females and a reduction of 60.996 s/year for males).

In other open-water long-distance swimming events, a more expressive improvement in female and male performance has been reported [5,10,13,14,25]. A potential explanation for these small performance improvements over the years could be the relatively short time frame in this specific sports discipline (2000–2020) compared to other open-water long distance swimming events such as the 'English Channel Crossing' [17,26]. It is also interesting to note a large variation in finishing times among the years in the 5, 10 and 25 km events, which may be attributable to the differences in sea or weather conditions. For example, if in one year the athletes swim against the current and in the other year they swim with the current, there can be a great impact on the difference in performance between years for both sexes [27].

Moreover, it is important to consider that the FINA OWS events (5 km, 10 km and 25 km) are measured distances with very little variation compared to the ultra-long solo OWS events. Therefore, as the distances are pre-determined for the 5 km, 10 km and 25 km, swimmers and their coaches are able to plan and execute training accordingly in order to complete the races in the shortest time possible. In contract, the ultra-long solo OWS events require swimmers to complete a distance set between two geographic points [28], and as such may be influenced by several environmental factors, thus changing the objective to reflect completing the challenge rather than defeating a field of other competitors [29,30].

Another important finding was that men were faster than women in all three disciplines. Generally, male performance is better than female performance in a variety of sports disciplines [31–34]. However, in some long-distance open-water swimming events, women were faster than men [20]. A potential explanation that women were slower than men in these 5 km, 10 km and 25 km FINA races could be the fact that these events are not long enough for potential physiological and body composition differences to influence the outcome [7,8]. Previous studies examining ultra-long OWS athletes hypothesized that body composition may have an important role in marathon swimming performance [7,8]. However, FINA races have banned the use of high-performance wetsuits which could potentially mitigate any performance advantage that may be conferred by sex during these events [27]. Moreover, as the events are much shorter than other solo OWS events, which limits water immersion time, which has been reported as a factor affect endurance during marathon swimming [35–37].

A limitation of the present study is that the present study did not assess the effect of age in performance [38]. Thus, the results show comparisons of the best times obtained among all athletes, but it is possible that if the differences in performance of each nationality by age group are studied, different results will be found. A further limitation is that environmental aspects such as temperatures were not considered since open-water swimming races can be characterized by extreme environmental conditions (e.g., water temperature, tides, currents, and waves) which might have an impact on performance, influencing both tactics and pacing [39]. In addition, physiological and anthropometric aspects [40] and race strategies [41,42] were not considered. Finally, the race time of the athletes who competed each year were analyzed, but we are not aware of the possibility that there were athletes who competed in more than one competition.

5. Conclusions

In summary, male swimmers from Europe (Germany, Italy and France), are dominating the 10 km FINA races, but there are no specific country dominations in 5 km or 25 km events for both sexes. The results do not change when all swimmers and only the top ten per country are considered. Future studies might investigate the aspect of nationality in other swimming disciplines such as in master swimming, elite pool swimming and ice swimming.

Author Contributions: Conceptualization, A.S., B.K., D.d.A.T.S. and M.S.A.; Formal analysis, M.S.A. Writing—review & editing, R.L.V., C.A.B.d.L., L.H. and T.R. All authors have read and agreed to the published version of the manuscript.

Funding: This research received no external funding.

Institutional Review Board Statement: The study was conducted according to the guidelines of the Declaration of Helsinki, and approved by the Institutional Review Board of Kanton St. Gallen Switzerland (protocol code EKSG 01-06-2010 and 1 June 2010 of approval).

Informed Consent Statement: Patient consent was waived due to publicly available data.

Data Availability Statement: Data were obtained from https://www.fina.org and are available from the authors upon request.

Conflicts of Interest: The authors declare no conflict of interest.

References

1. FINA. 6th FINA World Championships 1991. 2021. Available online: https://www.fina.org/competitions/1064/6th-fina-world-championships-1991 (accessed on 5 May 2021).
2. Swim England. An Introduction to Open Water Swimming. 2021. Available online: https://www.swimming.org/sport/open-water-swimming/ (accessed on 15 April 2021).
3. FINA. FINA Open Water Swimming Guide. 2018. Available online: https://resources.fina.org/fina/document/2021/02/03/8cd56ca-f5c2-4305-b5e7-aeb5a2c7caf3/ows_guide_new_lr2018.pdf (accessed on 5 April 2021).
4. FINA. Competition Results. 2021. Available online: www.fina.org/latest-results (accessed on 5 April 2021).
5. Knechtle, B.; Rosemann, T.; Rüst, C.A. Women cross the 'Catalina Channel' faster than men. *SpringerPlus* **2015**, *4*, 332. [CrossRef]
6. Knechtle, B.; Rosemann, T.; Lepers, R.; Rüst, C.A. Women Outperform Men in Ultradistance Swimming: The Manhattan Island Marathon Swim from 1983 to 2013. *Int. J. Sports Physiol. Perform.* **2014**, *9*, 913–924. [CrossRef]
7. Rüst, C.A.; Lepers, R.; Rosemann, T.; Knechtle, B. Will women soon outperform men in open-water swimming in the 'Maratona del Golfo Capri-Napoli'? *SpringerPlus* **2014**, *3*, 86. [CrossRef] [PubMed]
8. Nikolaidis, P.; Di Gangi, S.; De Sousa, C.V.; Valeri, F.; Rosemann, T.; Knechtle, B. Sex difference in open-water swimming—The Triple Crown of Open Water Swimming 1875–2017. *PLoS ONE* **2018**, *13*, e0202003. [CrossRef]
9. Nikolaidis, P.T.; De Sousa, C.V.; Knechtle, B. Sex difference in long-distance open-water swimming races—Does nationality play role? *Res. Sports Med.* **2018**, *26*, 332–344. [CrossRef] [PubMed]
10. Zingg, M.A.; Rüst, C.A.; Rosemann, T.; Lepers, R.; Knechtle, B. Analysis of sex differences in open-water ultra-distance swimming performances in the FINA World Cup races in 5 km, 10 km and 25 km from 2000 to 2012. *BMC Sports Sci. Med. Rehabil.* **2014**, *6*, [CrossRef] [PubMed]
11. Tipton, M.; Bradford, C. Moving in extreme environments: Open water swimming in cold and warm water. *Extrem. Physiol. Med.* **2014**, *3*, 12. [CrossRef]
12. Knechtle, B.; Nikolaidis, P.T.; Rosemann, T.; Rüst, C.A. Performance trends in 3000 m open-water age group swimmers from 25 to 89 years competing in the FINA World Championships from 1992 to 2014. *Res. Sports Med.* **2016**, *25*, 67–77. [CrossRef]
13. Allen, S.V.; Vandenbogaerde, T.J.; Hopkins, W.G. Career performance trajectories of Olympic swimmers: Benchmarks for talent development. *Eur. J. Sport Sci.* **2014**, *14*, 643–651. [CrossRef]
14. Allen, S.V.; Vandenbogaerde, T.J.; Hopkins, W.G. The performance effect of centralizing a nation's elite swim program. *Int. J. Sports Physiol. Perform.* **2015**, *10*, 198–203. [CrossRef]
15. Allen, S.V.; Vandenbogaerde, T.J.; Pyne, D.B.; Hopkins, W.G. Predicting a Nation's Olympic-Qualifying Swimmers. *Int. J. Sports Physiol. Perform.* **2015**, *10*, 431–435. [CrossRef]
16. Pyne, D.B.; Trewin, C.B.; Hopkins, W.G. Progression and variability of competitive performance of Olympic swimmers. *J. Sports Sci.* **2004**, *22*, 613–620. [CrossRef] [PubMed]
17. Rüst, C.A.; Knechtle, B.; Rosemann, T. The Relationship between Nationality and Performance in Successful Attempts to Swim across the 'English Channel'—A Retrospective Data Analysis from 1875 to 2012. *Med. Sport.* **2013**, *17*, 125–133. [CrossRef]

18. Knechtle, B.; Rosemann, T.; Rüst, C.A. Participation and performance trends by nationality in the 'English Channel Swim' from 1875 to 2013. *BMC Sports Sci. Med. Rehabil.* **2014**, *6*, 34. [CrossRef]
19. Nikolaidis, P.T.; Sousa, C.V.; Knechtle, B.; Nikolaidis, P.T.; Sousa, C.V.; Knechtle, B. The relationship of wearing a wetsuit in long-distance open-water swimming with sex, age, calendar year, performance, and nationality—Crossing the "Strait of Gibraltar". *Open Access J. Sports Med.* **2018**, *9*, 27–36. [CrossRef]
20. Knechtle, B.; Dalamitros, A.A.; Barbosa, T.M.; Sousa, C.V.; Rosemann, T.; Nikolaidis, P.T. Sex Differences in Swimming Disciplines—Can Women Outperform Men in Swimming? *Int. J. Environ. Res. Public Health* **2020**, *17*, 3651. [CrossRef]
21. Hill, L. Participation and Performance during the Extreme Open-Water 'Freedom Swim' Race from 2001 to 2018. *Eur. J. Phys. Educ. Sport Sci.* **2018**, *4*, 58–72.
22. Seffrin, A.; Lira, C.A.B.; Vancini, R.L.; Santos, D.A.T.; Moser, C.; Villiger, E.; Rosemann, T.; Knechtle, B.; Hill, L.; Andrade, M.S. Italians Are the Fastest 3000 m Open-Water Master Swimmers in the World. *Int. J. Environ. Res. Public Health* **2021**, *18*, 7606. [CrossRef] [PubMed]
23. Italian Open Water Tour. Available online: https://italianopenwatertour.com (accessed on 24 July 2021).
24. Open Water Schwimmen. Available online: www.openwaterschwimmen.com/news/categories/open-water-schwimmen (accessed on 24 July 2021).
25. Baldassarre, R.; Bonifazi, M.; Piacentini, M.F. Pacing profile in the main international open-water swimming competitions. *Eur. J. Sport Sci.* **2019**, *19*, 422–431. [CrossRef] [PubMed]
26. Eichenberger, E.; Knechtle, B.; Knechtle, P.; Rüst, C.A.; Rosemann, T.; Lepers, R. Best performances by men and women open-water swimmers during the 'English Channel Swim' from 1900 to 2010. *J. Sports Sci.* **2012**, *30*, 1295–1301. [CrossRef] [PubMed]
27. FINA. Open Water Swimming Manual 2020 Edition. 2020. Available online: https://resources.fina.org/fina/document/2021/02/03/84a6f630-7803-4915-8b27-a95e986cefc1/fina_ow_manual_2020_14may2020.pdf (accessed on 7 April 2021).
28. Bradford, C.D.; Gerrard, D.F.; Cotter, J.D. Open-Water Swimming. In *Heat Stress in Sport and Exercise*; Springer International Publishing: Cham, Switzerland, 2019; pp. 263–281.
29. Moles, K. The Social World of Outdoor Swimming: Cultural Practices, Shared Meanings, and Bodily Encounters. *J. Sport Soc. Issues* **2021**, *45*, 20–38. [CrossRef]
30. Throsby, K. *Immersion: Marathon Swimming, Embodiment and Identity*; Manchester University Press: Manchester, UK, 2016.
31. Suter, D.; Sousa, C.V.; Hill, L.; Scheer, V.; Nikolaidis, P.T.; Knechtle, B. Even pacing is associated with faster finishing times in ultramarathon distance trail running—The "ultra-trail du Mont Blanc" 2008–2019. *Int. J. Environ. Res. Public Health* **2020**, *17*, 7074. [CrossRef]
32. Knechtle, B.; Scheer, V.; Nikolaidis, P.T.; Sousa, C.V. Participation and performance trends in the oldest 100-km ultramarathon in the world. *Int. J. Environ. Res. Public Health* **2020**, *17*, 1719. [CrossRef] [PubMed]
33. Rüst, C.A.; Knechtle, B.; Rosemann, T.; Lepers, R. Men Cross America Faster Than Women—The "Race Across America" From 1982 to 2012. *Int. J. Sports Physiol. Perform.* **2013**, *8*, 611–617. [CrossRef] [PubMed]
34. Baumgartner, S.; Sousa, C.V.; Nikolaidis, P.T.; Knechtle, B. Can the Performance Gap between Women and Men be Reduced in Ultra-Cycling? *Int. J. Environ. Res. Public Health* **2020**, *17*, 2521. [CrossRef]
35. Knechtle, B.; Stjepanovic, M.; Knechtle, C.; Rosemann, T.; Sousa, C.V.; Nikolaidis, P.T. Physiological Responses to Swimming Repetitive "Ice Miles". *J. Strength Cond. Res.* **2021**, *35*, 487–494. [CrossRef]
36. Crow, B.T.; Matthay, E.C.; Schatz, S.P.; DeBeliso, M.D.; Nuckton, T.J. The Body Mass Index of San Francisco Cold-water Swimmers: Comparisons to U.S. National and Local Populations, and Pool Swimmers. *Int. J. Exerc. Sci.* **2017**, *10*, 1250. [PubMed]
37. Checinska-Maciejewska, Z.; Niepolski, L.; Checinska, A.; Korek, E.; Kolodziejczak, B.; Kopczynski, Z.; Krauss, H.; Pruszynska-Oszmalek, E.; Kolodziejski, P.; Gibas-Dorna, M. Regular cold water swimming during winter time affects resting hematological parameters and serum erythropoietin. *J. Physiol. Pharmacol.* **2019**, *70*, 747–756.
38. Baldassarre, R.; Bonifazi, M.; Zamparo, P.; Piacentini, M.F. Characteristics and Challenges of Open-Water Swimming Performance: A Review. *Int. J. Sports Physiol. Perform.* **2017**, *10*, 1275–1284. [CrossRef]
39. Baldassarre, R.; Pennacchi, M.; La Torre, A.; Bonifazi, M.; Piacentini, M.F. Do the Fastest Open-Water Swimmers have A Higher Speed in Middle- and Long-Distance Pool Swimming Events? *J. Funct. Morphol. Kinesiol.* **2019**, *4*, 15. [CrossRef]
40. VanHeest, J.L.; Mahoney, C.E.; Herr, L. Characteristics of elite open-water swimmers. *J. Strength Cond. Res.* **2004**, *18*, 302–305. [CrossRef] [PubMed]
41. Veiga, S.; Rodriguez, L.; González-Frutos, P.; Navandar, A. Race Strategies of Open Water Swimmers in the 5-km, 10-km, and 25-km Races of the 2017 FINA World Swimming Championships. *Front. Psychol.* **2019**, *10*, 654. [CrossRef] [PubMed]
42. Rodriguez, L.; Veiga, S. Effect of the Pacing Strategies on the Open-Water 10-km World Swimming Championships. *Int. J. Sports Physiol. Perform.* **2018**, *13*, 694–700. [CrossRef] [PubMed]

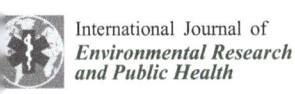

Review

Effect of Cycling Cadence on Neuromuscular Function: A Systematic Review of Acute and Chronic Alterations

Adrien Mater *, Pierre Clos and Romuald Lepers

INSERM UMR1093-CAPS, UFR des Sciences du Sport, Université Bourgogne Franche-Comté, F-21000 Dijon, France; pierre.clos@u-bourgogne.fr (P.C.); romuald.lepers@u-bourgogne.fr (R.L.)
* Correspondence: adrien.mater@u-bourgogne.fr; Tel.: +33-(0)660312007

Abstract: There is a wide range of cadence available to cyclists to produce power, yet they choose to pedal across a narrow one. While neuromuscular alterations during a pedaling bout at non-preferred cadences were previously reviewed, modifications subsequent to one fatiguing session or training intervention have not been focused on. We performed a systematic literature search of PubMed and Web of Science up to the end of 2020. Thirteen relevant articles were identified, among which eleven focused on fatigability and two on training intervention. Cadences were mainly defined as "low" and "high" compared with a range of freely chosen cadences for given power output. However, the heterogeneity of selected cadences, neuromuscular assessment methodology, and selected population makes the comparison between the studies complicated. Even though cycling at a high cadence and high intensity impaired more neuromuscular function and performance than low-cadence cycling, it remains unclear if cycling cadence plays a role in the onset of fatigue. Research concerning the effect of training at non-preferred cadences on neuromuscular adaptation allows us to encourage the use of various training stimuli but not to say whether a range of cadences favors subsequent neuromuscular performance.

Keywords: pedaling rate; pedaling frequency; fatigability; EMG; strength

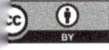

1. Introduction

Cycling is a common low-impact activity used for daily traveling, recreational practice, and professional competitive sport but also in rehabilitation programs. It appears that all cyclists spontaneously pedal across a narrow range of cadence. This is intriguing because work production per unit of time (i.e., power output), which is the product between pedaling rate and torque applied to the pedal, could theoretically be achieved using a wide range of cadence. Freely chosen cadences (FCC, or preferred cadence) are usually very close among individuals but influenced by practice level. Indeed, professional cyclists prefer cadences above 90 rpm, while active recreational cyclists rather use cadence around 80 rpm [1].

For a given power output, an upward shift of the pedaling cadence reduces the torque applied to the pedal, and vice versa, affecting the physiological and psychological demand of exercise [2]. Cadences can be considered low or high at a given power output when imposed pedaling frequencies were not included in a range of ±25 rpm relative to FCC, usually adopted during training or competition [3]. Sport scientists have been trying to understand why individuals select a cadence rather than another based on physiological, biomechanical, and perceptual parameters. Studies also described acute alterations induced by imposing a pedaling rate below or above the preferred one. A review summarized studies that focused on participants' responses to exercise, such as oxygen consumption, joint torque, blood lactate accumulation, muscular activation, and perception of effort [2]. The authors reported that all these factors were specifically affected by pedaling rate. Indeed, it appears that these variables follow a "J-curve" or "U-curve" in which the optimal cadence for blood lactate accumulation and oxygen consumption is lower than FCC. In contrast, for minimized mechanical joint torque, the optimal cadence seems above FCC. Then, preferred cadence seems to minimize perceived exertion and would reflect a trade-off between cadences below FCC, lowering oxygen consumption, and above FCC, minimizing mechanical load and thus the possible subsequent alterations of lower limb neuromuscular function.

Neuromuscular alterations could be the cause of a decrease in performance when the effort is prolonged. Indeed, a review investigated the role of pedaling rate on a time trial or time-to-exhaustion performances in relation to energy expenditure [4]. However, the disparity of exercise characteristics—intensities and durations—did not allow them to conclude about a cadence that would optimize performance. It nonetheless seems that cadence impacts performance, and this could occur through fatigue development. Fatigue is defined as "a disabling symptom in which physical and cognitive function is limited by interactions between performance fatigability and perceived fatigability" [5]. Mechanisms involved in the loss of maximal force are commonly investigated through neuromuscular function with the differentiation between muscular and neural components set below and above the neuromuscular junction, respectively.

Moreover, it is well known that fatigue is dependent on the characteristics of the task. Constant load exercise allows studying the impact of the duration and intensity of the task on neuromuscular function. Neural impairments are exacerbated as exercise duration increases (and the intensity that can be sustained decreases), whereas muscular disturbances are greater at higher intensities (and shorter durations of exercise) [6,7]. However, the effect of cadence on neuromuscular alteration after an acute cycling exercise remains to be clarified.

Interestingly, professional cyclists typically use cadences below FCC when training in order to increase muscle tension and provide resistance training-like adaptations, or above FCC to increase the metabolic demand and work on their pedaling gesture to improve their performance at FCC. While Hansen and Rønnestad [3] reported no evidence for a positive effect of training at low cadence, the authors did not emphasize the effect of cadence on chronic neuromuscular alterations while these could contribute to cycling performance [8]. This systematic review aimed to clarify how the utilization of different cycling cadences affects neuromuscular function (i) following a cycling bout, (ii) throughout a cycling exercise, and (iii) following a training period.

2. Materials and Methods

The present review was carried out following the "Preferred Reporting Items for Systematic review and Meta-analyses (PRISMA)" guidelines [9] by one scientist. The article search ended on 31 December 2020, and concerned all articles published since 1929. An advanced search was carried out in all files using key-word formulas on PubMed "(((cycling cadence) OR (Pedaling frequency) OR (Pedaling rate)) AND ((neuromuscular OR (jump) OR (training)))" and on Web of Science: "ALL = ((cycling cadence OR Pedaling frequency OR Pedaling rate) AND (neuromuscular OR jump OR training OR strength OR fatigue))." The research results were added and filtered in Mendeley software (version 1.19.4, 2008-19). Studies were included if they met the following inclusion criteria: (i) participants performed cycling at different cadences, and (ii) neuromuscular adaptations either induced by one fatiguing exercise session or a training intervention were reported. Articles were excluded if: (i) the text was not written in English or French, (ii) the studies did not focus on cycling exercise, or (iii) the studies did not present data on neuromuscular function. Risk of bias assessment was carried out using the Revised Cochrane Risk of Bias Tool for randomized trials (RoB 2.0) independently by two of the authors, following the guideline. Each study was analyzed throughout the five domains proposed by the tool and described as presenting "low risk", "some concerns", or a "high risk" of bias. The two investigators then discussed until they found a consensus upon the risk level. Results were then divided into two distinct sections: (1) adaptations caused by one bout of cycling and (2) chronic adaptations after a long-term intervention training. Moreover, to reduce the chance of missing relevant papers, studies' references were reviewed in order to find further studies of potential interest.

3. Results

A total of 4744 (PubMed: 4065, Web of Science: 1036) articles, including duplicates, were identified using electronic databases. After having filtered articles based on their titles and abstracts, 29 articles were included, among which 14 (12 focused on fatiguing bouts and two on training interventions) remained based on the inclusion criteria (including one conference presentation for which only the abstract was available) (Figure 1).

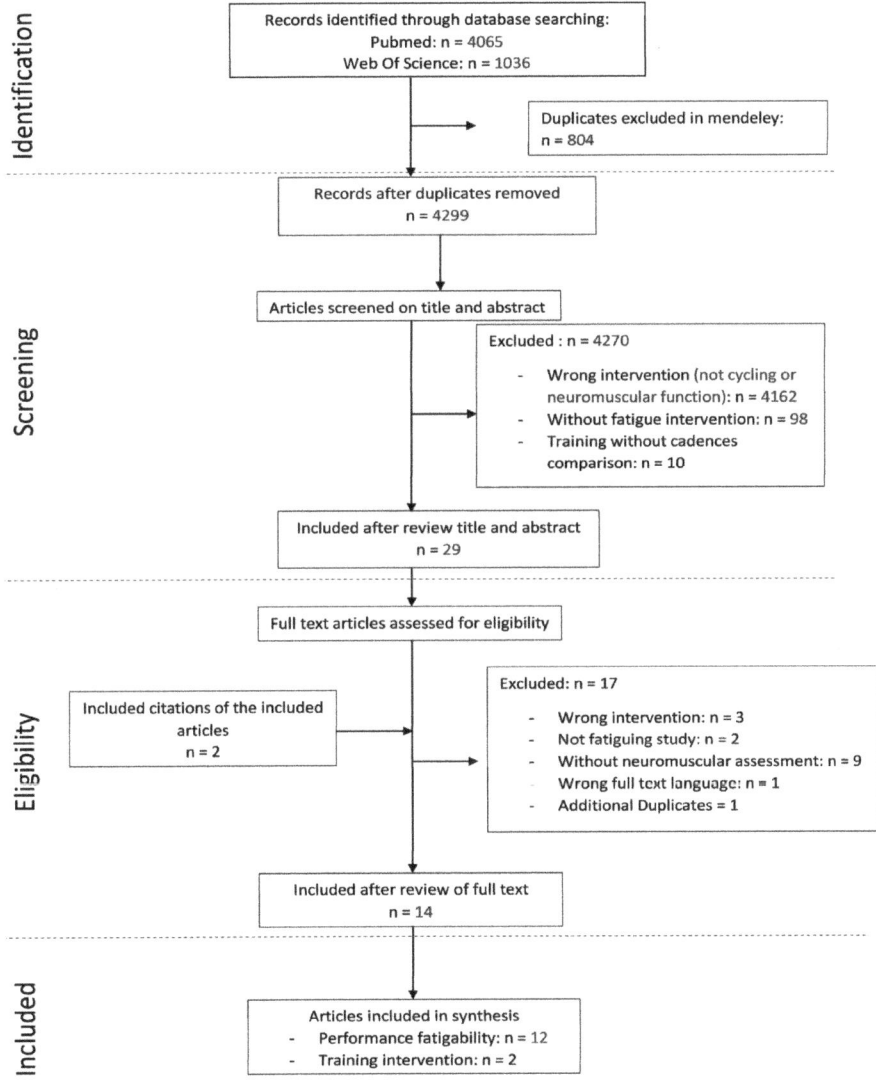

Figure 1. Flow diagram of the reviewing methods based on PRSIMA guidelines.

3.1. Risk of Bias

Only one in all 14 included studies evaluated with the RoB 2-tool had a high risk of bias that dealt with an overall high risk of bias. Some concern of bias present in the two first items came from the impossibility to blind participants and personnel from cycling intervention because they had to control their cadence. A similar result in the last items resulted from the fact that no indication was mentioned in studies about the selection of the reported results. Low risk of bias due to missing or measurement of outcome data were scored for all studies except one that performed the pre-test one day before the cycling exercise and not immediately before as advised, which means it scored as high risk (Figures 2 and 3).

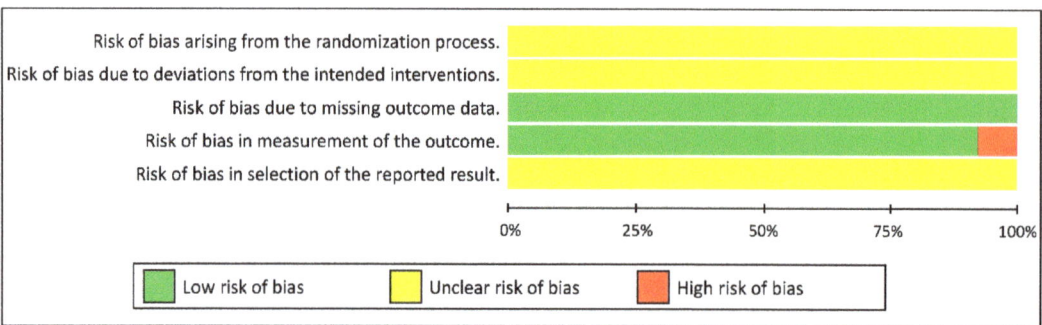

Figure 2. Risk of bias across studies.

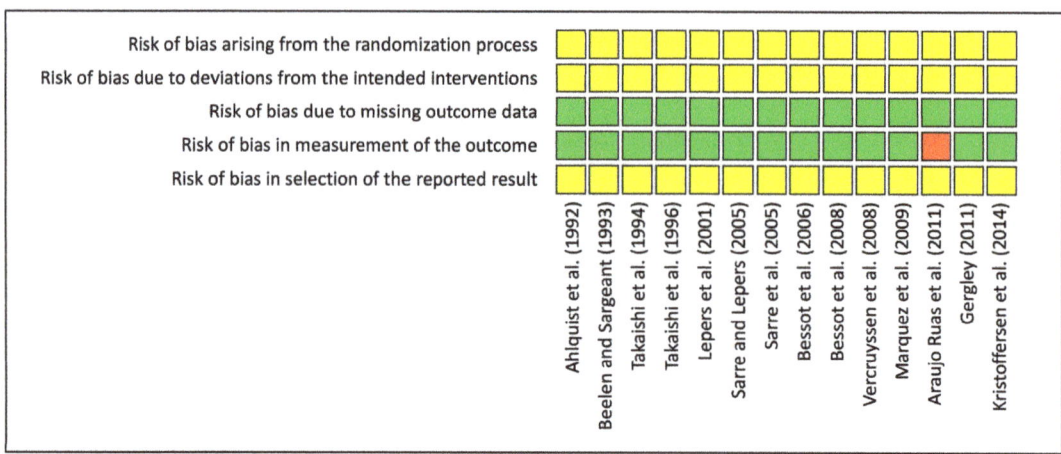

Figure 3. Risk of bias within studies.

3.2. Study Characteristics

Table 1 presents the main characteristics of studies that investigated neuromuscular impairments induced by one session at different pedaling cadences. Participants of seven studies were cyclists while others were merely healthy weightlifters or team sport players. Fatiguing bouts of pedaling lasted from ≈4 min—for a time-to-exhaustion—to 1 h at an intensity from ≈35% to 95% of peak power output (PPO) determined during an incremental test. In most studies, pedaling intensities were set as a percentage of PPO [10–14] or of maximal oxygen consumption (VO$_2$peak) [15–18]. One study compared cadences at both the same relative metabolic and mechanical work rate [19] and another at power outputs corresponding to the onset of blood lactate accumulation above 3.5 mmol.L^{-1} of lactate [20]

The utilized cadences ranged from 40 rpm to 110 rpm. A team opted for monitoring a large range of cadences without taking into account FFC [14,15] while all others favored cadences below and above the preferred cadence. In the latter case, cadences were considered as low or high with respect to FCC at the same power [3], except in the works of Beelen and Sargeant [19] and de Araujo Ruas et al. [20] who used the same absolute cadences for all participants.

Table 1. Effect of pedaling cadence on the acute neuromuscular alteration (FCC: freely chosen cadence, PPO: peak power output, rpm: rotation per minute, EMG: electromyogram, RMS: root mean square, MPF: mean power frequency, MVC: maximal voluntary contraction, CON120 and CON240: concentric contraction at 120 and 240°.s^{-1}, ISO: isometric contraction, VL: vastus lateralis, GL: gastrocnemius lateralis, RF: rectus femoris, iEMG: integrated electromyographic activity, HR$_{max}$: maximal heart rate, and RM: repetition maximal).

Study	Participants	Methods	Outcome
		During Cycling Exercise	
Takaishi et al. (1994)	8 healthy males Age: 20.7 ± 1.5 yrs Mass: 62.5 ± 3.1 kg	15 min at 75% VO$_2$peak (from 140 to 210 W) at 40, 50, 60, 70, or 80 rpm Measures: iEMG increase (iEMG slope) in VL during pedaling bout	iEMG followed a quadratic curve with a bottom at about 70 rpm iEMG slope 70 rpm < 50 rpm and 60 rpm, but no differences were found with 40 and 80 rpm
Takaishi et al. (1996)	6 cyclists with 3–4 yrs of road racing experience Age: 20.7 ± 1.5 yrs Mass: 62.5 ± 3.1 kg	15 min at 85% VO$_2$peak (from 200 to 240 W) at 50, 60, 70, 80, 90, or 100 rpm Measures: iEMG increase (iEMG slope) in VL during pedaling bout	iEMG slope demonstrated a quadratic curve with bottom near 80 rpm iEMG slope 80 rpm < than other cadences except 90 rpm iEMG slope 90 rpm < than at 100 rpm
Sarre and Lepers, (2005)	11 well-trained male cyclists with at least 4 yrs of racing experience Age: 27.8 ± 5.6 yrs Mass: 71.1 ± 7.8 kg PPO = 382 ± 43 W	60 min at 65% PPO at: FCC (88 ± 11 rpm) 50 rpm 110 rpm Measures: EMG RMS and MPF during pedaling bouts (VL, RF, GL, and BF muscles)	EMG RMS of muscles were differently affected by cadence: EMG RMS of VL and RF ↑ with time at 110 rpm only EMG RMS of BF ↓ at 50 rpm EMG MPF of VL, RF, GL did not change EMG MPF of BF ↑ whatever the cadence
Bessot et al. (2006)	11 male cyclists with 6.5 ± 1.7 yrs of racing experience and 9.8 ± 2.2 h of training per week Age: 19.1 ± 1.8 yrs Mass: 65.9 ± 6.5 kg	Time to exhaustion at 95% PPO at: FCC +20% (72 rpm) FCC −20% (108 rpm) Measures: EMG RMS increase (EMG slope) in VM and BF during pedaling bouts	Time to exhaustion was greater at FCC −20% than FCC + 20%; no difference between FCC and other cadences EMG RMS of VM ↑ regardless of cadence EMG RMS of BF ↑ FCC +20% > FCC −20%
Bessot et al., (2008)	9 competitive male cyclists with 9.8 ± 2.2 h of training per week Age: 21.4 ± 0.7 yrs Mass: 69.6 ± 6.8 kg PPO: 322 ± 32 W	21 min at 65% PPO FCC (86 ± 13 rpm) and 60, 75, 90, 105 rpm Measures: EMG RMS increase (EMG slope) in VM during pedaling bout	EMG slope 105 rpm > than at 75 rpm EMG slope 60 rpm > than at 75 and 90 rpm Optimal cadence to minimize EMG slope determined with regression analysis was 80 ± 7 rpm (not different from FCC)
Vercruyssen et al. (2008)	Well trained male cyclists Age: 25 ± 4 yrs Mass: 76 ± 6 kg VO$_2$peak = 64.7 ± 3.1 mL.kg^{-1}.min^{-1} PPO = 386 ± 38 W	6 min at 65 ± 7% VO$_2$peak at: 50 rpm 100 rpm Measures: iEMG and MPF EMG of VL and VM during pedaling bout	iEMG of VL and VM ↑ during 100 rpm bout only MPF of VL and VM did not change at any cadences
		Pre vs. Post Cycling Exercise	
Ahlquist et al. (1992)	8 physically active males (4 runners, 4 cyclists) Age: 20–40 yrs Mass: 81 ± 3 kg VO$_2$peak = 56.8 mL.kg^{-1}.min^{-1}	30 min at 85% VO$_2$peak (assessed at 75 rpm) at: 50 rpm 100 rpm Measures: muscle biopsy of VL—fiber glycogen depletion	No cadence effect on type I fiber Glycogen depletion 50 rpm > 100 rpm in type II fiber
Beelen and Sargeant (1993)	7 healthy males physically active Age: 27.9 ± 2.7 yrs Mass: 71.0 ± 11.6 kg	Pedaling 6 min at: 60 rpm and 90% VO$_2$peak (291 ± 31W) (A) 120 rpm and 90% VO$_2$peak (236 ± 30 W) (B) 60 rpm and same workrate as (B) (≈74 ± 11% of VO$_2$peak) Measures: 25 s of maximal sprint on cycle ergometer at 60 and 120 rpm	At same VO$_2$: ↓ peak power output or kinetic of power output during sprints without cadence effect At same workrate: Decrease in power output over the 25 s after bout at 120 rpm > 60 rpm

Table 1. Cont.

Study	Participants	Methods	Outcome
Lepers et al. (2001)	11 well-trained male cyclists with at least 4 yrs of racing experience Age: 28 ± 2 yrs Mass: 74 ± 5 kg Height = 183 ± 5 cm PPO = 384 ± 31 W VO$_2$peak = 64.1 ± 4.5 mL·kg^{-1}·min^{-1}	30 min of cycling at 80% of PPO at: FCC (86 ± 4 rpm) FCC +20% (103 ± 5 rpm) FCC −20% (69 ± 3 rpm) Measures: Neuromuscular function of knee extensors muscles	MVC ISO and MVC CON120 ↓ without cadence effect MVC CON240 did not change at any cadence Voluntary activation level ↓ without cadence effect Mechanical evoked torque ↓ whatever the cadence M-wave amplitude did not change at any cadences
Sarre et al. (2005)	11 well-trained male cyclists with at least 4 yrs of racing experience Age: 27.8 ± 5.6 yrs Mass: 71.1 ± 7.8 kg PPO = 382 ± 43 W	60 min at 65% PPO at: FCC (88 ± 11 rpm) 50 rpm 110 rpm Measures: Neuromuscular function of knee extensors and knee flexors muscles	MVC of knee extensors ↓ without cadence effect MVC of knee flexors ↓ after 50 and 110 rpm pedaling bout VAL ↓ without cadence effect EMG RMS/M-wave amplitude of VL and RF ↓ after the 110-rpm bout No change of EMG RMS/M-wave amplitude of VM Evoked torque ↓ whatever the cadence Area of M-waves of VL and VM ↓ after cycling at 50 rpm and FCC
Marquez et al. (2009)	10 physically team sport player males Age: 21 ± 4 yrs Mass: 75 ± 6 kg 9.8 ± 2.2 h of training per week PPO = 310 ± 38 W	15 min of cycling at 35% PPO at: FCC (71 rpm) FCC +20% (57 rpm) FCC −20% (85 rpm) Measures: CMJ before and immediately after pedaling bout	CMJ ↓ directly after bout at FCC and FCC −20% but remain unchanged after FCC +20% CMJ return to baseline after 1 min of rest at FCC and FCC −20%
Araujo Ruas et al. (2011)	13 weight lifter males Age: 23.0 ± 3.7 yrs Mass: 77.1 ± 8.8 kg 3 weight lifting sessions per week	30 min at onset of blood lactate accumulation (3.5 mmol·L^{-1}) at: 50 rpm (82.5% PPO) 100 rpm (71.9% PPO) Measures: 3 sets of 10 RM leg press or 3 sets of 10 maximal countermovement jump	Leg press repetitions ↓ after 100 rpm compared with control condition and 50 rpm Mean CMJ height for all sets did not differed between condition
Training Interventions			
Gergley et al. (2011)	14 young moderately trained males Age: 18–23 yrs	2 groups of concurrent training: 90 rpm (65% HR$_{max}$) + resistance training 70 rpm (65% HR$_{max}$) + resistance training 2 sessions per week during 9 weeks Measures: 1RM leg press	↑ lower body strength in 70 rpm + resistance training group only
Kristoffersen et al. (2014)	22 well trained male veteran cyclists Age: 47 ± 6 yrs Mass: 78 ± 7 kg VO2max: 57.9 ± 3.7 mL·kg^{-1}·min^{-1}	2 groups: 40 rpm—5 × 6 min at a HR of 73–82% HR$_{max}$ measured (total of 91 ± 31 h of training) FCC (about 95 rpm) - (total of 88 ± 34 h of training) 2 sessions per week during 12 weeks Measures: 1RM leg press and leg extension	No significant difference in either 1RM leg press or leg extension

Given the limited number of studies available on the neuromuscular alterations induced by chronic exposure to imposed low or high cadences, the two studies were presented at the end of Table 1. Kristoffersen et al. [21] and Gergley [22] recruited well trained master and young moderate-trained cyclists for an intervention of 12 and 9 weeks respectively. Participants trained twice a week with exercise intensity set from 65 to 82% of maximal heart rate. Cadences ranged from 40 to 90 rpm.

The methodology used to assess neuromuscular function differed between studies. First, studies compared values obtained before and after a cycling exercise or a training period. Maximal voluntary contractions (MVC) coupled with electrical stimulation, which was used in two studies [12,13], make it possible to distinguish between the neural and muscular components of performance fatigability [23]. An assessment with countermovement jump (CMJ), used in two others studies [14,20], provides the possibility to assess neuromuscular function in a more practical way [24]. Additional assessments were then used, such as the maximal power output during a 25 s cycling sprint [19] or the maximal number of leg press repetitions carried out with a given load [19,21]. Moreover, muscle biopsies served to determine glycogen depletion and distinguish the type of muscle fibers predominantly used during the exercise [18]. Second, using surface electromyography, studies evaluated the level of muscular activation during the exercise [10,11,15–17,25].

3.3. Main Outcomes

3.3.1. Acute Neuromuscular Alteration

Studies were further distinguished through two main methodologies: evaluating neuromuscular function during and/or after a cycling exercise. Ahlquist et al. [18] first compared the effect of 30 min of cycling at 85% VO_2peak at 50 or 100 rpm on glycogen depletion. They found that cadence did not affect glycogen depletion in type I fibers while cycling at 50 rpm led to a greater glycogen depletion in type II fibers than cycling at 100 rpm. Cycling at 80% PPO for 30 min led to a loss of isometric and concentric (up to $120°.s^{-1}$) knee extensors maximal voluntary contraction force (MVC) without a cadence effect when the pedaling rate was fixed at ±20% FCC [12]. This finding was similar when cycling was performed at 65% PPO for 30 min at 50 or 110 rpm, corresponding to −43% and +25% FCC [13]. Additionally, the latter study found that isometric knee flexors MVC decreased after pedaling at both low and high cadences but not at the preferred one. Moreover, these two studies applied percutaneous electrical stimulation on the femoral nerve to distinguish between muscular and neural components of force production failure. The maximal voluntary activation level decreased in both studies of Lepers et al. [12] and Sarre et al. [13] without difference between cadences. However, changes in the root mean square (RMS) of the electromyographic signal (EMG) during an MVC divided by the maximal muscle compound (M_{MAX}) amplitude—EMG_{MAX}/M_{MAX} ratio—which is used as a marker of neural drive, showed discrepancies between studies. This ratio decreased for the vastus lateralis (VL) and vastus medialis (VM) muscles after cycling at low and preferred cadences in the study of Lepers et al. [12]. It did not change at any cadences for the VM muscle and decreased for the VL and the rectus femoris (RF) muscles after high pedaling rate cycling in the study of Sarre et al. [13]. In both studies, the maximal torque evoked by motor nerve stimulation at rest decreased whatever the pedaling cadence. M_{MAX} amplitudes were reduced at FCC and low cadence in the study of Sarre et al. [13] but remained unchanged in that of Lepers et al. [12].

Neuromuscular function was also evaluated through high muscle coordination movements such as 25 s cycling sprints. Maximal power output during sprint and so-called rate of fatigue (decrement of power throughout the sprint) were affected by cycling 6 min at 90% VO_2peak without cadence effect when the pedaling rate was set at 60 and 120 rpm; power output at the high cadence represented 81% of that at the low cadence [19]. Nonetheless, when performed at an equal power output (236 ± 30 W), there was no difference in the peak of power output, but a greater power output decrement during the sprint occurred after cycling at a cadence of 120 compared with 60 rpm. Furthermore, modulating pedaling cadence yielded heterogeneous countermovement jump (CMJ) results. When it was performed after cycling at 35% PPO for 15 min, maximal CMJ height decreased immediately after bouts at FCC −20% and FCC, and returned to pre-exercise values after 1 min of rest, while it remained constant after cycling at FCC +20% [14]. However, when cycling exercise was performed at power outputs corresponding to the onset of blood lactate accumulation (82.5 and 71.9% PPO at 50 and 100 rpm, respectively), the subsequent average height of 10 CMJs was unaltered whatever the pedaling cadence [20]. The latter authors also reported fewer leg press repetitions after cycling at 100 rpm than the control or 50 rpm. Only one study examined the time-to-exhaustion at 95% PPO for different cadences [11]. It showed that FCC −20% yielded longer exercise durations than FCC +20%, while no differences were noticed with FCC.

A second way to assess modulations of neuromuscular function was the use of EMG during cycling. Bessot et al. [11] showed an increase in the EMG RMS of the VM muscle without difference for cadences corresponding to ±20% FCC during exercise. Conversely, both Sarre and Lepers [10] and Vercruyssen et al. [17] found that during 1 h of cycling at 65% PPO and 6 min at 65% VO_2peak, the EMG RMS of the VL and RF muscles as well as the integrated EMG of the VL and VM muscles raised with time at 110 and 100 rpm, respectively. Moreover, both studies conducted by Takaishi [15,16], which focused on the slope of integrated EMG drift of the VL muscle during 15 min of cycling at 75% and 85% VO_2peak, reported a quadratic curve with the lowest values at 70 and 80 rpm, respectively. Bessot et al. [25] also monitored the EMG RMS slope of the VM muscle during 21 min of cycling at 65% PPO. They found that the EMG RMS slope at 105 rpm was greater than at 75 rpm, and greater at 60 than 75 and 90 rpm. They also found that the lowest value of the mean quadratic regression was 80 ± 7 rpm, and did not differ from FCC. Additionally, two studies assessed the EMG of the biceps femoris. Bessot et al. [11] found a greater increase at 108 rpm than 72 rpm, while Sarre and Lepers [10] indicated a fall at 50 rpm only. Finally, EMG mean power frequency did not change in the VL, VM, RF, and gastrocnemius lateralis muscles [10,16] but increased for the biceps femoris muscle at all cadences [10].

3.3.2. Neuromuscular Adaptations Following a Training Period

The two interventions retained used different methodologies. Kristoffersen et al. [22] compared two groups of cyclists who added two 90-min sessions per week to their habitual training content. While the control group performed the additional training at moderate intensity (i.e., 73–85% of maximal heart rate) and FCC, the other group performed interval training (i.e., 5 × 6 min with 3 min of recovery) at the same relative intensity but at a cadence of 40 rpm. None of these interventions improved maximal strength assessed with leg extension and leg press movement. Gergley [22] compared two concurrent training programs with the same resistance training content but comprising cycling exercises that differed in terms of cadences (70 rpm or 90 rpm). They found that only the group performing concurrent training while cycling at 70 rpm improved its maximal leg press strength.

4. Discussion

This review aimed to summarize neuromuscular alterations following one bout of cycling or repetitive exposure to cycling performed at an imposed cadence, considered as low or high, primarily compared with the preferred one. Because of the heterogeneity of the variables measured and exercise characteristics (i.e., cadence, intensity, duration, and comparison criteria between cadences), the influence of pedaling cadence on neuromuscular function remains elusive yet offers perspectives for future research.

4.1. Methodological Considerations

Several precautions must be taken in the present review because of the relative heterogeneity of cadence for both acute and chronic interventions. Firstly, cycling exercises were always performed on a cycle ergometer that excluded contextual consideration, such as the effect of road gradient on cadence [26,27]. Then, the influence of the fitness level and sports background was limited because the freely chosen cadence (FCC) remains consistent within an individual [28], and all conditions (e.g., low cadence) were based on it. The most complicated factor to consider may be exercise intensity. Indeed, it is well known that FCC is intensity-dependent [29] and that, for a given percentage of peak oxygen consumption, shifting from one cadence to another affects power output. Consequently, the conclusions from studies testing the effect of pedaling cadences based on different intensity criteria (e.g., given power output or oxygen uptake) should be compared with caution [29]. Moreover, the cadences considered as low or high are heterogeneous because some investigators chose absolute and other relative (e.g., ±20% FCC) cadences below and above the preferred one [11,12]. For instance, when comparing cadences such as 110 or 50 rpm with FCC, the "high cadence" was 25% above FCC, whereas the "low" one was 43% below FCC [10]. Therefore, cadences considered as low or high can reside within the range of preferred cadences and thus may not affect neuromuscular function distinctly from FCC.

Based on the revised Cochrane assessment method, most studies present an unclear risk of bias. Only one study [20] exhibited a high risk of bias due to baseline measurements having been performed on a separate day and the time delay to perform the tests after the end of the cycling exercise. In addition, biases due to deviations from the intended interventions appear hard to control using such paradigms. Indeed, interventions could not be blind to participants because they were the ones who had to maintain the requested cadences.

4.2. Performance Fatigability

Cycling exercise can affect neuromuscular performance such as maximal voluntary isometric force [24], and a shift from the preferred pedaling cadence could exacerbate this phenomenon. Millet and Lepers [23] hypothesized that a shift from the preferred cadence could alter the recruitment of motor units and thus cause a greater maximal voluntary force decrease. This hypothesis came after Ahlquist et al. [18] found that a low-cadence cycling exercise induced a greater glycogen depletion of type II fibers than a higher pedaling rate. Their results suggested that the force applied on the pedals determines the recruitment of motor units. However, while no real consensus emerges from the presently reviewed studies, it appears that when participants were regular cyclists, modulating cadence did not impact neuromuscular performance as expected. Indeed, some authors suggested that trained cyclists can adjust cadences within a range near those usually used during training sessions and competitions without exhibiting more performance fatigability [12]. Moreover, two studies tested performance fatigability and neuromuscular function through isometric contractions, which could likely hide possible alterations at other knee angles or during a dynamic contraction [10,12]. Indeed, Clos et al. [30] showed that a subsequent isometric evaluation did not reflect differences in dynamic torque losses induced by eccentric and concentric tasks. To avoid this limitation, three studies performed dynamic assessments of neuromuscular performance [14,19,20]. Beelen and Sargeant [19] used a sprint on a cycle ergometer before and after fatiguing cycling exercises and, in addition to cycling sprints, de Araujo Ruas et al. [20] used more functional movements such as leg press repetitions with a load corresponding to 10 maximum repetitions and 10 countermovement jumps. Beelen and Sargeant [19] found greater fatigability (i.e., decrease in peak and average power output during the sprint)—after high- than low-cadence cycling at the same work rate. Interestingly, de Araujo Ruas et al. [20] also found a decrease in the number of leg press repetitions after pedaling at a high cadence and not after pedaling at a low cadence performed at a greater power output. These results seem to be in favor of a greater fatigability with high- than low-cadence cycling exercises in non-cyclists. Lastly, Marquez et al. [14] used an exercise intensity and duration typically used for warm-up (15 min at 35% PPO). Nonetheless, jump performance fell directly after cycling at low and preferred cadence, yet returned to baseline after 1 min of rest. Although this result differs from those of the two previously cited studies, it seems that when exercise intensity is sufficient, only high-cadence exercises alter dynamic neuromuscular performance such as cycling sprints and jumps in untrained cyclists.

Other makers of performance fatigability include impaired time trial or a time-to-exhaustion performance [5]. Findings from Bessot et al. [11] allowed us to suppose no clear effect of cadence because time-to-exhaustion was longer at low- compared with high-cadence cycling, but not different from FCC in any condition. A previous literature review supported the fact that cycling performance was altered by cadences higher than the preferred one [31], even if one study found a greater time-to-exhaustion duration at FFC compared with low cadence (50 rpm, without testing other cadences) [32].

4.3. Acute Neuromuscular Alterations

An upward drift of EMG RMS during a sustained task is commonly accepted as a marker of impaired muscle ability to produce power as additional motor units are probably recruited and/or firing rate increased despite a steady power output [33]. It appears that the cycling cadences used by all the studies included in this review induced an increase in central drive towards the knee extensors muscles, except the low cadence in the study of Vercruyssen et al. [17], and the low and preferred cadences in the study of Sarre and Lepers [10], where EMG remained constant. Divergences in the nature of cycling exercises (exhausting or not) and gaps between cadences used could lead to a misleading comparison of studies. However, muscular alterations and a decrease in maximal voluntary activation level after the exercise were not influenced by cadence [13,34]. A rise in knee extensor EMG RMS during the exercise was not related to subsequent muscular alterations. However central drive (EMG_{MAX}/M_{MAX} ratio) decreased after cycling at high cadence only [13], which could be explained by a compensatory increase in the neural drive (i.e., EMG RMS during the exercise, affecting the ability of supraspinal centers to drive the muscle. This is nonetheless speculatory, and it should be noted that changes in the maximal neural drive after cycling did not mirror changes in maximal voluntary activation (i.e., torque). Despite some discrepancies, the results suggest that pedaling at FCC minimizes the rise in EMG RMS throughout a cycling task. Findings from dynamic neuromuscular evaluations after the exercise suggest that non-preferred cadences impact neuromuscular function. These results were supported by the lower increase in EMG RMS at preferred cadences in both studies of Takaishi et al. [15,16] and one from Bessot et al. [25]. Of note, differences in FCC between these studies could be explained by the greater expertise of cyclists and power outputs selected in the second one [35].

The fall in knee flexors EMG RMS found at the low cadence in one study [10] may be explained by a decreased co-activation of this muscle group during the leg extension phase, allowing for a reduced knee extensors work. On the other hand, an increase in the activation of the biceps femoris at high cadence [11] might improve transition phases (at the end of downstroke and during the upstroke of the pedaling movement). It must be noted that despite distinct changes in knee flexors activation throughout low cadence cycling, both studies [10,11] tested trained cyclists. Then, this discrepancy may reflect different individual strategies prevailing in each one of the two moderate sample sizes (n = 11).

Complementary results concerning fiber recruitment patterns could be assessed with EMG methods. A rise in mean power frequency EMG during sustained task suggests recruiting additional muscle fibers and likely type II fibers [36]. Results indicate that motor unit recruitment during cycling did not change with cadence for most of the considered muscles (VL, VM, RF, and gastrocnemius lateralis) except for the biceps femoris, which showed an increased mean power frequency whatever the cadence used [10]. The confidence in the type of motor unit activated while pedaling could likely be improved using high-density EMG [37].

4.4. Training

Hansen and Rønnestad [3] already reviewed articles focusing on the effect of a training period at imposed cadences on cycling performance factors such as maximal power output and oxygen consumption or gross efficiency. Although muscular strength was considered as a performance factor and has mainly been focused on training for cyclists [8], only one study (out of seven in Ronnestad's review) considered it as the main outcome [21]. Then, we reported only one complete study and a conference paper that compared the effect of preferred and low cadences on lower limb muscle strength. It appears that although pedaling at 40 rpm must be considered as training at a low cadence, no effect was denoted on strength performance assessed with leg press and leg extension [21]. These results could be explained by the relatively low force development induced by sub-maximal low cadence cycling compared with heavy strength training, which is close to maximal lower limb force capacity. Indeed, the low-cadence exercises used in the studies of Gergley [22] and Kristoffersen et al. [21] were performed over long durations that were closer to endurance than resistance training efforts. Similarly, Koninckx et al. [38] compared 12 weeks of maximal cycling at a relatively low cadence for a sprint—80 rpm for about 825 W over 12 pedal revolutions—with resistance training. While the authors found no improvement in maximal isometric strength, the maximal power output during a 5 s sprint increased after both low-cadence and resistance training periods. However, despite a high torque applied on pedals, maximal sprint cycling training at low cadence did not affect isometric MVC. This result strengthens the point that, when possible, assessments of neuromuscular performance should be realized through functional tests (e.g., cycling sprint, jumping) and/or corresponding to a training regime. Finally, when coupled with resistance training, cycling sessions at a low cadence allowed for greater improvements in lower limb muscle strength than when pedaling at FCC [22]. As the results from training studies that modulated pedaling cadence are scarce, there is a need to multiply such investigations and broaden the training regimens to determine one or several optimal methods [3].

5. Conclusions

This review highlights that the role of cycling cadence in performance fatigability and neuromuscular alterations is unclear. It seems that a high cadence at a sufficiently high exercise intensity impairs dynamic neuromuscular performance more than low or preferred cadences, at least in untrained cyclists. One practical consequence of this is that inexperienced cyclists should probably not pedal above their spontaneously chosen cadence if their workout comprises subsequent explosive exercises. Above all, the findings show the relevance of using specific or functional tests for fatigability assessment and of paying attention to the selected population when comparing the impact of pedaling rates. Although research on the effect of cadence during a training period on neuromuscular function is still lacking, it seems essential for coaches to multiply/diversify training regimes even if it means leaving the strict framework of training on the bike. In this perspective, it could be interesting to associate so-called sub-maximal cycling strength training with resistance training. Finally, a method known as eccentric pedaling—resisting against the torque produced by an engine [39]—has recently been spreading in rehabilitation centers [40] and makes it possible to train lower limb muscles at significantly higher levels of force than those allowed by concentric pedaling, leading to superior voluntary force gains [41,42].

Author Contributions: Conceptualization, A.M., R.L.; methodology, A.M. and R.L.; validation, A.M., R.L. and P.C.; writing and editing, A.M., P.C. and R.L. All authors have read and agreed to the published version of the manuscript.

Funding: This research received no external funding.

Institutional Review Board Statement: Not applicable.

Informed Consent Statement: Not applicable.

Data Availability Statement: Not applicable.

Conflicts of Interest: The authors declare no conflict of interest.

References

Marsh, A.P.; Martin, P.E.; Sanderson, D.J. Is a joint moment-based cost function associated with preferred cycling cadence? *J. Biomech.* **2000**, *33*, 173–180. [CrossRef]
Ansley, L.; Cangley, P. Determinants of "optimal" cadence during cycling. *Eur. J. Sport Sci.* **2009**, *9*, 61–85. [CrossRef]
Hansen, E.A.; Rønnestad, B.R. Effects of cycling training at imposed low cadences: A systematic review. *Int. J. Sports Physiol. Perform.* **2017**, *12*, 1127–1136. [CrossRef] [PubMed]
Hansen, E.A.; Smith, G. Factors Affecting Cadence Choice During Submaximal Cycling and Cadence Influence on Performance Brief Review. *Int. J. Sports Physiol. Perform.* **2009**, *4*, 3–17. [CrossRef] [PubMed]
Enoka, R.M.; Duchateau, J. Translating fatigue to human performance. *Med. Sci. Sports Exerc.* **2016**, *48*, 2228–2238. [CrossRef] [PubMed]

6. Lepers, R.; Maffiuletti, N.A.; Rochette, L.; Brugniaux, J.; Millet, G.Y. Neuromuscular fatigue during a long-duration cycling exercise. *J. Appl. Physiol.* **2002**, *92*, 1487–1493. [CrossRef] [PubMed]
7. Thomas, K.; Elmeua, M.; Howatson, G.; Goodall, S. Intensity-Dependent Contribution of Neuromuscular Fatigue after Constant-Load Cycling. *Med. Sci. Sports Exerc.* **2016**, *48*, 1751–1760. [CrossRef]
8. Rønnestad, B.R.; Mujika, I. Optimizing strength training for running and cycling endurance performance: A review. *Scand. J. Med. Sci. Sports* **2014**, *24*, 603–612. [CrossRef]
9. Liberati, A.; Altman, D.G.; Tetzlaff, J.; Mulrow, C.; Gøtzsche, P.C.; Ioannidis, J.P.A.; Clarke, M.; Devereaux, P.J.; Kleijnen, J.; Moher, D. The PRISMA statement for reporting systematic reviews and meta-analyses of studies that evaluate health care interventions: Explanation and elaboration. *J. Clin. Epidemiol.* **2009**, *62*, e1–e34. [CrossRef]
10. Sarre, G.; Lepers, R. Neuromuscular function during prolonged pedalling exercise at different cadences. *Acta Physiol. Scand.* **2005**, *185*, 321–328. [CrossRef]
11. Bessot, N.; Nicolas, A.; Moussay, S.; Gauthier, A.; Sesboüé, B.; Davenne, D. The effect of pedal rate and time of day on the time to exhaustion from high-intensity exercise. *Chronobiol. Int.* **2006**, *23*, 1009–1024. [CrossRef]
12. Lepers, R.; Millet, G.Y.; Maffiuletti, N.A. Effect of cycling cadence on contractile and neural properties of knee extensors. *Med. Sci. Sports Exerc.* **2001**, *33*, 1882–1888. [CrossRef] [PubMed]
13. Sarre, G.; Lepers, R.; van Hoecke, J. Stability of pedalling mechanics during a prolonged cycling exercise performed at different cadences. *J. Sports Sci.* **2005**, *23*, 693–701. [CrossRef] [PubMed]
14. Marquez, G.J.; Mon, J.; Acero, R.M.; Sanchez, J.A.; Fernandez-Del-Olmo, M. Low-intensity cycling affects the muscle activation pattern of consequent countermovement jumps. *J. Strength Cond. Res.* **2009**, *23*, 1470–1476. [CrossRef] [PubMed]
15. Takaishi, T.; Yasuda, Y.; Ono, T.; Moritani, T. Optimal pedaling rate estimated from neuromuscular fatigue for cyclists. *Med. Sci. Sports Exerc.* **1996**, *28*, 1492–1497. [CrossRef]
16. Takaishi, T.; Yasuda, Y.; Moritani, T. Neuromuscular fatigue during prolonged pedalling exercise at different pedalling rates. *Eur. J. Appl. Physiol. Occup. Physiol.* **1994**, *69*, 154–158. [CrossRef]
17. Vercruyssen, F.; Missenard, O.; Brisswalter, J. Relationship between oxygen uptake slow component and surface EMG during heavy exercise in humans: Influence of pedal rate. *J. Electromyogr. Kinesiol. Off. J. Int. Soc. Electrophysiol. Kinesiol.* **2009**, *19*, 676–684. [CrossRef]
18. Ahlquist, L.E.; Bassett, D.R.; Sufit, R.; Nagle, F.J.; Thomas, D.P. The effect of pedaling frequency on glycogen depletion rates in type I and type II quadriceps muscle fibers during submaximal cycling exercise. *Eur. J. Appl. Physiol. Occup. Physiol.* **1992**, *65*, 360–364. [CrossRef]
19. Beelen, A.; Sargeant, A.J. Effect of prior exercise at different pedalling frequencies on maximal power in humans. *Eur. J. Appl. Physiol.* **1993**, *66*, 102–107. [CrossRef]
20. de Araujo Ruas, V.D.; Figueira, T.R.; Denadai, B.S.S.; Greco, C.C.; de Araújo Ruas, V.D.; Figueira, T.R.; Denadai, B.S.S.; Greco, C.C Effect of Cycling Exercise at Different Pedal Cadences on Subsequent Muscle Strength. *J. Exerc. Sci. Fit.* **2011**, *9*, 93–99. [CrossRef]
21. Kristoffersen, M.; Gundersen, H.; Leirdal, S.; Iversen, V.V. Low cadence interval training at moderate intensity does not improve cycling performance in highly trained veteran cyclists. *Front. Physiol.* **2014**, *5*, 34. [CrossRef] [PubMed]
22. Gergley, J.C. Concurrent Training: A Comparison of High and Low Cadence Cycle Ergometry on Lower-body Strength in Young Moderately Trained Males. *Med. Sci. Sports Exerc.* **2011**, *43*, 836. [CrossRef]
23. Millet, G.Y.; Lepers, R. Alterations of Neuromuscular Function after Prolonged Running, Cycling and Skiing Exercises. *Sport Med.* **2004**, *34*, 105–116. [CrossRef]
24. Oliver, J.; Lloyd, R.; Whitney, A. Monitoring of in-season neuromuscular and perceptual fatigue in youth rugby players. *Eur. J Sport Sci.* **2015**, *15*, 514–522. [CrossRef] [PubMed]
25. Bessot, N.; Moussay, S.; Laborde, S.; Gauthier, A.; Sesbouee, B.; Davenne, D. The role of the slope of oxygen consumption and EMG activity on freely chosen pedal rate selection. *Eur. J. Appl. Physiol.* **2008**, *103*, 195–202. [CrossRef] [PubMed]
26. Lucía, A.; Hoyos, J.; Chicharro, J.L. Preferred pedalling cadence in professional cycling. *Med. Sci. Sports Exerc.* **2001**, *33*, 1361–1366. [CrossRef]
27. Vogt, S.; Roecker, K.; Schumacher, Y.O.; Pottgiesser, T.; Dickhuth, H.-H.; Schmid, A.; Heinrich, L. Cadence-power-relationship during decisive mountain ascents at the Tour de France. *Int. J. Sports Med.* **2008**, *29*, 244–250. [CrossRef] [PubMed]
28. Albin, E.; Ann, H.; Ohnstad, E. Evidence for freely chosen pedalling rate during submaximal cycling to be a robust innate voluntary motor rhythm. *Exp. Brain Res.* **2008**, *186*, 365–373. [CrossRef]
29. Macintosh, B.R.; Neptune, R.R.; Horton, J.F. Cadence, power, and muscle activation in cycle ergometry. *Med. Sci. Sport. Exerc* **2000**, *32*, 1281–1287. [CrossRef] [PubMed]
30. Clos, P.; Garnier, Y.; Martin, A.; Lepers, R. Corticospinal excitability is altered similarly following concentric and eccentric maximal contractions. *Eur. J. Appl. Physiol.* **2020**, *120*, 1457–1469. [CrossRef]
31. Vercruyssen, F.; Brisswalter, J. Which factors determine the freely chosen cadence during submaximal cycling? *J. Sci. Med. Sport* **2010**, *13*, 225–231. [CrossRef]
32. Nickleberry, B.L.; Brooks, G.A. No effect of cycling experience on leg cycle ergometer efficiency. *Med. Sci. Sports Exerc.* **1996**, *28*, 1396–1401. [CrossRef]
33. Taylor, J.L.; Gandevia, S.C. A comparison of central aspects of fatigue in submaximal and maximal voluntary contractions. *J. Appl. Physiol.* **2008**, *104*, 542–550. [CrossRef]

4. Lepers, R.; Millet, G.Y.; Maffiuletti, N.A.; Hausswirth, C.; Brisswalter, J. Effect of pedalling rates on physiological response during endurance cycling. *Eur. J. Appl. Physiol.* **2001**, *85*, 392–395. [CrossRef] [PubMed]
5. Lucia, A.; Balmer, J.; Davison, R.C.R.; Perez, M.; Santalla, A.; Smith, P.M. Effects of the rotor pedalling system on the performance of trained cyclists during incremental and constant-load cycle ergometer tests. *Int. J. Sports Med.* **2004**, *25*, 479–485. [CrossRef] [PubMed]
6. Linnamo, V.; Moritani, T.; Nicol, C.; Komi, P.V. Motor unit activation patterns during isometric, concentric and eccentric actions at different force levels. *J. Electromyogr. Kinesiol.* **2003**, *13*, 93–101. [CrossRef]
7. Heckman, C.J.J.; Enoka, R.M. Motor unit. *Compr. Physiol.* **2012**, *2*, 2629–2682. [CrossRef] [PubMed]
8. Koninckx, E.; Van Leemputte, M.; Hespel, P. Effect of isokinetic cycling versus weight training on maximal power output and endurance performance in cycling. *Eur. J. Appl. Physiol.* **2010**, *109*, 699–708. [CrossRef] [PubMed]
9. Knuttgen, H.G.; Patton, J.F.; Vogel, J.A. An ergometer for concentric and eccentric muscular excercise. *J. Appl. Physiol. Respir. Environ. Exerc. Physiol.* **1982**, *53*, 784–788. [CrossRef] [PubMed]
10. Hoppeler, H. Moderate Load Eccentric Exercise; A Distinct Novel Training Modality. *Front. Physiol.* **2016**, *7*, 483. [CrossRef] [PubMed]
11. Clos, P.; Laroche, D.; Stapley, P.J.; Lepers, R. Neuromuscular and perceptual responses to sub-maximal eccentric cycling. *Front. Physiol.* **2019**, *10*, 354. [CrossRef] [PubMed]
12. Barreto, R.V.; de Lima, L.C.R.; Denadai, B.S. Moving forward with backward pedaling: A review on eccentric cycling. *Eur. J. Appl. Physiol.* **2020**, *121*, 381–407. [CrossRef] [PubMed]

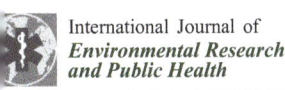

Article

How Task Constraints Influence the Gaze and Motor Behaviours of Elite-Level Gymnasts

Joana Barreto [1,*], Filipe Casanova [2,3], César Peixoto [4], Bradley Fawver [5,6] and Andrew Mark Williams [6]

1. Universidade de Lisboa, Faculdade de Motricidade Humana, Laboratório de Perícia no Desporto, CIPER, Cruz Quebrada Dafundo, 1495-751 Lisboa, Portugal
2. Faculty of Physical Education and Sport, University Lusófona of Humanities and Technology, 1749-024 Lisbon, Portugal; p5661@ulusofona.pt
3. Center of Research, Education, Innovation and Intervention in Sport (CIFI2D), Faculty of Sport, University of Porto, 4200-450 Porto, Portugal
4. Universidade de Lisboa, Faculdade de Motricidade Humana, Laboratório de Perícia no Desporto, Cruz Quebrada Dafundo, 1495-751 Lisboa, Portugal; cpeixoto@fmh.ulisboa.pt
5. US Army Medical Research Directorate-West, Walter Reed Army Institute of Research, Joint Base Lewis McChord, Pierce, WA 98433, USA; bradley.j.fawver.ctr@mail.mil
6. Department of Health and Kinesiology, College of Health, University of Utah, Salt Lake City, UT 84112, USA; Mark.Williams@health.utah.edu
* Correspondence: joana.cpbarreto@gmail.com; Tel.: +351-910213883

Abstract: Perception-action coupling is fundamental to effective motor behaviour in complex sports such as gymnastics. We examined the gaze and motor behaviours of 10 international level gymnasts when performing two skills on the mini-trampoline that matched the performance demands of elite competition. The presence and absence of a vaulting table in each skill served as a task-constraint factor, while we compared super-elite and elite groups. We measured visual search behaviours and kinematic variables during the approach run phase. The presence of a vaulting table influenced gaze behaviour only in the elite gymnasts, who showed significant differences in the time spent fixating on the mini-trampoline, when compared to super-elite gymnasts. Moreover, different approach run characteristics were apparent across the two different gymnastic tasks, irrespective of the level of expertise, and take-off velocity was influenced by the skill being executed across all gymnasts. Task constraints and complexity influence gaze behaviours differed across varying levels of expertise in gymnastics, even within a sample of international level athletes. It appears that the time spent fixating their gazes on the right areas of interest during the approach run is crucial to higher-level performance and therefore higher scores in competition, particularly on the mini-trampoline with vaulting table.

Keywords: expertise; inertial sensors; kinematic analysis; perception-action coupling; performance; visual fixation

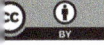

1. Introduction

Gymnasts perform highly complex skills on diverse apparatus, each with specific characteristics and requirements [1]. Within the Teamgym discipline, athletes perform skills using only the mini-trampoline (MT) and using the mini-trampoline with vaulting table (MTVT). Both skills require continuous perception-action coupling in order to visually regulate motor behaviour, particularly during the approach run [2–7]. The mechanisms underlying performance are believed to vary by apparatus and skill complexity, notably with the inclusion of a vaulting table on MTVT skills; however, our understanding of how task constraints influence gaze and motor behaviours during the approach run to the MT and MTVT remains limited.

The need for on-line visual regulation during the approach run when vaulting has been previously confirmed [4], with the springboard and vaulting table considered important sources of visual information [2,3,7]. Gymnasts regulate the approach run based on a visual strategy using time-to-contact information [6]. The application of direct measures of gaze behaviour (e.g., eye-tracking systems) in recent work [8–12] has allowed consideration of the spotting hypothesis: gymnasts fixate their gaze on specific locations in their environment when performing complex techniques, but these behaviours are dependent on the experimental condition/task and performer's level of expertise. In a recent study with elite-level gymnasts (i.e., national team members), we demonstrated that gymnasts used different visual strategies when performing on an MT alone compared to the MTVT [12]. These data collectively suggest that elite gymnasts develop a unique visual strategy to optimally select and process relevant visual information from their environment, especially when different constraints are presented (e.g., vaulting table).

Several limitations in the existing literature prompted the present study. First, the tasks used in previous work [3,4,6–8,13,14] were relatively simple (e.g., single back somersault on trampoline and handspring on vault) compared to the techniques typically performed at the elite level. Second, the selection of indirect measures of gaze behaviour did not allow effective inferences about gaze and motor behaviours during skill execution. Lastly, comparisons across groups of true experts are generally lacking in this field of literature.

To address these gaps, we measured gaze and motor behaviours while international level gymnasts of varying levels of expertise (i.e., super elite and elite) performed mini-trampoline skills either in the absence (i.e., MT) or presence (i.e., MTVT) of a vaulting table. This approach is novel in addressing two key gaps in the existing literature: (1) measuring perceptual and motor variables during the execution of complex skills; and (2) the recruitment of a cohort on truly elite (national team) athletes, although in regards to the latter at the cost of a reduced sample size.

The purpose of this study is to investigate if task constraints (i.e., presence and absence of vaulting table) influence gaze and motor behaviours of elite-level gymnasts. First, we expected that gaze behaviours would be influenced by task constraints independently of participants' levels of expertise [15]. More specifically, gymnasts were expected to fixate on the most relevant environment locations during both skills: (a) greater fixation number and longer dwell times on the mini-trampoline when performing the MT skill; and (b) a significant increase in the proportion of fixation number and dwell times on the vaulting table when performing the MTVT skill [2,3]. Second, we predicted that super elite gymnasts would exhibit longer final fixations on areas of interest (AOI; either mini-trampoline or vaulting table), compared to their less-elite counterparts; and the number of fixations was expected to be positively associated with superior performance, since a faster visual search rate in more-expert gymnasts has been reported in other related tasks [16–18]. Third, we predicted that motor behaviour, more specifically take-off velocity, would be influenced by task constraint with all participants increasing their take-off velocity on MTVT, due to the higher complexity of the task. Finally, we expected that greater take-off velocity would be associated with better scores [19–22].

2. Materials and Methods

2.1. Sample

Altogether, 10 elite Teamgym gymnasts, all from the Teamgym national team participated in the study. Five international Teamgym judges from Portugal, Italy and the Czech Republic scored execution on MT and MTVT according to the Teamgym Code of Points [23]. Based on the scores from judges, the participants were separated into two groups: super elite (i.e., with higher scores) gymnasts ($n = 5$; mean age: 27.8 ± 3.35 years mean experience: 13.4 ± 2.32 years); and elite (i.e., with lower scores) gymnasts ($n = 5$ mean age: 22.6 ± 2.30 years, mean experience: 8.2 ± 1.04 years). The study was conducted in accordance with the Declaration of Helsinki and approved by the Faculty Ethics Committee (1/2020; 24/01/2020). Gymnasts reported normal or corrected to normal vision and signed an informed consent prior to starting experimental procedures.

2.2. Tasks

Participants performed two separate skills on two apparatus: tucked barani out on MT (Figure 1A) and handspring tucked barani out on MTVT (Figure 1B). The manipulation of task constraints (i.e., apparatus) was represented by the presence (MTVT) or absence (MT) of a vaulting table. Both skills have similar movement patterns and are usually performed at elite level in this discipline.

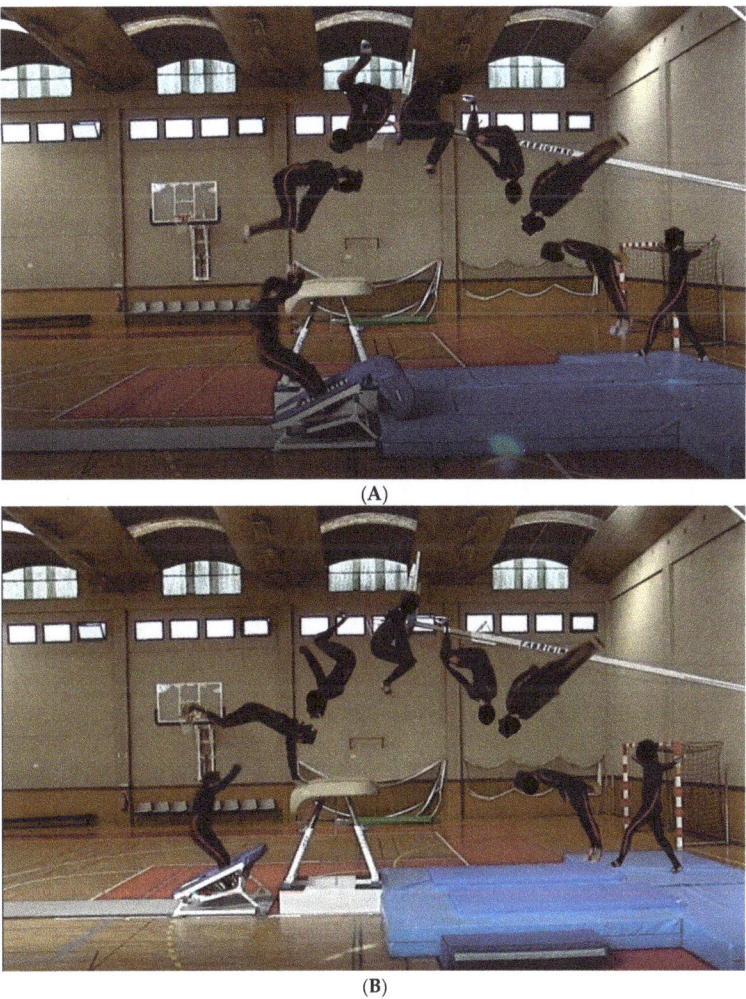

Figure 1. (**A**) Task performed on mini-trampoline (MT): tucked barani out. After a maximum 25 m approach run, the gymnast performs a take-off from the mini-trampoline followed by a double somersault in a tucked position (720° on transversal axis rotation), and a half twist (180° on longitudinal axis rotation) before landing. (**B**) Task performed on mini-trampoline with vaulting table (MTVT): handspring tucked barani out. After a maximum 25 m approach run, the gymnast performs a take-off from the mini-trampoline followed by a forward entrance placing their hands in vaulting table (support phase), one and a half somersault in a tucked position (total of 720° on transversal axis rotation) and a half twist (180° on longitudinal axis rotation) before landing.

2.3. Instruments and Procedure

Gaze data were sampled frame-by-frame at 50 Hz using a Tobii Pro Glasses 2 (Tobii Pro AB, Stockholm, Sweden) mobile eye-tracking system (ETS), which uses a binocular eye movement system to measure the relative position of the pupil and corneal reflection and overlays point-of-gaze onto a video image of the scene. Tobii Glasses Controller Software running on a Dell Venue 11 Pro 7130, Windows 8/8.1 Pro tablet was used to manage eye movement recording, with images transferred to a computer and analysed using Tobii Pro Lab (Version 1.142, Tobii Pro AB, Stockholm, Sweden). The eye-movement system was calibrated by asking each participant to stand still and visually fixate on the centre of calibration card 1.25 m away for five seconds. After calibration, participants fixated on nine different points in the environment at various distances, heights, and widths.

A visual fixation was defined as a period of at least 100 ms when the eye remained stationary within $\pm 0.5°$ of movement tolerance [24]. Visual gaze behaviours were analysed to obtain search rate and dwell time data for dependent measures. Specifically, we quantified search rate from recordings of the mean number of visual fixations, the mean fixation duration in milliseconds, and the total number of fixation locations per AOI. We defined dwell time as the proportion of time spent fixating on each of eight different locations/AOIs as a percent of the total fixation time (see Figure 2). The AOIs included: (a) the first 10 m of approach run or 'Start Run'; (b) between 10 and 20 m of approach run or 'Mid Run'; (c) the last 5 m of approach run or 'End Run'; (d) the floor area surrounding or 'Floor'; (e) the mini-trampoline; (f) the vaulting table if present; (g) the landing mat; and (h) the front wall. The final fixation dwell time relative to the total duration of the approach run was calculated, as well as the final fixation duration before mini-trampoline take-off (if >100 ms).

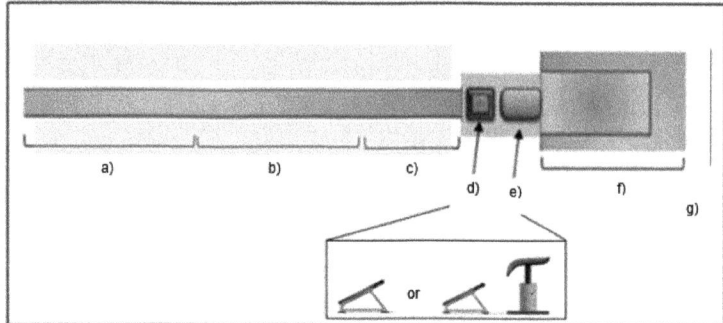

Figure 2. The experimental setup, apparatus, and areas of interest (AOIs) considered for analysis. AOIs included: (**a**) Start Run (10 × 2 m); (**b**) Mid Run (10 × 2 m); (**c**) End Run (5 × 2 m—grey areas); (**d**) mini-trampoline; (**e**) vaulting table; (**f**) landing mat (4 × 7 m); and (**g**) front wall. Lateral detailed view is presented at the bottom of the figure for each apparatus and AOIs: mini-trampoline without vaulting table (MT) and mini-trampoline with vaulting table (MTVT). Adapted from Hughes et al. (2013).

We recorded kinematic data using a system of seventeen inertial measurement sensors (Xsens MVN Link; Xsens Technologies, Enschede, The Netherlands) at a rate of 240 Hz. The placement of sensors and calibration conformed to the manufacturer's recommendation. Kinematic data were processed in multilevel high definition using MVN Analyse software (Version 2019.2.1, Xsens Technologies, Enschede, The Netherlands). We used acceleration peaks, representing foot impacts on the mat carpet, to define the number of steps of the approach run and contact with mini-trampoline [25]. We calculated segment position and orientations using MVN Fusion Engine for Xsens, and these data were imported into Visual 3D (Version 6, C-Motion, Inc., Germantown, MD, USA) for dependent measure computation. We derived specific measures from the kinematic post-processing including

(a) take-off velocity in meters per second; (b) step length—mean length of the last nine steps before take-off in meters; (c) hurdle length—mean length between the last step and take-off on mini-trampoline in meters; and (d) step frequency—the number of steps per minute. Both systems were synchronized using an LED connected through a trigger signal.

Experimental tasks were performed in a sports hall according to Teamgym directives [26]. All trials were recorded using a video camera (Casio EXILIM EX-F1, 60 Hz) placed perpendicular to the MT/MTVT. Participants performed a twenty-minute warm-up and several practice trials before instrument calibration was performed.

Participants performed four trials of each skill as if they were in a competition, starting with MT, and were informed that trials would be evaluated by international Teamgym judges. Participants chose the distance of the run-up, which was marked with black tape every five meters. We repeated instrument calibrations before each trial. Following the completion of all trials, participants were fully debriefed. According to judges' scores, we considered the best two trials performed on each apparatus for analysis (MT and MTVT) as well as computing a total score on each apparatus.

2.4. Statistical and Data Analysis

A between and within-participants research design was carried out. Gaze and kinematic trial durations were normalized to 100 data points to improve comparison between groups. We performed Intraclass Correlation Coefficient (ICC) and Confidence Intervals (CI) estimates for judges' ratings. Linear mixed-effect regressions (LMERs) were utilized to examine the effects of Expertise level (Group: super elite, elite) × Task/Skill (Apparatus: MT, MTVT) on vaulting scores and whether these factors were associated with different process-tracing measures of performance (e.g., gaze behaviour, kinematics). In each model, Group and Apparatus were fixed effects, while random effects included Participant and Participant × Group. The normality of residuals was inspected using Q–Q plots, with all models exhibiting normality visually and according to the Kolmogorov–Smirnov test (all $p < 0.05$). Given the elite nature of the participants, and therefore smaller sample size available, data normality was confirmed using equivalent. We also conducted non-parametric tests of normality using the Shapiro–Wilk test. We evaluated heterogeneity using Levene's test. In the case of deviations with respect to these tests, the measure of interest was transformed (e.g., log, mean-centred) prior to analysis.

We calculated the significance of individual parameters for each model using a t-test with a Welch–Satterthwaite approximation and report 95% confidence intervals for all analyses. We also report partial-eta squared (η^2) effect sizes for main effects, interactions, and univariate follow-up tests, and Cohen's d effect sizes are reported for pairwise comparisons. The significance level for all statistical tests was set at $\alpha = 0.05$. Analyses were conducted using SPSS v25.0 (SPSS Inc., Chicago, IL, USA; IBM Corp, Armonk, NY, USA) or R-Studio v3.6.1.

3. Results

3.1. Performance

The ICC estimates and 95% confident intervals for judges' scores indicated good reliability [27], with an absolute agreement value of 0.863 ($CI_{95\%} = 0.813, 0.904$). The more-elite or super elite group (mean final score = 9.492 pts ± 0.05, out of 10) generally outperformed the less elite group (mean final score = 9.112 pts ± 0.17); however, a significant Group × Apparatus interaction was documented for score, $\beta = 0.356$ (0.07, 0.64), $t(28.0) = 2.446$, $p = 0.021$, $\eta^2 = 0.150$. Post hoc tests revealed that when performing on MTVT, the super elite group scored significantly higher (mean score = 9.32 pts ± 0.14) compared to the elite group (mean score = 8.77 pts ± 0.37; $\beta = 0.542$ (0.24, 0.84), $t(8) = 3.529$, $p = 0.007$, $\eta^2 = 0.491$, $d = 1.97$), but this effect was not evident on the MT ($p = 0.126$, $d = 0.96$). Scores were significantly higher for MT compared to MTVT for both the super elite ($\beta = 0.320$ (0.17, 0.47), $t(18) = 4.123$, $p < 0.001$, $\eta^2 = 0.486$, $d = 1.85$) and elite groups ($\beta = 0.676$ (0.43, 0.92), $t(14) = 5.588$, $p < 0.001$, $\eta^2 = 0.656$, $d = 2.30$). In summary, expertise level was positively associated with vaulting scores overall, which was driven by the more difficult constraints present during the MTVT task.

3.2. Gaze Behaviour

The mean ± SD values for search rate and gaze behaviour variables are presented as a function of apparatus in Table 1. A significant Group × Apparatus interaction was obtained for dwell time percent on the mini-trampoline, $\beta = 20.040$ (6.30, 33.78), $t(28) = 8.133$, $p = 0.009$, $\eta^2 = 0.205$ (Figure 3A). Post hoc tests revealed that when performing the MTVT task, the elite participants spent significantly less time (~16%) fixating on the mini-trampoline (mean dwell time = 33.08% ± 8.98) compared to the super elite group (mean dwell time = 49.46% ± 13.38; $\beta = 16.379$ (4.61, 28.15), $t(10) = 3.012$, $p = 0.013$, $\eta^2 = 0.372$, $d = 1.46$). However, there were no main effects of Group for dwell time on the mini-trampoline when executing the MT skill ($p = 0.593$, $d = 0.27$). Dwell time on the mini-trampoline was significantly greater (~21%) for the elite group when performing the MT skill compared to MTVT skill, $\beta = 21.63$ (13.24, 30.03), $t(14) = 5.208$, $p < 0.001$, $\eta^2 = 0.633$, $d = 2.05$. In summary, participants in the elite group tended to fixate less on the mini-trampoline when performing the MTVT task (~33%), whereas dwell time on the mini-trampoline did not differ across groups for both apparatuses (~49–55%). Although the super elite group appeared to spend less time fixating the vaulting table when performing the MTVT skill (mean dwell time = 17.08% ± 6.86) when compared to the elite group (mean dwell time = 26.80% ± 10.75), this effect did not reach the threshold for significance, $\beta = 9.720$, $p = 0.083$, $\eta^2 = 0.228$, $d = 1.08$.

Table 1. The scores and gaze behaviour measures (mean ± SD) by group for vaulting skills executed using the mini trampoline without the vaulting table (MT) and with a vaulting table (MTVT).

	MT		MTVT	
	Super Elite	Elite	Super Elite	Elite
Score	9.64 ± 0.20	9.45 ± 0.19	9.32 ± 0.14	8.77 ± 0.37 [a,b]
Fixations mid run (#)	1.10 ± 0.74	1.20 ± 0.79	1.50 ± 0.85	1.50 ± 0.71
Fixations end run (#)	2.00 ± 1.70	1.80 ± 0.79	1.80 ± 1.55	1.50 ± 1.08
Fixations MT (#)	3.30 ± 2.21	3.20 ± 1.48	3.10 ± 1.73	3.10 ± 1.66
Fixations VT (#)	—	—	1.40 ± 0.52	2.20 ± 1.55
Total fixations (#)	8.70 ± 2.58	7.60 ± 1.84	8.10 ± 1.91	9.00 ± 1.89
Avg. fixation duration (ms)	291.47 ± 83.85	383.21 ± 112.20 [a]	357.78 ± 98.05	286.81 ± 96.10 [a]
Dwell time mid run (%)	12.56 ± 11.31	14.31 ± 9.51	14.11 ± 11.86	17.05 ± 9.88
Dwell time end run (%)	22.29 ± 14.07	19.28 ± 13.38	19.36 ± 13.61	15.49 ± 7.79
Dwell time MT (%)	51.05 ± 15.44	54.71 ± 11.90 [b]	49.46 ± 13.08 [b]	33.08 ± 8.98 [a,b]
Dwell time VT (%)	—	—	17.08 ± 6.86	26.80 ± 10.75
Final fixation dwell (%)	17.60 ± 11.81	21.20 ± 14.07	15.4 ± 6.64	16.4 ± 5.02
Final fixation duration (ms)	488.00 ± 429.49	822.00 ± 487.12	522.00 ± 225.77	550.00 ± 165.80

Note: # = number; MT = mini-trampoline; VT = vaulting table; [a] denotes a significant Group × Apparatuses interaction; [b] denotes a significant difference between apparatus.

A significant Group × Apparatus interaction was documented for mean fixation duration, $\beta = 162.70$ (48.07, 277.34), $t(28) = 2.776$, $p = 0.010$, $\eta^2 = 0.154$ (Figure 3B). Post hoc tests revealed that this effect was driven by participants in the elite group demonstrating average fixation durations that were approximately 100 ms longer when performing the MT (mean fixation time = 383.21 ms ± 112.20) compared to MTVT (mean fixation time = 291.47 ms ± 83.85; $\beta = 96.40$ (19.96, 172.83), $t(14) = 2.574$, $p = 0.022$, $\eta^2 = 0.304$, $d = 0.923$). Finally, there were no significant main effects of Group or Apparatus, or interaction effects, for the total number of fixations ($p > 0.085$), dwell time on the Mid Run ($p > 0.676$), dwell time on the End Run ($p > 0.693$), final fixation dwell time ($p > 0.686$), or final fixation duration ($p > 0.144$).

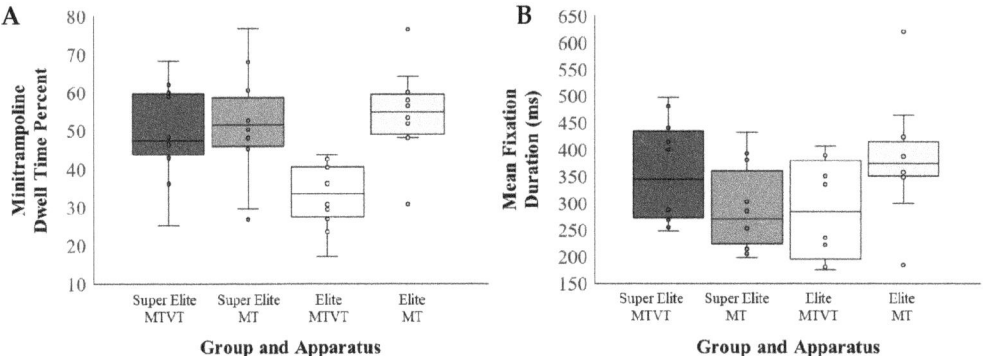

Figure 3. Gaze measures by group (super elite vs. elite) and apparatus (MTVT vs. MT): (**A**) dwell time percent on the mini-trampoline during the approach run, as a function of total fixation time; (**B**) mean fixation duration in milliseconds.

3.3. Motor Behaviour

The mean ± SD values for movement kinematics during the approach run and take-off are presented in Table 2. No main effect of Group was found for take-off velocity on either the MTVT ($p = 0.175$) or MT skills ($p = 0.193$), $d = 0.621$; however, a significant Group × Apparatus interaction was documented for take-off velocity, $\beta = 0.766$ (0.15–1.38), $t(27.99) = 2.462$, $p = 0.020$, $\eta^2 = 0.162$ (Figure 4A). The super elite group displayed significantly greater take-off velocity (~0.5 m/s) when performing the MTVT compared to MT, $\beta = 0.533$ (0.15, −1.38), $t(18) = 3.863$, $p = 0.001$, $\eta^2 = 0.453$, $d = 1.72$. The same but larger effect of apparatus (~1.3 m/s greater velocity for MTVT) was documented in the elite group, $\beta = 1.299$ (0.75, −1.85), $t(14) = 4.815$, $p < 0.001$, $\eta^2 = 0.603$, $d = 1.76$.

Table 2. The movement behaviour (mean ± SD) for expert and less-expert performers across skills executed using the mini-trampoline without a vaulting table (MT) and with a vaulting table (MTVT).

Measure	MT		MTVT	
Step Length Variables	**Super Elite**	**Elite**	**Super Elite**	**Elite**
Step −8 to −9 (m)	1.04 ± 0.24	1.09 ± 0.31	0.85 ± 0.33	1.22 ± 0.16
Step −7 to −8 (m)	1.09 ± 0.28	1.18 ± 0.34	1.09 ± 0.54	1.22 ± 0.31
Step −6 to −7 (m)	1.09 ± 0.33	1.26 ± 0.29	1.25 ± 0.28	1.29 ± 0.24
Step −5 to −6 (m)	1.27 ± 0.21	1.29 ± 0.26	1.33 ± 0.26	1.40 ± 0.09
Step −4 to −5 (m)	1.38 ± 0.18	1.49 ± 0.35	1.39 ± 0.17	1.42 ± 0.10
Step −3 to −4 (m)	1.47 ± 0.21	1.45 ± 0.20	1.47 ± 0.12	1.51 ± 0.10
Step −2 to −3 (m)	1.47 ± 0.12	1.50 ± 0.21	1.50 ± 0.11	1.58 ± 0.13
Step −1 to −2 (m)	1.41 ± 0.14	1.37 ± 0.10	1.46 ± 0.08	1.44 ± 0.20
Take-off to step −1 (m)	3.10 ± 0.28	2.97 ± 0.22	3.22 ± 0.19	3.03 ± 0.18
Avg. step length (m)	1.28 ± 0.17	1.33 ± 0.09	1.29 ± 0.16	1.39 ± 0.07
Step Velocity Variables	**Super Elite**	**Elite**	**Super Elite**	**Elite**
Step −9 (m/s)	3.33 ± 0.87	4.52 ± 0.96	4.14 ± 0.88	5.09 ± 0.57
Step −8 (m/s)	4.06 ± 0.77	5.01 ± 0.91	4.80 ± 0.77	5.58 ± 0.52
Step −7 (m/s)	4.58 ± 0.65	5.42 ± 0.81	5.32 ± 0.57	5.99 ± 0.40
Step −6 (m/s)	5.10 ± 0.61	5.77 ± 0.76	5.79 ± 0.52	6.35 ± 0.34
Step −5 (m/s)	5.55 ± 0.50	6.05 ± 0.65	6.14 ± 0.40	6.57 ± 0.26
Step −4 (m/s)	5.96 ± 0.49	6.27 ± 0.55	6.77 ± 0.26	7.04 ± 0.19
Step −3 (m/s)	6.29 ± 0.45	6.49 ± 0.46	6.77 ± 0.26	7.04 ± 0.19
Step −2 (m/s)	6.64 ± 0.45	6.74 ± 0.38	7.15 ± 0.29	7.32 ± 0.21
Step −1 (m/s)	6.90 ± 0.46	6.80 ± 0.30	7.33 ± 0.22	7.37 ± 0.25
Take-off velocity (m/s)	4.71 ± 0.26 [b]	4.24 ± 0.87 [b]	5.24 ± 0.35 [b]	5.53 ± 0.56 [b]
Avg. step velocity (m/s)	5.37 ± 0.54	5.89 ± 0.63	5.99 ± 0.46	6.47 ± 0.26
Step frequency (steps/min)	204.60 ± 13.38	213.90 ± 12.18 [a]	208.30 ± 13.58	229.40 ± 16.97 [a]

Note: Mean step length and velocity calculated from last nine steps before take-off; [a] denotes significant main effect of group; [b] denotes significant Group × Apparatus interaction.

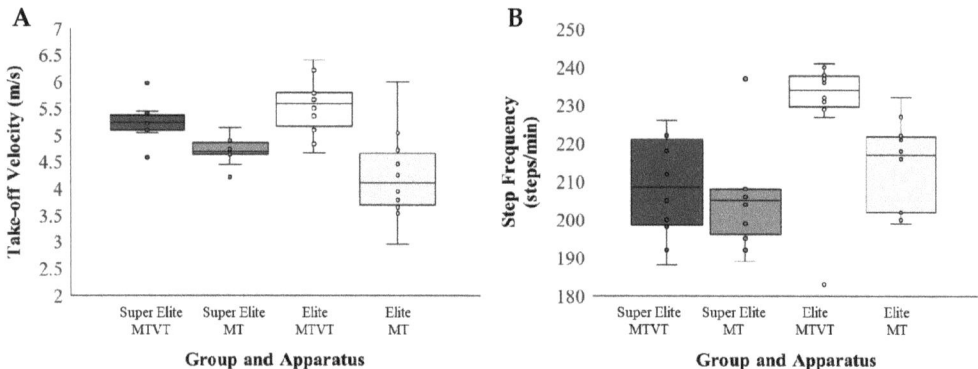

Figure 4. Kinematic measures by group (super elite vs. elite) and apparatus (MTVT vs. MT): (**A**): take-off velocity in meters per seconds; (**B**) step frequency in steps per minute.

A significant main effect of Group was documented for step frequency, $\beta = 32.9$ (9.35, 56.45), $t(28) = 2.649$, $p = 0.012$, $\eta^2 = 0.190$, indicating that the elite group demonstrated significantly more steps/minute (mean step frequency = 221.65 steps/min ± 16.43) compared to the super elite group (mean step frequency = 206.45 steps/min ± 13.26) (Figure 4B). Although it appeared that these effects were isolated to the elite group displaying a greater number of approach-run steps on MT in particular, the Group × Apparatus interaction did not reach the threshold for significance, $\beta = 11.80$, $p = 0.096$. Additionally no main effects of Group, Apparatus or their interactions were reported (all p's > 0.175).

4. Discussion

We examined the influence of task constraints (i.e., the presence (MTVT) or absence (MT) of a vaulting table) on gaze and motor behaviours in elite, international level gymnasts of varying levels of expertise. Contrary to our hypothesis that gaze behaviours would be influenced by task constraints independently of participants' levels of expertise, results showed that task constraints influence the gaze behaviours of elite participants to a greater degree than super elite gymnasts (Table 1). Specifically, elite gymnasts significantly reduced the amount of time fixating the mini-trampoline when performing on MTVT, while the super elite gymnasts did not differ in the time fixating the mini-trampoline in both task. As we hypothesized, motor behaviour was influenced by the task constraints (Table 2) with both groups significantly increasing their take-off velocity during the MTVT skill compared to MT. Furthermore, the elite participants demonstrated increased step frequency in MTVT compared to MT. Groups did not differ in performance scores in MT, but the super elite participants' scores on MTVT were significantly higher than their elite counterparts. Finally, the two groups did not differ in gaze behaviours in MT, and no differences were documented between groups for the number of total fixations, final fixation dwell and duration during both skills, in opposition to what was hypothesized.

While super elite participants generally outperformed their elite counterparts, groups did not differ in performance scores on the MT skill, and decomposition of the interaction effect revealed that this was driven by performance in the more difficult MTVT skill. These findings suggest that simple tasks, typically mastered earlier in sport development, are not sufficient to detect expertise differences amongst elite level gymnasts.

Expertise level did not alter the preference of gymnasts to direct gaze behaviour predominantly towards the mini-trampoline (dwell time on MT = 51.05 ± 15.44% vs 54.71 ± 11.90%). The amount of gaze time directed to the mini-trampoline was possibly driven by the need to regulate current position and therefore control distance and time-to contact for the take-off phase [2–4,6,7,13]. Participants with less expertise spent significantly less time directing gaze to the mini-trampoline during the MTVT task compared to the MT skill (see Table 1). A meta-analysis [17] reported that gaze behaviour is indeed moderated by task complexity, and several published reports have corroborated the malleability of visual regulation using other related tasks [17,28–31]. The emergence of different visual behaviours depends on task characteristics and complexity, although the more-expert group demonstrated similar gaze behaviours when performing on MT and MTVT. It appears that expertise may lead to an improvement in how vision is used to process information from the environment [32,33], thereby allowing super-elite competitors to find common, efficient ways to use the visual system during similar, but different, complex motor tasks.

From a technical point of view, MTVT skills present additional constraints specifically during the first flight phase (i.e., from mini-trampoline to vaulting table) and the second flight phase (i.e., from take-off from vaulting table to landing) [21,34,35]. The elite group may have more difficulty during these phases of movement, resulting in a reduction in time directing gaze to the mini-trampoline during the approach run, in order to find their hand placement location on the vaulting table. We suggest that differences in level of expertise indicate that even elite gymnasts of significant skill-level (e.g., national team athletes) must learn how to efficiently use attention in order to focus on the right cues for the right amount of time during more complex vaults. As a result, super-elite gymnasts have the ability to direct their gaze predominantly to the mini-trampoline (as in MT task) to constantly perceive information and adjust their approach run, because they are not reliant on as much information extracted from the vaulting table. It is also possible that super-elite participants were using their peripheral vision to obtain visual information from the proximal edge of the vaulting table, while directing their focal gaze to the mini-trampoline [36]. The elite group seem to perceive visual information to adjust their approach run (with mini-trampoline still being the most fixated), as well as directing their gaze to the vaulting table to precisely place their hands (i.e., the elite group spent ~10% more time on average fixating on the vaulting table). Therefore, in applied practice, one strategy to improve MTVT skill execution would be to train hand location on the vaulting table so gymnasts can learn to relate kinaesthetic feedback with the use of limited (or peripheral) visual information from the vaulting table. Additionally, and since the mini-trampoline is the most relevant visual AOI for these tasks, we suggest the implementation of strategies such as using colours to increase attunement to this AOI. In this way, we are manipulating the task constraint to lead gymnasts to improve their gaze behaviours and motor performance.

Take-off velocity did not differ across groups, but all participants demonstrated greater take-off velocity during the MTVT (see Table 2), highlighting that motor behaviour is influenced by task constraints. As we predicted, greater velocities during the approach run and take-off have been shown to be associated with better performances and higher scores on vaulting [19,21,22,37]. The higher level of complexity on the MTVT task likely explains this discrepancy in take-off velocities between apparatuses [20,37]. Additionally, the elite group displayed significantly increased step frequency on MTVT, which has been demonstrated to be positively correlated with approach run velocity for handspring entries on the vaulting table [38]. Given the higher scores observed for the super-elite group on the MTVT compared to the elite gymnasts, in future, researchers should investigate other kinematic parameters in elite-level gymnasts that might be stronger determinants of performance outcomes on complex skills using a vaulting table.

Several limitations are worth acknowledging. First, the sample size in this study was relatively small, but gymnasts were all international level performers from the same team (Teamgym national team). We felt that securing samples of super elite and elite gymnasts would generate more insightful and impactful findings compared to using more diverse skill groupings, as per the more typical expert vs. novice design. Second, repeated trials were time consuming and quickly led to participant fatigue; therefore, we limited participants to four trials on each apparatus and took the two best trials for analysis. In future research, it would be beneficial to analyse central-peripheral awareness [36,39] and the location of the hands on the vaulting table (i.e., the distance between the edge of the vaulting table and hands), in groups with various levels of expertise. Furthermore, analysis of kinematic parameters during the approach run and contacts with the mini-trampoline and vaulting table, namely, joint angles and angular velocity, may provide detailed insight into how task constraints influence performance across various levels of expertise in gymnastics. These approaches may facilitate the design of training programs that focus on the most relevant AOIs from the environment, but essentially on its relationship with motor behaviour. In this way, gymnasts can improve their ability to select important visual information to improve motor performance.

5. Conclusions

We provide novel knowledge about how task constraints influence gaze and motor behaviours in elite, international level gymnasts when performing skills with similar technical structures but different levels of complexity. We also addressed how these factors change as a function of expertise. When performing skills that require a vaulting table, the amount of gaze time directed to AOIs from the environment distinguishes super elite from elite gymnasts. In contrast, the motor behaviours were less indicative of gymnast expertise level overall, and expertise level was less predictive of performance on the relatively-easier MT skill. These findings underscore the importance of visual perception for effective motor regulation and performance during vaulting skill execution in international level gymnasts.

Author Contributions: Conceptualization, J.B., F.C., C.P., B.F. and A.M.W.; methodology, J.B. and B.F.; software, J.B., F.C. and B.F.; investigation, J.B.; writing—original draft preparation, J.B. and B.F. writing—review and editing, F.C., C.P. and A.M.W.; supervision, C.P., F.C. and A.M.W. All authors have read and agreed to the published version of the manuscript.

Funding: This work was supported by the Fundação para a Ciência e Tecnologia, under Grant UIDB/00447/2020 to CIPER-Centro Interdisciplinar para o Estudo da Performance Humana (unit 447).

Institutional Review Board Statement: The study was conducted according to the guidelines of the Declaration of Helsinki, and approved by the Ethics Committee of the Faculty of Human Kinetics–University of Lisbon (1/2020, 24/01/2020).

Informed Consent Statement: Informed consent was obtained from all subjects involved in the study.

Data Availability Statement: The correspondent author should be contacted for more details on data.

Conflicts of Interest: The authors report no conflict of interest or disclosures. Material has been reviewed by the Walter Reed Army Institute of Research. There is no objection to either its presentation, publication, or both. The opinions or assertions contained herein are the private views of the authors and are not to be construed as official, or as reflecting the true views of the Department of the Army or the Department of Defense. The investigators have adhered to the policies for protection of human subjects as prescribed in AR 70-25.

References

1. Jemni, M.; Sands, W.A.; Salmela, J.H.; Holvoet, P.; Gateva, M. *The Science of Gymnastics*, 1st ed.; Routledge: Oxon, UK, 2011; pp. 32–37.
2. Heinen, T.; Vinken, P.; Jeraj, D.; Velentzas, K. Movement Regulation of Handsprings on Vault. *Res. Q Exerc. Sport* **2013**, *84*, 68–78. [CrossRef]
3. Heinen, T.; Jeraj, D.; Thoeren, M.; Vinken, P.M. Target-directed running in gymnastics: The role of the springboard position as an informational source to regulate handsprings on vault. *Biol. Sport* **2011**, *28*, 215–221. [CrossRef]
4. Bradshaw, E. Gymnastics: Target-directed running in gymnastics: A preliminary exploration of vaulting. *Sport Biomech.* **2004**, *3*, 125–144. [CrossRef]
5. Bradshaw, E.; Sparrow, W. The approach, vaulting performance, and judge's score in women's artistic gymnastics. In Proceedings of the Biomechanics Symposia, San Francisco, CA, USA, 26 June 2001.
6. Haigis, T.; Schlegel, K. The regulatory influence of the visual system: An exploratory study in gymnastics vaulting. *Sci. Gymnast. J.* **2020**, *12*, 61–73.
7. Heinen, T.; Brinker, A.; Mack, M.; Hennig, L. The role of positional environmental cues in movement regulation of Yurchenko vaults in gymnastics. *Sci. Gymnast. J.* **2017**, *9*, 113–126.

Natrup, J.; Bramme, J.; Lussanet, M.; Joris, K.; Lappe, M.; Wagner, H. Gaze behavior of trampoline gymnasts during a back tuck somersault. *Hum. Mov. Sci.* **2020**, *70*, 102589. [CrossRef]

Natrup, J.; de Lussanet, M.; Boström, K.; Lappe, M.; Wagner, H. Gaze, head and eye movements during somersaults with full twists. *Hum. Mov Sci.* **2021**, *75*, 102740. [CrossRef]

Heinen, T.; Velentzas, K.; Vinken, P. Functional Relationships Between Gaze Behavior and Movement Kinematics When Performing High Bar Dismounts—An Exploratory Study. *Hum. Mov.* **2012**, *13*, 218–224. [CrossRef]

Heinen, T. Evidence for the spotting hypothesis in gymnasts. *Motor Control.* **2011**, *15*, 267–284. [CrossRef] [PubMed]

Barreto, J.; Casanova, F.; Peixoto, C. Gaze behaviour in elite gymnasts when performing mini-trampoline and mini-trampoline with vaulting table—A pilot study. *Sci. Gymnast J.* **2020**, *12*, 287–297.

Heinen, T. Movement Regulation of Gymnastics Skills under varying Environmental Constraints. *Eur. J. Hum. Mov.* **2017**, *39*, 96–115.

Heinen, T.; Jeraj, D.; Vinken, P.; Velentzas, K. Land where you look?—Functional relationships between gaze and movement behaviour in a backward salto. *Biol. Sport.* **2012**, *29*, 177–183. [CrossRef]

Heinen, T.; Velentzas, K.; Vinken, P. Analyzing Gaze Behavior in Complex (Aerial) Skills. *Int. J. Sport Sci. Eng.* **2012**, *06*, 165–174.

Mann, D.T.; Williams, A.M.; Ward, P. Perceptual-cognitive expertise in sport: A meta-analysis. *J. Sport Exerc. Psychol.* **2007**, *29*, 457–478. [CrossRef]

Gegenfurtner, A.; Lehtinen, E.; Säljö, R. Expertise Differences in the Comprehension of Visualizations: A Meta-Analysis of Eye-Tracking Research in Professional Domains. *Educ. Psychol. Rev.* **2011**, *23*, 523–552. [CrossRef]

Brams, S.; Ziv, G.; Levin, O.; Spitz, J.; Wagemans, J.; Williams, A.M.; Helsen, W.F. The relationship between gaze behavior, expertise, and performance: A systematic review. *Psychol. Bull.* **2019**, *145*, 980–1027. [CrossRef]

Takei, Y. Three-dimensional analysis of handspring with full turn vault: Deterministic model, coaches' beliefs, and judges' scores. *J. Appl. Biomech.* **1998**, *14*, 190–210. [CrossRef]

Fujihara, T. Revisiting run-up velocity in gymnastics vaulting. In Proceedings of the 34th International Conference on Biomechanics in Sports, Tsukuba, Japan, 18–22 July 2016.

Fernandes, S.M.B.; Carrara, P.; Serrão, J.C.; Amadio, A.C.; Mochizuki, L. Kinematic variables of table vault on artistic gymnastics. *Rev. Bras. Educ. Física Esporte.* **2016**, *30*, 97–107. [CrossRef]

Van der Eb, J.; Filius, M.; Rougoor, G.; Niel, C.; Water, J. Optimal Velocity Profiles for Vault. In Proceedings of the 30th Annual Conference of Biomechanics in Sports, Melbourne, Australia, 2–6 July 2012.

Sjostrand, P.; Lemmetty, H.; Hughes, K.; Gryga, P.; Jónsdóttir, S. 2017–2021 Code of Points Seniors and Juniors Teamgym. Unpublished work. 2019.

Vater, C.; Roca, A.; Williams, A.M. Effects of anxiety on anticipation and visual search in dynamic, time-constrained situations. *Sport Exerc. Perform Psychol.* **2016**, *5*, 179–192. [CrossRef]

Mo, S.; Chow, D.H.K. Accuracy of three methods in gait event detection during overground running. *Gait Posture.* **2018**, *59*, 93–98. [CrossRef]

Hughes, K.; Lemmetty, H.; Sjostrand, P.; Dvoracek, R.; Gryga, P. Directives for Equipment (European Union of Gymnastics). Unpublished work. 2013. Available online: https://www.british-gymnastics.org/technical-information/discipline-updates/teamgym/4298-2013-2016-teamgym-equipment-directives/file (accessed on 12 February 2019).

Koo, T.K.; Li, M.Y. A Guideline of Selecting and Reporting Intraclass Correlation Coefficients for Reliability Research. *J. Chiropr. Med.* **2016**, *15*, 155–163. [CrossRef] [PubMed]

Witkowski, M.; Tomczak, E.; Łuczak, M.; Bronikowski, M.; Tomczak, M. Fighting Left Handers Promotes Different Visual Perceptual Strategies than Right Handers: The Study of Eye Movements of Foil Fencers in Attack and Defence. *Biomed. Res. Int.* **2020**, *2020*, 1–11. [CrossRef]

Kurz, J.; Hegele, M.; Reiser, M.; Munzert, J. Impact of task difficulty on gaze behavior in a sequential object manipulation task. *Exp. Brain Res.* **2017**, *235*, 3479–3486. [CrossRef]

Zeuwts, L.; Vansteenkiste, P.; Deconinck, F.; van Maarseveen, M.; Savelsbergh, G.; Cardon, G.; Lenoir, M. Is gaze behaviour in a laboratory context similar to that in real-life? A study in bicyclists. *Transp. Res. Part F Traffic Psychol. Behav.* **2016**, *43*, 131–140. [CrossRef]

Pelz, J.; Rothkopf, C. *Oculomotor Behavior in Natural and Man-Made Environments*, 1st ed.; Elsevier: Oxford, UK, 2007; pp. 661–676.

Haider, H.; Frensch, P.A. The role of information reduction in skill acquisition. *Cogn. Psychol.* **1996**, *30*, 304–337. [CrossRef]

Haider, H.; Frensch, P.A. Eye Movement during Skill Acquisition: More Evidence for the Information-Reduction Hypothesis. *J. Exp. Psychol. Learn Mem. Cogn.* **1999**, *25*, 172–190. [CrossRef]

Farana, R.; Vaverka, F. The effect of biomechanical variables on the assessment of vaulting in top-level artistic female gymnasts in world cup competitions. *Acta Univ. Palacki. Olomuc Gymnica.* **2012**, *42*, 49–57. [CrossRef]

Penitente, G. Performance analysis of the female yurchenko layout on the table vault. *Int. J. Perform Anal. Sport* **2014**, *14*, 84–97. [CrossRef]

Vater, C.; Kredel, R.; Hossner, E.J. Examining the functionality of peripheral vision: From fundamental understandings to applied sport science. *Curr. Issues Sport Sci.* **2017**, *1*, 1–11. [CrossRef]

37. Krug, J.; Knoll, K.; Kothe, T.; Zocher, H.D. Running approach velocity and energy transformation in difficult vaults in gymnastics. In Proceedings of the ISBS '98 XVI International Symposium on Biomechanics in Sports, Konstanz, Germany, 21–25 July 1998.
38. Schärer, C.; Lehmann, T.; Naundorf, F.; Taube, W.; Hübner, K. The faster, the better? Relationships between run-up speed, the degree of difficulty (D-score), height and length of flight on vault in artistic gymnastics. *PLoS ONE* **2019**, *14*, 1–12. [CrossRef]
39. Potgieter, K.; Ferreira, J.T. The effects of visual skills on rhythmic gymnactics. *South Afr. Optom.* **2009**, *68*, 137–154.

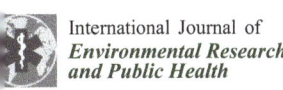

International Journal of *Environmental Research and Public Health*

Article

Running around the Country: An Analysis of the Running Phenomenon among Brazilian Runners

Mabliny Thuany [1], Beat Knechtle [2,*], Thomas Rosemann [3], Marcos B. Almeida [4] and Thayse Natacha Gomes [4]

1. Centre of Research, Education, Innovation and Intervention in Sport (CIFI2D), Faculty of Sports, University of Porto, 4200-450 Porto, Portugal; mablinysantos@gmail.com
2. Medbase St. Gallen Am Vadianplatz, Vadianstrasse 26, 9001 St. Gallen, Switzerland
3. Institute of Primary Care, University of Zurich, 8091 Zurich, Switzerland; thomas.rosemann@usz.ch
4. Department of Physical Education, Federal University of Sergipe, São Cristóvão 49100-000, SE, Brazil; mb.almeida@gmail.com (M.B.A.); thayse_natacha@hotmail.com (T.N.G.)
* Correspondence: beat.knechtle@hispeed.ch; Tel.: +41-(0)-71-226-93-00

Abstract: Differences in economic and social aspects between Brazilian states/regions can determine participation in running. The purpose of this study was to identify the occurrence of the OUTrun (i.e., Out Running), mapping the main routes carried out by runners, as well as the factors associated with this behavior between different Brazilian regions. The sample comprised 1053 runners of both sexes (women: 426; men: 627) who answered an online questionnaire, providing information related to individual, socioeconomic (SES), and training characteristics. A logistic regression analysis was computed, considering the regions. South and Southeast regions received the largest number of runners; runners from the North and Northeast regions were those who left their states the most to compete. Factors related to the OUTrun were the preferred distance, SES, and age. The results provide information to facilitate access to running events and can provide benefits related to making the practice accessible to a larger number of people.

Keywords: running; economic factors; sport events

1. Introduction

Considered the main physical activity trend for the year 2020 [1], road running stands out among the most practiced sports in the world [2]. Data covering 96% of the United States's race events, and 91% of the race results from Canada, Australia, and a portion of Africa, Asia, and South America between the years 1986 and 2018, showed an increase of 57.8% in the number of participants in these events [3]. In the Brazilian context, data covering races hosted in São Paulo and Rio de Janeiro showed an increase in participation and number of events during the last years [4]. Moreover, regarding economic factors, Brazilian data from 2019 showed that there were about 4 million runners who comprised a market of about BRL 3.1 billion/year in 2019 (about USD 12.4 billion/year) [5]. Individual costs are related to the purchase of sports equipment (e.g., shoes, Global Positioning System watches, clothing, etc.), knowledge about running (e.g., subscriptions to websites and specialized magazines), involvement in running groups/clubs, and especially participation in running events [5,6].

Despite the growth in the number of running events at a national level [7], the distribution of these events between the Brazilian states is not similar, with a huge discrepancy observed. The Southeast region concentrates the highest number of these events, as well as the most important and traditional events (e.g., São Silvestre, São Paulo Marathon, Rio de Janeiro Marathon, Pampulha International Tour, ten miles Garoto race) [8,9]. Therefore, there is a tendency for runners from the different Brazilian states going to this region to take part in these races, in a phenomenon that can be called "Out Running" (OUTrun), in which runners "exit" from their states of residence and "enter into" other places (state and/or countries) to participate in race events.

Although usually considered as a cheap and affordable practice, a deep look at the context of running reveals changes in the profile of its practitioners, and its "accessibility" can be questioned [10,11]. In general, studies showed that economic factors may be related to the involvement/practice in road running [12]. For example, in the Brazilian scenario, more than 600 races are held annually [13], whose registration prices can exceed BR 200.00/person (about USD 35.00/person). Notwithstanding that this is not cheap or accessible for a large portion of the Brazilian population (and even for most runners), these events attract runners and usually reach their registration goals [14].

Economic and sociodemographic factors are also associated with running practice [12,15]. Moreover, individuals with higher socioeconomic status and education level and aged between 30 and 40 years are more likely to engage in the practice of the modality [2,12]. Thus, given the geographic extension of the country, which leads to differences in economic and social aspects between states/regions [16,17], the purpose of this study was to identify, between Brazilian regions, the occurrence of the OUTrun, mapping the main routes carried out by runners, as well as the factors associated with this behavior. Based on previous studies, we hypothesized that economic level must be associated with participation in running events.

2. Materials and Methods

2.1. Design and Sample

The present study is part of the InTrack Project [18], a cross-sectional research project developed with the aim to identify the predictors of runner's performance in non-professional runners. To take part in the study, runners must have answered the online questionnaire sent via social media, and available from September 2019 to March 2020, and be aged ≥ 18 years. From the 1173 answered questionnaires, 104 runners were excluded from the analysis because they did not report having taken part in any official race event in the last 12 months, and 16 were excluded because they did not answer all the mandatory questions. Thus, the final sample, for the present study, comprised 1053 runners of both sexes (women: 426; men: 627), from all the five Brazilian regions (Southeast: 409; Northeast: 350; South: 130; Midwest: 90; North: 74). This study was conducted in accordance with the Declaration of Helsinki and was approved by the Ethics Committee of the Federal University of Sergipe, Brazil (protocol n° 3.558.630).

2.2. Procedures and Data Collection

The information was collected through the online questionnaire "Profile characterization and associated factors for runner's performance" [19]. The questionnaire allowed obtaining information related to (1) runner identification (age and sex), (2) anthropometric variables (height and weight), (3) sociodemographic profile (neighborhood, income, educational level, and marital status), (4) perception about the environment (natural or built) influence on the practice, (5) training variables (volume and frequency/week, sessions/day, practice time, pace (min/km), involvement in official races in the last 12 months, involvement in a running club, the use of a personal coach to guide the practice, motivation for the practice, and preferred distance), and (6) the family environment (family composition, family members engaged in running practice, involvement in sports during childhood, and family support for sporting involvement during childhood). The Intraclass Correlation Coefficient demonstrated that items were classified as "excellent" ($R \geq 0.75$), and the Kappa Coefficient presented concordance "substantial" to "almost perfect".

2.2.1. Individual Characteristics

Sex, age, and state of residence were self-reported.

Anthropometric characteristics—height (cm) and body mass (kg)—were self-reported, as performed in previous studies [20]. Body mass index (BMI) was computed through the standardized formula (body mass (kg)/height (m)^2).

Socioeconomic status (SES): runners were asked to provide an estimate of their monthly income, on a Likert scale, based on Brazilian minimum wage in 2019 [21]. Furthermore, answers were organized into two categories: "$\leq$5 minimum wages" ($\leq$4990.00 BRL or about $\leq$1.205 USD) and ">5 minimum wages" (>4990.00 BRL or about >1.205 USD).

Educational level: runners provided information regarding the highest education level achieved, being classified as "<elementary school", "elementary school", "high school", or "university degree".

2.2.2. Training Characteristics

Running pace: participants were asked to provide information regarding their running pace (min/km) in their preferred distance.

Volume/km: the mean weekly value was reported (in kilometers) by runners.

Practice time: runners were categorized into two groups, namely "$\leq$1 year" of practice and ">1 year" of practice.

Preferred distance: runners answered their preferred running distance, and they were categorized as "short distance" runners (until 10 km) or "long-distance" runners (above 10 km).

OUTrun phenomenon: information about runners' participation in any race event in the last 12 months was provided by participants. We considered OUTrun when this participation occurred in a different state (or country) from the one of their residence.

2.3. Statistical Analysis

The information collected was presented as mean (and standard deviation) or frequency (%). Logistic regression analysis was computed to identify the predictors associated with the OUTrun phenomenon (chance to exit from their state of residence to participate in race events in another state or country), and models were built for each region. The variables included as predictors were sex (female or male), age, SES ("$\leq$5 minimum wages", or ">5 minimum wages"), and preference distance ("short distance" or "long distance"). For categorical variables, the first category reported was the reference group during data analysis. All the analyses were performed in SPSS 24.0 software (IBM Corp., Armonk, NY, USA), with a significant level set at 95%. The Gephi software (version 0.9.2) (Gephi, WebAtlas, Paris, France) was used to build the networks established by runners related to their travels between states (or countries).

3. Results

Table 1 presents descriptive information. The sample presented a mean running pace of 5:30 min/km and a mean BMI of 24.4 kg/m^2. The mean age of the sample was 38.6 $\pm$ 8.4 years for women and 37.6 $\pm$ 9.9 years for men. The runners were from all states of the country, except Rondônia. Most of the runners reported living in the Southeast (38.2%) and Northeast (33.8%) regions.

The North, Northeast, and Midwest regions showed the highest percentage of runners who leave their states of residence to take part in races hosted in other states, and, except for the Northeast region, the majority of runners who traveled from their states to compete prefer long distances instead of short distances (Table 2). Taking sex into account, 68.1% and 57.1% of the women and men, respectively, reported preferring short distances.

Table 1. Descriptive statistics of runners, by region.

Variables	Brazil	Midwest (n = 90)	Northeast (n = 350)	North (n = 74)	Southeast (n = 409)	South (n = 130)
Sex						
Woman	426 (40.5%)	41 (45.6%)	135 (38.6%)	32 (43.2%)	160 (39.1%)	58 (44.6%)
Man	626 (59.4%)	49 (54.4%)	214 (61.1%)	42 (56.8%)	249 (60.9%)	72 (55.4%)
Age (years)	38.0 (9.3)	39.2 (9.7)	37.8 (9.9)	35.6 (10.4)	38.6 (8.9)	37.6 (8.6)
BMI (kg.m^2)	24.4 (3.3)	24.0 (3.3)	24.4 (3.2)	25.1 (3.8)	24.6 (3.3)	24.0 (3.1)
Running pace (min/km)	5:30 (1:09)	05:38 (1:19)	05:38 (1:19)	5:38 (1:26)	05:28 (1:06)	05:14 (55.7)
Volume/km	35.4 (29.5)	36.0 (27.4)	31.1 (26.1)	34.1 (21.6)	39.7 (35.1)	34.5 (22.5)
SES						
≤5 minimum wages	552 (52.4%)	32 (36%)	179 (51.1%)	45 (62.5%)	242 (59.4%)	55 (43.7%)
>5 minimum wages	485 (46.1%)	57 (64%)	166 (47.4%)	27 (37.5%)	164 (40.1%)	71 (56.3%)
Educational level						
<Elementary school	8 (0.8%)	1 (1.1%)	1 (0.3%)	0	6 (1.5%)	0
Elementary school	42 (4.0%)	4 (4.4%)	10 (2.9%)	3 (4.1%)	23 (5.6%)	2 (1.5%)
High school	239 (22.7%)	13 (14.4%)	78 (22.3%)	18 (24.3%)	107 (26.2%)	23 (17.7%)
University degree	758 (72.0%)	70 (77.8%)	261 (74.6%)	52 (70.3%))	271 (66.3%)	104 (80.0%)
Missing	6 (0.6%)	2 (2.2%)		1 (1.4%)	2 (0.5%)	1 (0.8%)
Practice time						
Until 1 year	167 (15.9%)	16 (17.8%)	65 (18.6%)	11 (14.9%)	70 (17.1%)	5 (3.8%)
>1 year	886 (84.1%)	74 (82.2%)	285 (81.4%)	63 (85.1%)	339 (82.9%)	125 (96.2%)

Table 2. Percentage of runners who reported to travel abroad their states of residence to take part in running events, by region and distance of preference.

Region	Total *	Distance of Preference		
		Short Distances **	Long Distances **	Missing **
Southeast	54 (13.4%)	9 (17.0%)	44 (81.5%)	1 (1.9%)
Northeast	82 (24.5%)	41 (50.0%)	40 (48.8%)	1 (1.2%)
North	18 (25.5%)	6 (33.3%)	12 (66.7%)	
Midwest	21 (24.4%)	4 (19.0%)	17 (81.0%)	
South	23 (18.1%)	11 (47.8%)	12 (52.2%)	

* Percentage values based on the total runners in each region; ** percentage values based on the number of runners who left their states to compete.

Figure 1 presents the networks derived from the origin-destination dyad related to runner's participation in racing events. In general, there was a greater outflow of runners from the states of São Paulo, Rio de Janeiro, Sergipe, Minas Gerais, Paraná, and Espírito Santo (indicated by the grey circles), while Santa Catarina, São Paulo, Rio de Janeiro, Rio Grande do Sul, Distrito Federal, and Espírito Santo states were those where runners arrive the most (coming from other states) to take part in running events (represented by the biggest circles). Furthermore, it is also possible to observe the runners' "way out" to get involved in races in other countries, namely Argentina, Chile, Uruguay, the United States, Germany, Spain, France, Greece, and Portugal, highlighting the international facet related to the practice.

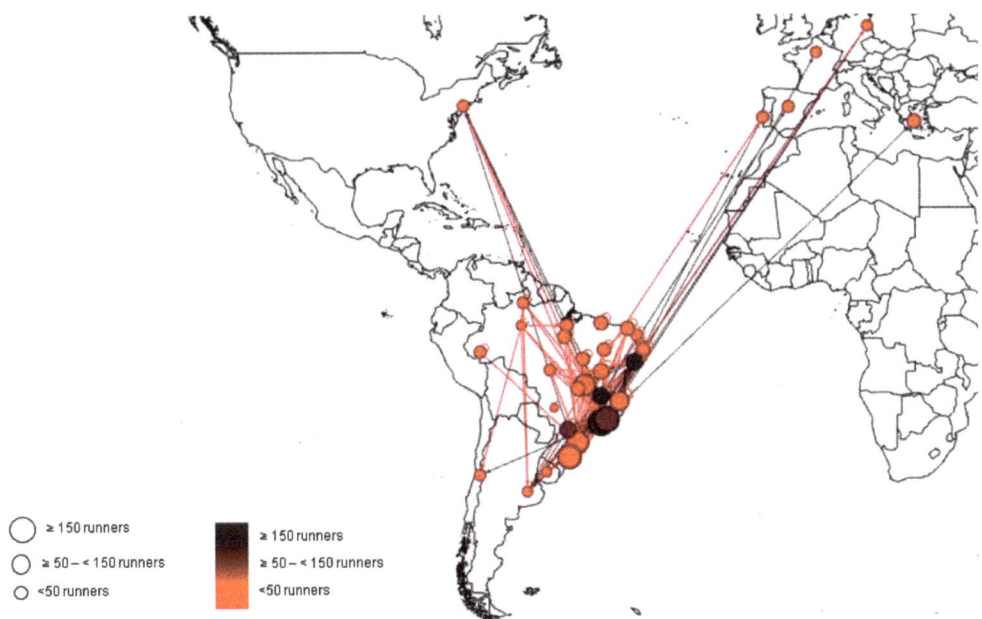

Figure 1. Network derived from runners exit and entrance in states (or countries) to take part in road running events.

Table 3 presents the results of logistic regression analysis. Except for the South region, the preferred distance was a significant predictor for participation in the racing events in other states/countries, indicating that runners who preferred long-distance running tend to travel abroad to compete more than those who indicated short running distances as their preferred ones (Midwest: OR = 6.28, p = 0.017; North: OR = 10.10, p = 0.002; Northeast: OR = 1.95, p = 0.017; Southeast: OR = 7.02, p < 0.001). In addition, in the Southeast and Northeast regions, the higher the SES, the higher the chances of runners traveling abroad to take part in running events (Northeast: OR = 2.06, p = 0.017; Southeast: OR = 3.09, p = 0.002). Moreover, it highlights the role played by sex in the South region (OR = 0.32, p = 0.030) in the studied phenomenon (Table 3).

Table 3. Results from the logistic regression for the predictors associated with traveling abroad to take part in race events.

Variables	Midwest	North	Northeast	Southeast	South
	OR (95% CI)				
Sex (male)	0.70 (0.18–2.76)	1.72 (0.39–7.70)	1.49 (0.84–2.66)	0.64 (0.32–1.29)	0.32 (0.12–0.90) *
Age (years)	0.97 (0.90–1.05)	1.08 (0.99–1.17)	1.02 (0.99–1.05)	1.00 (0.96–1.04)	0.97 (0.91–1.04)
SES (>5 minimum wages)	5.18 (0.49–55.31)	1.57 (0.33–7.42)	2.06 (1.14–3.72) *	3.09 (1.50–6.39) *	1.56 (0.53–4.57)
Distance (long distance)	6.28 (1.38–28.53) *	10.10 (2.33–43.83) *	1.95 (1.13–3.38) *	7.02 (2.97–16.63) *	2.67 (0.98–7.33)

$p < 0.05$ *.

4. Discussion

The purpose of this study was to identify the occurrence of OUTrun, mapping the main routes carried out by runners, as well as the factors associated with this phenomenon. The main finding of the study was that the states of São Paulo, Rio de Janeiro, Sergipe, Minas Gerais, Paraná, and Espírito Santo are those with the highest number of runners who reported traveling from their states of residence to compete, while the states of Santa Catarina, São Paulo, Rio de Janeiro, Rio Grande do Sul, Distrito Federal, and Espírito Santo were those where runners arrived the most to take part in running events.

Results are associated with a large number of running events and some of the most important Brazilian road running races, which are hosted in South and Southeast regions, especially in the states of Rio de Janeiro, São Paulo, Rio Grande Sul, and Minas Gerais [13]. In a multilevel approach previously performed, it was observed that runners from states with more athletics events were those with the best performance [15]. Although the present study did not investigate differences in runners' performance, an association between sports events, sports participation, and sports performance seems to exist [12]. Furthermore, a previous study conducted in Brazil reported these regions as having the friendliest environment, which may be related to a higher opportunity for citizens to take part in outdoor physical activities and training practice, which can lead to increases in demand for race events. In addition, as an outdoor event, long-distance running (half marathon and marathon) performance tend to be associated with a natural environment (e.g., climate, weather, wind, altitude), and the North and Northeast Brazilian regions are those with the highest annual average temperature, meaning that this could impact in the runners' choice in the place to compete.

About a quarter of the runners from the North, Northeast, and Midwest regions leave their states to participate in events in states from other regions, especially in long-distance running events. One possible reason is the fact that long-distance running races, such as marathons, are less frequent in some states. This can be observed in the calendar of running events for the year 2020, which indicated that of the 17 official marathons planned to occur in Brazil, only one of them was supposed to be hosted in the North region (Amazonas) and five in the Northeast region, while the state of São Paulo was supposed to host at least two of them [22].

In this context, an increase in the number of runners participating in long-distance running, namely half-marathon running, has been observed worldwide [23]. Moreover, the profile of these runners has aroused the attention of the tourism market ("Maratourism") with several companies providing logistic advisory services to runners, helping them in their movement to the place of the competition, as well as providing accommodation options and, eventually, leisure entertainment during the time the runner spends in the city of the event. This service moves the local economy in several segments: hotel chain, transportation, restaurants, and business [5].

As hypothesized, SES was associated with the OUTrun. However, this result was only observed in runners from the Southeast and Northeast regions, where individuals with higher monthly incomes were more likely to participate in events outside their state of residence. According to Berger et al. [24], adherence to a given behavior/practice is associated with individual economic issues, in association with the available time and the personal feeling about the relevance of the sports practice. This information confirms findings from previous studies. For example, a previous study, investigating the demographic and economic model in different practices (sports participation, cycling, swimming, running, fitness, gymnastics, walking, football, dancing, and tennis) showed that the model can be used to predict participation in several sports. Especially in running, higher economic level and working time were associated with involvement in the modality [12,15]. Furthermore, evidence suggests an inverse relationship between event registration fees (registration fees and other associated costs) and the number of participants in the events [11], in opposition to the idea that the modality is accessible to everyone, regardless of their economic conditions, for example [10].

The relevance of economic conditions in running practice is further reinforced when it is noted that the registration fee in a single event of the modality (with an average registration fee of BRL 101/person or USD 19.33) could represent about 10% of the Brazilian minimum wage in the year 2020 [21]. In addition, other costs related to involvement in the events cannot be disregarded, which may become a barrier to participation in running events. As mentioned above, most long-distance running events require runners to travel from their state of residence to take part in the events, which demands high costs, in association with the higher registration fees. In the present study, runners who indicated long-distance running races as their preference were more likely to leave their states to compete.

Despite the reduction in the ratio between sexes over the years, the male frequency is still higher in absolute terms than the female in competitions [7,25]. Although in the present study men reported a greater preference for long-distance running events than women, sex was found to be a significant predictor of the occurrence of OUTRun only in the South region, where men were less likely to compete in other states/countries than women. Since male runners seemed to prefer long-distance running events, the fact that the South region hosts some Brazilian half-marathon, marathon, and ultramarathon races, runners who deserve to take part in events in such distances do not need to travel abroad to perform.

Although the increase in the number of participants in the modality could be seen throughout the country [4], there were differences regarding the practice preference between the regions. For example, in the Midwest Region, about 8% of the adults indicated running as their preferred sports practice, while in the South Region, only 3.6% of the adults indicated such a preference [26]. Even so, the South region receives a large number of runners from other states, who usually travel to this region to take part in the marathons held in Porto Alegre and Florianopolis, which, due to the topography of the area where they occur, are considered some of the best races for professional runners obtain their best scores [27–29], which is highlighted by the high frequencies of the best times achievement, among Brazilian marathoners, observed in these events (61% for men and 51% for women).

Regarding the limitations of the present study, it is worth mentioning differences in the sample size between the regions; however, the purpose of the study was not to obtain a representative sample in all states or regions. In addition, questions related to the individual investment in practice could help to elucidate issues related to individual and local economic aspects. Despite the previous validation of the instrument used, and the fact that the online survey has been used in previous studies, we are aware of the bias associated with sample selection, due to the strategy used to publicize the questionnaire. Given this limitation, we suggest caution in the generalization of the information. Finally, to our knowledge, this is the first study that highlights the main networks established between road running and the factors associated with OUTrun. Future studies should compare performance at races with different costs of participation (e.g., free and paid events) and should investigate states variables (e.g., economic, cultural, social, and tourist potential characteristics) that are possibly associated with race events distribution, as well as differences in performance between athletes in different races.

5. Conclusions

OUTrun was more frequent in runners from São Paulo (Southeast), Rio de Janeiro (Southeast), Sergipe (Northeast), Minas Gerais (Southeast), Paraná (South), Espírito Santo (Southeast), and Rio Grande do Sul (South), while Santa Catarina (South), São Paulo, Rio de Janeiro, Rio Grande do Sul, Distrito Federal (Midwest), and Espírito Santo were the states that received most of the runners. Regarding the factors associated with OUTrun, different variables were significantly associated with it for different regions. Except for the South region, the distance preference (long distance) was shown to be a significant predictor, increasing the chances of runners traveling to participate in these events in another city/country. Economic level was also associated with OUTrun in Northeast and Southeast regions, while sex was a significant predictor in the South region. The present study can be used by stakeholders and sports events organizers to develop strategies to make these events more accessible, and allowing the benefits associated with the sport practice to reach a larger number of people, regardless of their SES or place of residence.

Author Contributions: Conceptualization, M.T. and T.N.G.; methodology, M.T., T.N.G., and M.B.A.; formal analysis, M.T. and T.N.G.; writing—original draft preparation, M.T. and T.N.G.; writing—review and editing, M.T., B.K., T.R., M.B.A., and T.N.G. All authors have read and agreed to the published version of the manuscript.

Funding: This research received no external funding.

Institutional Review Board Statement: This study was conducted in accordance with the Declaration of Helsinki, and was approved by the Ethics Committee of the Federal University of Sergipe Brazil (protocol n° 3.558.630).

Informed Consent Statement: Informed consent was obtained from all subjects involved in the study

Data Availability Statement: Data are available from the authors upon request.

Conflicts of Interest: The authors declare no conflict of interest.

References

1. Thompson, W.R. Worldwide survey of fitness trends for 2020. *Health Fit. J.* **2020**, *23*, 10–18. [CrossRef]
2. Nilson, F.; Lundkvist, E.; Wagnsson, S.; Gustafsson, H. Has the second 'running boom' democratized running? A study on the sociodemographic characteristics of finishers at the world's largest half marathon. *Sport Soc.* **2019**, *24*, 659–669. [CrossRef]
3. Andersen, J.J. The State of Running 2019. Available online: https://runrepeat.com/state-of-running (accessed on 17 August 2020)
4. Thuany, M.; Gomes, T.N.; Estevam, L.C.; Almeida, M.B.D. Crescimento do número de corridas de rua e perfil dos participantes no Brasil. In *Atividade Física, Esporte e Saúde: Temas Emergentes*; Rbf Editora: Belém, PA, Brazil, 2021; Volume 1.
5. Sebrae. Tendências do Mercado de Corrida de Rua. Available online: https://sebraeinteligenciasetorial.com.br/produtos/boletins-de-tendencia/tendencias-do-mercado-de-corridas-de-rua/5b5a1605d0a9751800f2af49 (accessed on 4 December 2019)
6. Runner's World. How Much Does Running Cost over A Lifetime? Available online: https://www.runnersworld.com/news/a20832909/how-much-does-running-cost-over-a-lifetime/ (accessed on 17 April 2021).
7. Federação Paulista de Atletismo. Demonstrativo de Corridas de Rua nos Últimos Anos no Estado de São Paulo. Available online: http://www.atletismofpa.org.br/source/Demonstrativo-de-Corridas-de-Rua-nos-Ultimos-Anos-no-Estado-de-Sao-Paulo-2017.pdf (accessed on 10 November 2019).
8. Balu, D. Os Maiores Eventos de Corrida de Rua do Brasil—2018. Available online: https://blogrecorrido.com/2019/01/22/os-maiores-eventos-de-corrida-de-rua-do-brasil-2018/ (accessed on 10 May 2021).
9. Balu, D. As 50 Maiores Corridas de Rua do Brasil (2017). Available online: https://blogrecorrido.com/2018/01/15/as-50-maiores-corridas-de-rua-do-brasil-2017/ (accessed on 10 May 2021).
10. Thuany, M.; Gomes, T.N. Is Running Accessible for Everyone? Encyclopedia: Basel, Switzerland, 2020.
11. Van Dyck, D.; Cardon, G.; Bourdeaudhuij, I.d.; Ridder, L.d.; Willem, A. Who participates in running events? 10 Socio-demographic characteristics, psychosocial factors and barriers as correlates of non-participation—a pilot study in Belgium. *Int J Env. Res Public Health.* **2017**, *14*, 1–14. [CrossRef] [PubMed]
12. Breuer, C.; Hallmann, K.; Wicker, P. Determinants of sport participation in different sports. *Manag. Leis.* **2013**, *16*, 269–286 [CrossRef]
13. Ticket. Perfil do Corredor Brasileiro. Available online: https://blog.ticketagora.com.br/infografico-o-perfil-dos-corredores-2019 (accessed on 27 February 2020).
14. Dallari, M.M. Corrida de rua: Um fenômeno sociocultural contemporâneo. Ph.D. Thesis, University of São Paulo, São Paulo Brazil, 2009.
15. Thuany, M.; Gomes, T.N.; Hill, L.; Rosemann, T.J.; Knechtle, B.; Almeida, M.B. Running performance variability among runners from different brazilian states: A multilevel approach. *Int. J. Environ. Res. Public Health* **2021**, *18*, 3781. [CrossRef] [PubMed]
16. Instituto Brasileiro de Geografia e Estatística—IBGE. Painel de Indicadores. Available online: https://www.ibge.gov.br/indicadores.html (accessed on 19 August 2020).
17. Programa das Nação Unidas para o Desenvolvimento (PNUD); Instituto de Pesquisa Econômica Aplicada (IPEA); Fundação João Pinheiro (FJP). Atlas do Desenvilvimento Humano no Brasil. Available online: http://atlasbrasil.org.br/2013/pt/home (accessed on 12 January 2020).
18. InTrack Project. Welcome to InTrack Project. Available online: https://intrackproject.wixsite.com/website (accessed on 10 May 2021).
19. Thuany, M.; Gomes, T.N.; Almeida, M.B. Validação de um instrumento para caracterização e verificação de fatores associados ao desempenho de corredores de rua. *Sci. Plena* **2020**, *16*, 1–7. [CrossRef]
20. Nikolaidis, P.T.; Knechtle, B. Validity of Recreational Marathon Runners' Self-Reported Anthropometric Data. *Percept. Mot. Skill* **2020**, *127*, 1068–1078. [CrossRef] [PubMed]
21. Brasil, R.F. Decreto n° 9.661, de 1° de Janeiro de 2019. In *Diário Oficial da União*; Presidency of the Republic, General Secretaria Brasilia, Brazil, 2019.
22. Contrarelógio. Ranking dos Melhores Maratonistas Brasileiros em 2019. Available online: https://www.contrarelogio.com.br (accessed on 10 October 2020).
23. Vitti, A.; Nikolaidis, P.T.; Villiger, E.; Onywera, V.; Knechtle, B. The "New York City Marathon": Participation and performance trends of 1.2M runners during half-century. *Res. Sports Med.* **2019**, *28*, 121–137. [CrossRef] [PubMed]
24. Berger, I.E.; O'Reilly, N.; Parent, M.M.; Se´guin, B.; Hernandez, T. Determinants of sport participation among Canadian adolescents. *Sport Manag. Rev.* **2008**, *11*, 277–307. [CrossRef]

5. Fonseca, F.S.; Cavalcante, J.A.M.; Almeida, L.S.C.; Fialho, J.V.A.P. Análise do perfil sociodemográfico, motivos de adesão, rotina de treinamento e acompanhamento profissional de praticantes de corrida de rua. *Rev. Bras. Ciência e Mov.* **2019**, *27*, 189–198. [CrossRef]
6. Brasil. *Diesporte–Diagnóstico Nacional do Esporte*; Ministério do Esporte: São Paulo, Brasília, 2015; Volume 1, p. 44.
7. Confederação Brasileira de Atletismo. Ranking Brasileiro 2020. Available online: https://www.cbat.org.br/novo/?pagina=ranking_quadro (accessed on 7 March 2020).
8. Confedereção Brasileira de Atletismo (CBAt). Ranking Brasileiro de Corredores de rua 2019. Available online: http://www.cbat.org.br/novo/?pagina=ranking (accessed on 12 August 2019).
9. Thuany, M.; Gomes, T.N.; Souza, R.F.; Almeida, M. *Onde Estão os Melhores Corredores do Brasil? Dados não Publicados*; Encyclopedia: Basel, Switzerland, 2020.

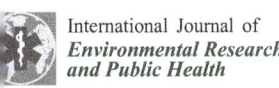

Reply to Laby, D.M.; Appelbaum, L.G. Comment on "Nascimento et al. Citations Network Analysis of Vision and Sport. *Int. J. Environ. Res. Public Health* 2020, 17, 7574"

Henrique Nascimento [1,2], Clara Martinez-Perez [1,*], Cristina Alvarez-Peregrina [2] and Miguel Ángel Sánchez-Tena [1,3]

1 ISEC Lisboa, Instituto de Educação e Ciência de Lisboa, 1750-179 Lisboa, Portugal; henrique.nascimento@iseclisboa.pt (H.N.); masancheztena@ucm.es (M.Á.S.-T.)
2 Faculty of Biomedical and Health Science, Universidad Europea de Madrid, 28670 Madrid, Spain; cristina.alvarez@universidadeuropea.es
3 Department of Optometry and Vision, Faculty of Optics and Optometry, Universidad Complutense de Madrid, 28670 Madrid, Spain
* Correspondence: claramarperez@hotmail.com

Introduction

In response to a comment, in this study [1] we have performed a citation network analysis, not a bibliometric analysis. Carrying out this type of analysis at some point in time will permit knowledge of the existing bibliography networks, which establish the citations in academic publications that represent a specialty and a scientific community. In turn, the structures and characteristics of said specialty and community can be studied. By making comparisons between time periods, the historical development of the specialty and the community can be modeled. In the analysis of dating networks, a set of objects (documents, authors, journals, or groups of them) that represent a research field is selected. The strengths of the interrelationships (or levels of connection) between these data are analyzed using various scores that come from citation counts, structures, and characteristics of the corresponding research fields and academic communities. To reveal the structures underlying these relationships, multivariate statistical analyses are often applied using citation scores as measures of similarity. For this reason, network visualization tools are also frequently used to produce visual maps of these relationships [2].

Depending on the units of analysis (documents or groups of them by authors, journals, research fields, nations, etc.) and the thresholds of citation scores, both macrostructures (general maps of the entire scientific effort with each node in the La network representing a discipline) and microstructures (structures of a single specialty with each node of the network representing a single document) of science can be mapped and studied, allowing the user to access general descriptions of the fields of investigation, as well as exploring the underlying structures [3].

There are three types of commonly used citation-based measures of the strength of the interrelation between two objects [3]:

- Interleaved citation count—the number of times two objects have cited each other;
- Co-citation counts—the number of documents that have cited two objects together;
- Bibliographic coupling frequencies (BCF)—the number of cited references that have two objects in common.

Therefore, we agree with the given comments. However, it was not the analysis that was carried out in our study [1], and that is why the data cited in the comment were not obtained.

Conflicts of Interest: The authors declare no conflict of interest.

References

1. Nascimento, H.; Martinez-Perez, C.; Alvarez-Peregrina, C.; Sánchez-Tena, M.Á. Citations Network Analysis of Vision and Sport. *Int. J. Environ. Res. Public Health* **2020**, *17*, 7574. [CrossRef] [PubMed]
2. Rangeon, S.; Gilbert, W.; Bruner, M. Mapping the World of Coaching Science: A Citation Network Analysis. *J. Coach. Educ.* **2012**, *5*, 83–108. [CrossRef]
3. Zhao, Y.; Zhao, R. An evolutionary analysis of collaboration networks in scientometrics. *Scientometrics* **2016**, *107*, 759–772. [CrossRef]

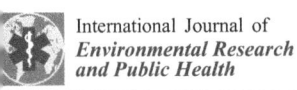

Comment

Comment on Nascimento et al. Citations Network Analysis of Vision and Sport. *Int. J. Environ. Res. Public Health* 2020, 17, 7574

Daniel M. Laby [1,*] and Lawrence G. Appelbaum [2]

1. ChampionsEdge, LLC, New York, NY 10022, USA
2. Department of Psychiatry and Behavioral Sciences, Duke University School of Medicine, Durham, NC 27710, USA; greg@duke.edu
* Correspondence: drlaby@sportsvision.nyc

In October 2020, the paper "Citations Network Analysis of Vision and Sport [1]" was published in the *International Journal of Environmental Research and Public Health*. Using the Web of Science database, the authors used several search terms (sport, vision, and eye) to identify sports vision publications, the most frequently cited publication, as well as the journals that published the most articles in sports vision, among other measures. Although publications by authors in a growing field are critical to the growth of that field, the accuracy and completeness of the publications are perhaps more critical.

As frequent contributors to the field of sports vision, and with over half a century of combined experience, we read, with great interest, the above publication, and looked forward to gaining a greater understanding of the scope and breath of publications. Unfortunately, after critically reviewing the manuscript, we noted several potential fatal flaws in the methodology and resulting interpretation of results by the authors.

Perhaps, and possibly most importantly, the authors failed to include many publications in the field of sports vision. This may have been caused by the very narrow search terms used in the initial Web of Science search, as well as restricting the search to a single database. For example, a PubMed search for the terms, "sport" and "eye" reveals ~3300 citations. A larger number is noted in a search of the Google Scholar database. The use of only three keywords also removed from the analysis the many publications that do not include those terms. For example, a search of the PubMed database with the terms "baseball" and "eye" revealed 142 publications, a search of "soccer" and "eye" revealed 148 citations and a search of "rugby" and "eye" revealed 182 publications, as examples.

When conducting a survey of the literature, with the intention of noting the frequency of publications, authorship as well as journal frequency, it is imperative that the pool of analyzed publications be as complete as possible and be created by multiple search criteria, as well as multiple search engines. It appears that the authors did not conduct a sufficiently comprehensive search of the sports vision literature; thus, severely under-representing the field, and as a result skewing their results and interpretation.

The restrictive analysis created several issues with regard to study results. For example, Table 4 in the manuscript, listing the "top 10 authors with the largest number of publications" notes Mann, D.L. as the author "with the largest number of publications in sports vision" with a total of 10, and at the other end of the table, they note Kredel, R. as having three publications. A count of all the sports vision papers authored by Mann, D.L., listed in PubMed, totals about four-times the number listed in the table. Likewise, there are many authors in the sports vision field who have published many more publications than those listed in the "top 10" table in this publication (e.g., Gray, R., Abernethy, B., Laby, D.M., Kirschen, D., Williams, M., Appelbaum, L.G., etc.).

The authors note that the most cited publication in the field of sports vision was by Williams et al. in 2002 regarding Quiet Eye duration. The authors note that this article was cited 55 times. We found it interesting that the creator of the "Quiet Eye" concept, Prof Joan Vickers, was not even included in the list of top 10 authors, despite her articles in the field having been cited hundreds of times each. For example, her 1996 article, titled "Visual control when aiming at a far target [2]", which escaped the keyword search by the authors despite describing the gaze characteristics of basketball athletes, has been cited more than 600 times. Additionally, many other of her foundational publications, that have been cited hundreds of times, were not included in the author's publication, most likely because of the very narrow and incomplete search of the literature.

Lastly, the authors failed to include, or make note of, recent literature reviews in the field of sports vision, which would have been helpful in their data acquisition and resulting analysis. For example, in a 2016 publication, Appelbaum and Erickson [3] reviewed different sports vision training interventions. In that publication, the authors cite almost 175 publications relevant to their review. Clearly, the overwhelming majority of these publications, although certainly overlapping with other fields, should have been considered by the authors as publications in the field of sports vision. Interestingly, the Web of Science lists 59 citations for this publication, more than double the number noted by the authors for the publication by Williams [4]. Moreover, the first two words in the title of this article are "Sports Vision" opening questions as to how this paper escaped the keyword search performed in this citation network analysis.

As the authors correctly note, sports vision is a relatively new specialty. A specialty that is comprised of a varied and cross-disciplinary population of ophthalmologists, optometrists, as well as vision scientists and other researchers and practitioners. The growing field depends on the scientific study and reporting of data, which is completed in adherence to scientific norms, is well executed, and properly reviewed prior to publication to be of benefit to the field. We commend the authors on their intention to contribute to the field but note several serious flaws that indicate this is a poor representation of the desired literature. We would encourage the authors to conduct a more comprehensive review but in the interest of completeness, we crafted this letter so that readers are aware of the shortcomings in this published article.

Conflicts of Interest: The authors declare no conflict of interest.

References

1. Nascimento, H.; Martinez-Perez, C.; Alvarez-Peregrina, C.; Sánchez-Tena, M.Á. Citations Network Analysis of Vision and Sport. *Int. J. Environ. Res. Public Health* **2020**, *17*, 7574. [CrossRef] [PubMed]
2. Vickers, J.N. Visual control when aiming at a far target. *J. Exp. Psychol. Hum. Percept. Perform.* **1996**, *22*, 342–354. [CrossRef] [PubMed]
3. Appelbaum, L.G.; Erickson, G. Sports vision training: A review of the state-of-the-art in digital training techniques. *Int. Rev. Sport Exerc. Psychol.* **2018**, *11*, 160–189. [CrossRef]
4. Williams, A.M.; Singer, R.N.; Frehlich, S.G. Quiet Eye Duration, Expertise and Task Complexity in Near and Far Aiming Tasks. *J. Mot. Behav.* **2002**, *34*, 197–207. [CrossRef] [PubMed]

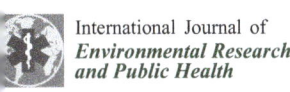

Article

Effects of Padel Competition on Brain Health-Related Myokines

Francisco Pradas [1], María Pía Cádiz [2], María Teresa Nestares [3], Inmaculada C. Martínez-Díaz [4] and Luis Carrasco [4,*]

[1] Training, Physical Activity and Sports Performance Research Group (ENFYRED), Faculty of Health and Sports Sciences, Pabellón Polideportivo Río Isuela, E-22001 Huesca, Spain; franprad@unizar.es
[2] Department of Pedagogy, Faculty of Educational Sciences, San Sebastián University, Bellavista 7, Recoleta Piso 6, Santiago 1457, Chile; maria.cadiz@uss.cl
[3] Department of Physiology, Faculty of Pharmacy, University of Granada, Cartuja University Campus, E-18071 Granada, Spain; nestares@ugr.es
[4] Department of Physical Education and Sport, University of Seville, E-41013 Seville, Spain; martinezdiaz@us.es
* Correspondence: lcarrasco@us.es

Abstract: Padel is becoming one of the most widespread racket sports that may have potential health benefits. Considering that several myokines mediate the cross-talk between skeletal muscles and the brain, exerting positive effects on brain health status, this study was designed to evaluate the responses of brain-derived neurotrophic factor (BDNF), leukemia inhibitory factor (LIF), and irisin (IR) to padel competition in trained players and to determine whether these responses were sex-dependent. Twenty-four trained padel players (14 women and 10 men with a mean age of 27.8 ± 6.3 years) participated voluntarily in this study. Circulating levels of BDNF, LIF, and IR were assessed before and after simulated padel competition (real playing time, 27.8 ± 8.49 min; relative intensity, 75.2 ± 7.9% maximum heart rate). Except for BDNF responses observed in female players (increasing from 1531.12 ± 269.09 to 1768.56 ± 410.75 ng/mL), no significant changes in LIF and IR concentrations were reported after padel competition. In addition, no sex-related differences were found. Moreover, significant associations between IR and BDNF were established at both pre- and post-competition. Our results suggest that while competitive padel practice stimulates BDNF response in female players, padel competition failed to boost the release of LIF and IR. Future studies are needed to further explore the role of these exercise-induced myokines in the regulation of brain functions and to identify the field sports that can contribute to myokine-mediated muscle–brain crosstalk.

Keywords: padel; sports competition; myokines; BDNF; leukemia inhibitory factor; irisin

1. Introduction

Padel is a particular racket sport that has grown in popularity and is currently being practiced by millions of people worldwide [1]. Padel is played in doubles on a rectangular court (20 × 10 m) divided into two fields by a central net that is lower than the tennis one. Moreover, this court is completely surrounded by a suitable combination of concrete walls and fence wire, which prevent the ball from exiting the playing area [2,3].

As in other racket sports, several studies have been focused on the assessment of players' court-movement patterns and the physiological demands of padel competition. Cardiorespiratory responses (oxygen consumption and mean heart rate) as well as perceived exertion rates are similar to those previously found in tennis. However, they are lower compared to those assessed in squash and badminton [1]. More specifically, and considering that padel practice is characterized by alternated intervals of intense and moderate-low exercise intensity, the mean VO_2 measured during an official competition (lasting around 1 h) reached values below 50% of maximum VO_2 (VO_{2max}), whereas the mean HR represented approximately 74% of maximum HR (HR_{max}) [2]. Thus, moderate energy expenditure (with aerobic metabolism as the main energy source) and an easy and accessible technique seem to be the two key factors behind the extended practice of padel

However, although padel practice keeps increasing there remains a lack of information about its impact on players' health. According to the reviewed scientific literature, there are not many studies dealing with the physiological, health-related effects of high-level padel competition [2]. To our knowledge, only one very recent study has been aimed at analyzing the changes in hematological and biochemical parameters induced by competitive padel practice. As can be observed, high-level padel competition provokes a significant increase in muscle damage biomarkers (e.g., creatine kinase) as well as remarkable decreases in blood electrolytes concentrations [4]. Nevertheless, apart from these intensity-related effects it would be necessary to conduct studies focused on determining the stimulating effects of competitive padel practice on different health-related benefits through specific biomarkers

Brain-derived neurotrophic factor (BDNF) is an important neurotrophin that plays important roles in the plasticity of several regions of the central nervous system (CNS) during development, adulthood, and aging [5]. Nevertheless, it has been suggested that BDNF is expressed in non-neurogenic tissues (including skeletal muscle), so that BDNF may play a role not only in CNS plasticity but also as a metabolic regulator of skeletal muscle (enhancing glucose consumption and fat oxidation). In any case, of all neurotrophins BDNF seems to be the most susceptible to regulation by exercise and physical activity [6]. In fact, the response of BDNF to acute exercise has been investigated using different exercise protocols and, consequently, different results have been reported (from a lack of response to increases anywhere between 11.7 and 410.0% with respect to basal levels) [7].

The skeletal muscle acts as a secretory organ that, in addition to BDNF, produces cytokines and other muscle fiber-derived peptides called myokines [8]. In general, myokines are muscle-derived molecules that exert physiological functions on maintaining systemic homeostasis. Thus, myokines regulate whole-body metabolism, bone growth, satellite cell proliferation, and muscle hypertrophy in an autocrine, paracrine, or endocrine manner [9,10]. Irisin (IR) and leukemia inhibitory factor (LIF) are two novel myokines that are associated with brain and muscle adaptations. A recent study has reported that IR is involved in whole-body metabolism regulation by stimulating FFA, oxidation, and lipolysis and inducing fat browning. Moreover, IR stimulates glucose uptake and regulates muscle growth [11]. Although the primary source of IR is skeletal muscle, another source of this myokine is the brain. Therefore, IR could play roles in mediating the effects of physical activity on the brain [12]. On the other hand, LIF is produced by skeletal muscle and affects intact muscles as well as isolated muscle cells. Among its various roles, the most important role of LIF in muscle satellite cell is the proliferation of proper muscle hypertrophy and regeneration [10,13].

However, considering the beneficial effects of BDNF, LIF, and IR on brain health status, there is a lack of information about the magnitude of their responses to field sports activities [14]. As it has been reported in a recent study, the amount of evidence for the effects of exercise on the blood concentration of BDNF is moderate [15]. Moreover, studies on the response of IR to exercise have not been conclusive [16], and although LIF seems to play an autocrine role within the skeletal muscle tissue, it has been difficult to determine changes in their circulating levels in response to exercise.

Thus, taking into account the increasing popularity of padel and the potential brain health effects of BDNF, LIF, and IR, this study was designed to evaluate the responses of these myokines to padel competition in trained players and to determine whether they are sex-dependent.

2. Materials and Methods

2.1. Participants

A total of 24 trained padel players (14 female and 10 male young-adult players) with more than five years of experience in the professional circuit World Padel Tour participated voluntarily in this study. The characteristics of the subjects can be seen in Table 1. All of the participants gave their informed consent for inclusion prior to participation. The study was conducted in accordance with the Declaration of Helsinki, and the protocol was approved by the Ethics Committee of the Department of Health and Consumption of the Government of Aragon, Spain (code: 21/2012; date: 19 December 2012).

Table 1. Padel players' characteristics.

	Females	Males	Total	Sig. (CI = 95%)
Age (years)	29.1 ± 3.8 (26.5–31.6)	26.3 ± 8.2 (20.4–32.2)	27.8 ± 6.3 (24.9–30.6)	$p = 0.323$
Height (cm)	167.1 ± 5.7 (163.3–170.9)	177.1 ± 2.8 (175.1–179.1)	171.9 ± 6.8 (168.8–174.9)	$p < 0.001$
Weight (kg)	60.7 ± 4.5 (57.6–63.7)	76.7 ± 6.2 (72.2–81.1)	68.3 ± 9.7 (63.8–72.7)	$p < 0.001$
BMI (kg/m^2)	21.7 ± 1.0 (21.0–22.4)	24.4 ± 1.8 (23.1–25.7)	23.0 ± 1.9 (22.1–23.9)	$p < 0.001$
Body fat (%)	20.2 ± 2.1 (18.8–21.7)	13.4 ± 5.1 (9.7–17.0)	16.9 ± 5.1 (14.6–19.3)	$p = 0.001$
Muscle mass (%)	37.1 ± 2.9 (35.1–39.0)	43.3 ± 2.2 (41.7–44.9)	40.1 ± 4.1 (38.2–41.9)	$p < 0.001$
VO$_{2max}$ (mL/kg/min)	47.5 ± 4.9 (44.2–50.8)	57.5 ± 5.7 (53.4–61.6)	52.3 ± 7.3 (48.9–55.6)	$p < 0.001$
HR$_{max}$ (bpm)	186.2 ± 7.8 (181.0–191.5)	188.3 ± 10.7 (180.7–195.3)	187.2 ± 9.1 (183.1–191.4)	$p = 0.622$

CI, confidence interval; BMI, body mass index; VO$_{2max}$, maximum oxygen consumption; HR$_{max}$, maximum heart rate measured in the graded exercise test. Numbers in brackets represent the mean 95% CI of the mean. Italics are used to highlight statistical significance.

The calculations for sample size and power were based on BDNF responses to moderate and vigorous exercise reported by a previous study [17]. Considering the large effect sizes (ES) shown by these authors (e.g., Cohen's d range of 0.63–1.16), the a priori sample size calculation (G*Power v.3.1) with ES = 0.64 established that a sample of 22 would be sufficient to obtain a statistical power of 0.8 ($p < 0.05$). Therefore, our sample size of 24 allowed us to overcome a power of 85%.

2.2. Experimental Approach

Participants were involved in two separate testing sessions with at least seven days between them (Figure 1). In the first session, subjects' body composition analysis was assessed (bioelectrical impedance, TANITA BC–418MA, Amsterdam, The Netherlands) and a graded exercise test was also performed. The second session consisted of participating in a simulated competition following the International Padel Federation rules.

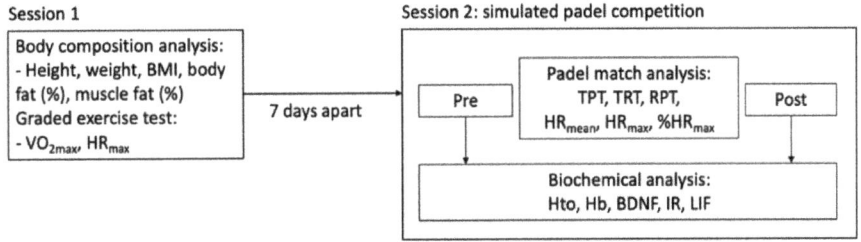

Figure 1. Study protocol.

For each session (conducted between 9:00 a.m. and 12:00 a.m.), participants were instructed to avoid strenuous physical activity during the previous 24 h and to abstain from food (overnight fasting), caffeine, and alcohol 12 h before testing. Padel matches were held on outdoor courts with a relative environmental humidity and temperature of 45.7 ± 7.3% and 24.1 ± 7.1 degrees Celsius, respectively.

2.2.1. Session 1: Determination of Cardiorespiratory Fitness

Players' maximum oxygen consumption (VO_{2max}) and maximum heart rate (HR_{max}) were assessed in the first session using an incremental running test on a treadmill (Pulsar HP Cosmos, Nussdorf, Germany) equipped with a gas analyzer (Oxycon Pro. Jaegger, Germany) and heart rate monitor (Cosmos, Nussdorf, Germany). After a warm-up period of 5 min of brisk walking (6 km/h), the initial speed was set at 8 km/h, increasing by 1 km/h every minute until volitional exhaustion. The treadmill slope was kept at 1°. VO_{2max} was defined following the ACSM criteria [18], whereas HR_{max} determined as the highest HR value observed during the running test.

2.2.2. Session 2: Simulated Padel Competition Analysis

All matches were played to the best of three sets. If the situation of six equal games was reached, a tie breaker was played. Before each match, players performed a standardized 15 min warm-up. Total playing time (TPT, full time of the match from the beginning to the end, considering the periods of game and rest), total resting time (TRT, sum of periods in which the ball was not in play), and real playing time (RPT, total playing time minus total resting time) were measured (s) for each match. Moreover, players' HR was continuously recorded during the competition (Polar Team System, Kempele, Finland) as average values over 5 s.

Blood sampling. In the second session, two 5-mL blood samples (pre- and post-padel competition) were drawn from the antecubital vein of each participant. Blood samples were collected in Vacutainer tubes (BD Vacutainer, Plymouth, UK) containing ethylenediaminetetraacetic acid (EDTA) as an anticoagulant. The first sample was collected 90 min before the competition (fasting conditions), and the second was collected within 10 min after the matches. Blood samples were immediately put on ice and transferred to a laboratory for processing.

Hematological and biochemical assessment. Hematological parameters (red blood cells, hematocrit, and hemoglobin) were determined using the Coulter counter model Ac·T diff (Beckman Coulter Inc., Brea, CA, USA). BDNF concentrations were measured using the BDNF Exam Immunoassay System kit (R&D Corp., Minneapolis, MN, USA) according to the manufacturer's instructions. Whole blood LIF concentrations were determined by enzyme linked immunosorbent assay (ELISA) using a human LIF ELISA kit (PromoKine, Heidelberg, Germany) following the manufacturer's instructions. On the other hand, IR blood levels were measured using a commercial kit (Wuhan Fine Biological Technology Co., Ltd., Wuhan, China). Absorbances for LIF and IR were measured in duplicate using a spectrophotometric microplate reader at a wavelength of 450 nm (Biotek, Winooski, VT, USA).

Lastly, considering that the players were allowed to hydrate ad libitum during the competition (with bottled mineral water), changes in plasma volume were calculated using hematocrit and hemoglobin values following the methods of Dill and Costill [19]. Moreover, blood levels of BDF, LIF, and IR were individually corrected according to the formula described by Matomäki et al. [20].

The data are expressed as mean ± standard deviation (sd). The Shapiro–Wilk test was applied to test for a normal distribution of variables. Parametric and non-parametric tests (ANOVA-time × sex interaction-, Wilcoxon signed-rank, and Mann–Whitney tests) were used where appropriate to determine both intragroup and intergroup differences between the pre- and post-competition time points. Moreover, effect size (ES) was calculated using both partial eta squared ($\eta^2 p$) and the d-value proposed by Cohen [21]. Thus, the ES was interpreted as trivial when $\eta^2 p < 0.01$ and $d < 0.19$; small when $\eta^2 p = 0.01$ and $d = 0.20$

medium when $\eta^2p = 0.06$ and $d = 0.50$; and large when $\eta^2p = 0.14$ and $d = 0.80$. Bivariate correlations were also performed using both Pearson's *r* and Spearman's *rho*, which was set at 0.500 for a positive correlation. For all tests, a *p*-value of <0.05 was used to indicate statistical significance.

3. Results

3.1. Participants' Characteristics and Cardiorespiratory Fitness

Body composition variables showed significant sexual dimorphism. Moreover, VO_{2max} was significantly higher in male than in female players (Table 1).

3.2. Characteristics of Simulated Padel Competition

As it can be seen in Table 2, one of the most peculiar characteristics of padel competition was the 1:1.5 ratio established between TPT and TRT. Although TPT and TRT showed sex-related differences (both variables were higher in males), no differences were found in RPT.

Table 2. Characteristics of simulated padel competition.

	Females	Males	Total	Sig. (CI = 95%)
TPT (s)	3495.9 ± 1165.1 (2521.9–4469.9)	4760.0 ± 1074.7 (3766.0–5753.9)	4085.8 ± 1264.8 (3385.4–4786.3)	*p* = 0.05
RPT (s)	1490.8 ± 480.7 (1088.9–1892.7)	1872.5 ± 496.1 (1413.7–2331.3)	1668.9 ± 509.8 (1386.6–1951.2)	*p* = 0.155
TRT (s)	1961.7 ± 687.2 (1387.2–2536.3)	2825.7 ± 647.1 (2227.3–3424.1)	2364.9 ± 783.9 (1930.8–2799.0)	*p* = 0.027
HR_{mean} (bpm)	142.4 ± 11.8 (135.9–149.0)	145.4 ± 18.2 (134.3–156.4)	143.8 ± 14.9 (138.0–149.6)	*p* = 0.615
HR_{max} (bpm)	167.8 ± 11.4 (161.4–174.1)	173.8 ± 17.8 (163.1–184.6)	170.6 ± 14.8 (164.9–176.3)	*p* = 0.289
% HR_{max}	77.2 ± 5.8 (73.1–81.4)	72.7 ± 9.8 (64.5–81.0)	75.2 ± 7.9 (71.3–79.2)	*p* = 0.245
PV changes (%)	+1.5 ± 2.7 (−0.1–3.1)	+0.5 ± 1.6 (−0.6–1.7)	+1.1 ± 2.3 (−0.6–3.1)	*p* = 0.351

CI, confidence interval; TPT, total playing time; RPT, real playing time; TRT, total resting time; HR_{mean}, mean heart rate assessed during padel competition; HR_{max}, maximum heart rate assessed during padel competition; %HR_{max}, percentage of HR_{mean} on reference HR_{max} (graded exercise test); PV, plasma volume. Numbers in brackets represent the 95% CI of the mean. Italics are used to highlight statistical significance.

On the other hand, HR_{mean} and HR_{max} during padel competition were similar in both males and females. Likewise, considering that HR_{max} measured during maximal exercise test did not report sex differences, the percentage of HR_{mean} on reference HR_{max} (graded exercise test) did not show any statistical significance. Regarding PV changes, a slight but not statistically significant increase (+1.1 ± 2.3% for the total group; CI-95%: −0.6 to 3.1) was observed (Table 2).

3.3. BDNF, LIF, and IR Responses

Although no sex-related differences were found, padel competition induced a significant increase in circulating BDNF levels in female players (from 1531.12 ± 269.09 to 1768.56 ± 410.75 ng/mL; CI-95%: −507.20 to 32.32; Z = −2.27, *p* < 0.05, d = 1.527). In contrast, BDNF concentrations measured in males after exercise were lower than those found before (1523.01 ± 307.10 and 1295.51 ± 288.88 ng/mL, respectively). However, no significant differences were observed (CI-95%: −52.61 to 507.61; Z = −0.866, *p* = 0.186, d = 0.476; Figure 2).

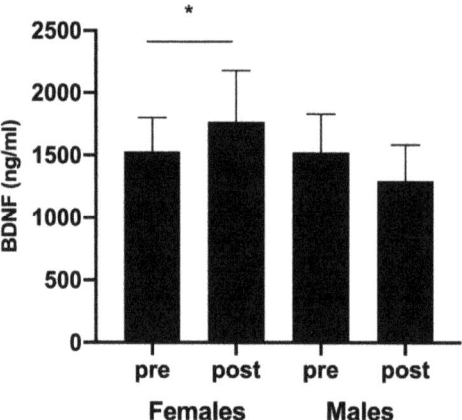

Figure 2. Blood BDNF concentrations (ng/mL) measured before and after padel competition. * $p < 0.05$.

3.4. Statistical Analysis

Regarding LIF responses, no significant differences were observed when sex ($F(3,43) = 0.590$; $p = 0.447$, $\eta^2p = 0.014$), time ($F(3,43) = 0.004$; $p = 0.952$, $\eta^2p < 0.01$), and sex × time interaction ($F(3,43) = 0.318$; $p = 0.576$, $\eta^2p < 0.01$) analyses were performed. Nevertheless, post-exercise LIF concentrations showed a slight decrease in females (from 8.48 ± 5.25 to 7.28 ± 3.76 ng/mL after competition; CI-95%: -2.35 to 4.75) but a nonsignificant increase in males (from 5.91 ± 3.95 to 6.88 ± 4.46 ng/mL, respectively; CI-95%: -4.93 to 2.99) (Figure 3).

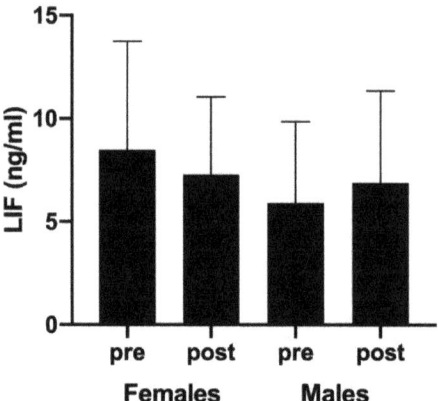

Figure 3. Blood LIF levels (ng/mL) measured before and after padel competition.

On the other hand, intergroup analysis revealed no significant sex-related differences for IR responses (CI-95%: -158.64 to 111.78, $Z = -0.205$, $p = 0.837$, $d = 0.084$ and CI-95%: -142.48 to 92.88, $Z = -0.312$, $p = 0.755$, $d = 0.096$ before and after padel competition respectively). Moreover, unlike BDNF and LIF, the same decreasing trend of IR levels was observed in both female and male players after padel competition. Nevertheless, no significant differences regarding pre-competition levels were found (CI-95%: -89.3 to 118.49, $Z = -0.594$, $p = 0.552$, $d = 0.322$ for females, and CI-95%: -142.36 to 168.68, $Z = -0.051$, $p = 0.959$, $d = 0.027$ for males; Figure 4).

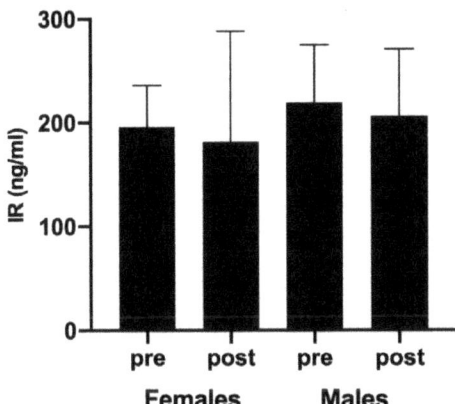

Figure 4. Blood IR concentrations (ng/mL) measured before and after padel competition.

Finally, a correlation analysis reported significant associations between BDNF and IR for the entire group in both before (rho = 0.461; p = 0.024), and after competition (rho = 0.665; p < 0.001).

4. Discussion

The main aims of this study were to evaluate the responses of BDNF, LIF, and IR to padel competition in trained players and to determine whether these responses were sex-dependent. To our knowledge, there have not been many studies evaluating the responses of neurotrophic factors and specific myokines to competitive sports practice. As has been indicated, padel is increasingly practiced by more people, so it is important to define all of its potential health benefits.

According to previous findings, as was expected, the padel players evaluated in our study showed sexual dimorphism in body composition [22] and cardiorespiratory variables [23]. Moreover, sex-related differences were also observed in padel competition characteristics. TPT and RPT were higher in male than in female players. However, RPT did not show any differences between groups. While these sex-related effects were in accordance with the findings of a very recent study [4], they were contrary to those reported by Torres-Luque et al. [24], who found higher TPT and RPT in female players. In any case, TPT in our study was established approximately between 55 and 80 min, which is in line with these previous reports.

On the other hand, we assessed cardiovascular responses to padel competition using HR_{mean} during matches and its percentage on HR_{max} measured during a graded exercise test. Our results are similar to those previously described by Castillo-Rodriguez et al. [1], who reported a HR_{mean} equivalent to 77% of HR_{max} during padel competition. Only one previous study [4] has considered the impact of padel practice on the hemodynamic variables that could modulate other physiological and/or biochemical responses in padel players. Accordingly, it seems necessary to check PV changes associated with intense outdoor exercise, especially if athletes need to hydrate to replace the water lost through sweating and to maintain an adequate thermoregulation. Thus, taking into account that our padel players kept hydrated during the competition, it was necessary to calculate PV changes to avoid any hemoconcentration or hemodilution that could affect the results. Nevertheless, although a mean increase of 1.1% in PV was measured after padel competition, biochemical data were individually corrected.

Biochemical analysis was focused on BDNF, LIF, and IR, a group of myokines that, among others, could explain the underlying biological mechanisms of neuroprotective and regenerative potential effects of exercise in both CNS and the periphery [25]. In fact, increased levels of multiple myokines that have beneficial endocrine effects play crucial roles in the interactions between skeletal muscle and other organs in response to exercise [11]. Nonetheless, our study showed that, with some exceptions, padel competition fails to induce remarkable changes in circulating levels of these biomarkers. Moreover, it is important to note that their responses were characterized by large interindividual variability.

The response of BDNF to acute exercise has been investigated by several authors using different exercise protocols and, consequently, different results have been reported [7]. In our study, padel competition induced only a slight but significant increase in the circulating BDNF concentrations of female players. This attenuated response is in line with those observed in previous studies in which low or moderate-intensity exercise was used [26,27]. The magnitude of BDNF increase seems to be exercise intensity-dependent, since high-intensity exercises induced huge BDNF responses [7,28], whereas low or moderate-intensity exercises were insufficient to do so [26]. Thus, padel competitions that consisted of 55–80 min of discontinuous exercise (RPT from 22 to 33 min) performed at 72–77% of HR_{max} may fail to stimulate large BDNF responses.

Although LIF is a myokine mainly associated with muscle regeneration, various studies have demonstrated the importance of LIF at various stages of neurogenesis and its involvement in both neuronal cell differentiation and neuritic outgrowth [29]. Previous studies demonstrated that aerobic exercise induces the expression of LIF in human skeletal muscle [13,30]. However, our results reported no changes in LIF circulating levels after padel competition. Moreover, we did not observe differences regarding the players' sex. Similar results were found by Donnikov et al. [31], who reported a slight decrease in LIF concentrations in a group of athletes after a six hour marathon ultra-race. This lack of LIF responses to exercise could be explained by many different hypotheses. First, as it has been previously observed, exercise-induced LIF responses are characterized by a remarkable interindividual variability. In fact, both increases and decreases in circulating post-exercise LIF levels have been measured in athletes [31]. Second, LIF seems to be muscle-specific, as LIF was undetectable in plasma. It is possible that LIF is secreted to the interstitial space between muscle fibers and does not easily reach circulation. Third, considering the short blood half-life of LIF (6–8 min), it could be difficult to detect accumulated circulating levels of LIF protein during prolonged exercise [32]. Finally, it seems that resistance exercises (mainly eccentric muscle contractions) regulate LIF secretion better than aerobic exercises [13], which would also explain the attenuated LIF responses observed here.

Previous studies have confirmed that IR may stimulate both neuronal proliferation and differentiation [33,34]. Furthermore, IR contributes to the neuroprotective effect of exercise against brain disorders [35]. Although the primary source of IR in humans is skeletal muscle, which produces over 70% of the total circulating level of IR, other non-muscle sources of this myokine (such as the brain) play roles in mediating the effects of physical activity on the brain [12]. In any case, previous results reported that plasma IR levels were elevated in humans following exercise [36]. Thus, it was to be expected that circulating IR levels were increased after padel competition. However, we observed no effect of exercise on IR blood concentrations, since post-exercise values were similar to those measured before padel matches. At the same time, no sex-related differences were detected when both pre and post-exercise IR levels were contrasted between male and female players. These results are in line with those obtained by Pekkala et al. [37] and Tsuchiya et al. [38], who did not find changes in IR concentrations after 1 h of aerobic cycling at intensities of 50% and 65% VO_{2max}, respectively. In this sense, it seems that exercise-related IR response is intensity dependent, since various studies have demonstrated significant IR acute responses when both trained and untrained subjects performed high-intensity exercises [39,40]. Moreover, after comparing resistance exercise with interval- and endurance-type exercise protocols, Huh et al. [41] reported that, as occurs with LIF, strengthening exercise induced a greater IR response than continuous cardiovascular ones.

Nevertheless, contrary to the findings of Briken et al. [25], correlation analyses revealed significant associations between IR and BDNF in both pre- and post-exercise evaluations. On the basis of these associations, it is important to consider that exercise-related IR response is stimulated by an increased expression of PGC1-α, a regulator of mitochondrial biogenesis. PGC1-α is an inducer of fibronectin type III domain-containing protein 5 (FNDC5) expression, a single-pass membrane-spanning protein. Upon exercise, the ectodomain of FNDC5-IR is released into the bloodstream. Interestingly, FNDC5 was shown to mediate beneficial CNS effects of endurance exercise by upregulating BDNF expression [42]. In any case, future studies should explore this type of relationship and its potential benefits for brain health.

Lastly, as with the majority of studies performed on sports competition, there are some limitations inherent to the design used that should be noted. First, simulated padel competition could be quite different from real padel competition. Second, taking into account the interindividual variability shown by the outcome variables, the sample size was relatively small. However, considering the recruiting difficulties inherent to competitive athletes, the participants in our study were homogeneous in terms of padel competitive category and training status.

5. Conclusions

Our results suggest that competitive padel practice induces a slight but significant response of BDNF in female players. However, padel competition failed to stimulate the release of LIF and IR. Padel competition characteristics and relative playing intensity could explain this lack of stimulating effect. In addition, IR and BDNF showed an interesting association that needs to be studied in future research. Nevertheless, with respect to practical applications the findings of our study suggest that padel could be included as a part of programs promoting brain health, especially for women.

Author Contributions: Conceptualization, F.P., M.P.C., I.C.M.-D. and L.C.; methodology, F.P., M.P.C., I.C.M.-D. and L.C.; investigation, F.P., M.P.C. and I.C.M.-D.; formal analysis, F.P., M.T.N., L.C., M.P.C. and I.C.M.-D.; writing—original draft preparation, F.P., M.P.C. and I.C.M.-D.; writing—review and editing, F.P. and M.P.C.; supervision, F.P. and L.C. All authors have read and agreed to the published version of the manuscript.

Funding: This research received no external funding.

Institutional Review Board Statement: The study was conducted according to the guidelines of the Declaration of Helsinki and approved by the Ethics Committee of the Department of Health and Consumption of the Government of Aragón, Spain (code: 21/2012).

Informed Consent Statement: Informed consent was obtained from all subjects involved in the study.

Data Availability Statement: The data presented in this study are available upon request from the corresponding author.

Acknowledgments: The authors gratefully acknowledge the technical support of the Sport Medicine Lab, Huesca, Government of Aragón.

Conflicts of Interest: The authors declare no conflict of interest.

References

Castillo-Rodríguez, A.; Alvero-Cruz, J.R.; Hernández-Mendo, A.; Fernández-García, J.C. Physical and physiological responses in paddle tennis competition. *Int. J. Perform. Anal. Sport* **2014**, *14*, 524–534. [CrossRef]

Carrasco, L.; Romero, S.; Sañudo, B.; De Hoyo, M. Game analysis and energy requirements of paddle tennis competition. *Sci. Sports* **2011**, *26*, 338–344. [CrossRef]

Courel-Ibáñez, J.; Martinez, B.J.S.A.; Marín, D.M. Exploring game dynamics in padel. *J. Strength Cond. Res.* **2019**, *33*, 1971–1977. [CrossRef] [PubMed]

Pradas, F.; García-Giménez, A.; Toro-Román, V.; Sánchez-Alcaraz, B.J.; Ochiana, N.; Castellar, C. Effect of a padel match on biochemical and haematological parameters in professional players with regard to gender-related differences. *Sustainability* **2020**, *12*, 8633. [CrossRef]

Cardenas-Aguayo, M.d.C.; Kazim, S.F.; Grundke-Iqbal, I.; Iqbal, K. Neurogenic and neurotrophic effects of BDNF peptides in mouse hippocampal primary neuronal cell cultures. *PLoS ONE* **2013**, *8*, e53596. [CrossRef]

Knaepen, K.; Goekint, M.; Heymann, E.M.; Meeusen, R. Neuroplasticity: Exercise-induced response of peripheral brain-derivied neurotrophic factor. *Sports Med.* **2010**, *40*, 765–801. [CrossRef]

7. Martínez-Díaz, I.C.; Escobar, M.C.; Carrasco, L. Acute Effects of High-Intensity Interval Training on Brain-Derived Neurotrophic Factor, Cortisol and Working Memory in Physical Education College Students. *Int. J. Environ. Res. Public Health* **2020**, *17*, 8216. [CrossRef]
8. Giudice, J.; Taylor, J.M. Muscle as a paracrine and endocrine organ. *Curr. Opin. Pharm.* **2017**, *34*, 49–55. [CrossRef]
9. Li, H.; Chen, Q.; Li, C.; Zhong, R.; Zhao, Y.; Zhang, Q.; Zhang, Y. Muscle-secreted granulocyte colony-stimulating factor functions as metabolic niche factor ameliorating loss of muscle stem cells in aged mice. *EMBO J.* **2019**, *38*, e102154. [CrossRef]
10. So, B.; Kim, H.J.; Kim, J.; Song, W. Exercise-induced myokines in health and metabolic diseases. *Integr. Med. Res.* **2014**, *3*, 172–179. [CrossRef]
11. Chen, W.; Wang, L.; You, W.; Shan, T. Myokines mediate the cross talk between skeletal muscle and other organs. *J. Cell Physiol.* **2020**, *236*, 2393–2412. [CrossRef] [PubMed]
12. Dun, S.L.; Lyu, R.M.; Chen, Y.H.; Chang, J.K.; Luo, J.J.; Dun, N.J. Irisin-immunoreactivity in neural and non-neural cells of the rodent. *Neuroscience* **2013**, *240*, 155–162. [CrossRef] [PubMed]
13. Broholm, C.; Pedersen, B.K. Leukaemia inhibitory factor—an exercise-induced myokine. *Exerc. Immunol. Rev.* **2010**, *16*, 77–85. [PubMed]
14. Fatouros, I.G. Is irisin the new player in exercise-induced adaptations or not? A 2017 update. *Clin. Chem. Lab. Med.* **2018**, *56*, 525–548. [CrossRef]
15. Kim, S.; Choi, J.Y.; Moon, S.; Park, D.H.; Kwak, H.B.; Kang, J.H. Roles of myokines in exercise-induced improvement of neuropsychiatric function. *Eur. J. Physiol.* **2019**, *471*, 491–505. [CrossRef]
16. Arias-Loste, M.T.; Ranchal, I.; Romero-Gómez, M.; Crespo, J. Irisin, a link among fatty liver disease, physical inactivity and insulin resistance. *Int. J. Mol. Sci.* **2014**, *15*, 23163–23178. [CrossRef]
17. Rojas-Vega, S.; Struder, H.K.; Wahrmann, B.V.; Schmidt, A.; Bloch, W.; Hollmann, W. Acute BDNF and cortisol response to low intensity exercise and following ramp incremental exercise to exhaustion in humans. *Brain Res.* **2006**, *1121*, 59–65. [CrossRef] [PubMed]
18. American College of Sports Medicine. *ACSM's Guidelines for Exercise Testing and Prescription*, 7th ed.; Lippincott Williams & Wilkins: New York, NY, USA, 2006.
19. Dill, D.B.; Costill, D.L. Calculation of percentage changes in volumes of blood, plasma, and red cells in dehydration. *J. Appl. Physiol.* **1974**, *37*, 247–248. [CrossRef]
20. Matomäki, P.; Kainulainen, H.; Kyröläinen, H. Corrected whole blood biomarkers–the equation of Dill and Costill revisited. *Physiol. Rep.* **2018**, *6*, e13749. [CrossRef] [PubMed]
21. Cohen, J. *Statistical Power Analysis for the Behavioral Sciences*; Lawrence Earlbaum Associates: Hillsdale, MI, USA, 1988.
22. Pradas, F.; González-Jurado, J.A.; García-Giménez, A.; Gallego Tobón, F.; Castellar Otín, C. Anthropometric characteristics of elite paddle players. A pilot study. *Rev. Int. Med. Cienc. Act. Fís. Dep.* **2019**, *19*, 181–195.
23. Borges, C.; Del Vecchio, F.B. Physical fitness of amateur paddle tennis players: Comparisons between different competitive levels. *Motricidade* **2018**, *14*, 42–51.
24. Torres-Luque, G.; Ramirez, A.; Cabello-Manrique, D.; Nikolaidis, T.P.; Alvero-Cruz, J.R. Match analysis of elite players during paddle tennis competition. *Int. J. Perform. Anal. Sport* **2015**, *15*, 1135–1144. [CrossRef]
25. Briken, S.; Rosenkranz, S.C.; Keminer, O.; Patra, S.; Ketels, G.; Heesen, C.; Hellweg, R.; Pless, O.; Schulz, K.H.; Gold, S.M. Effects of exercise on Irisin, BDNF and IL-6 serum levels in patients with progressive multiple sclerosis. *J. Neuroimmunol.* **2016**, *299*, 53–58. [CrossRef] [PubMed]
26. Ferris, L.; Williams, J.S.; Shen, C.L. The Effect of acute exercise on serum brain-derived neurotrophic factor levels and cognitive function. *Med. Sci. Sports Exerc.* **2007**, *39*, 728–734. [CrossRef] [PubMed]
27. Schmolesky, M.T.; Webb, D.L.; Hansen, R.A. The effects of aerobic exercise intensity and duration on levels of brain-derived neurotrophic factor in healthy men. *J. Sports Sci. Med.* **2013**, *12*, 502–511.
28. Gustafsson, G.; Lira, C.M.; Johansson, J.; Wisén, A.; Wohlfart, B.; Ekman, R.; Westrin, A. The acute response of plasma brain derived neurotrophic factor as a result of exercise in major depression. *Psychiatry Res.* **2009**, *94*, 1159–1160.
29. Ostasov, P.; Houdek, Z.; Cendelin, J.; Kralickova, M. Role of leukemia inhibitory factor in the nervous system and its pathology. *Rev. Neurosci.* **2015**, *26*, 443–459. [CrossRef]
30. Broholm, C.; Mortensen, O.H.; Nielsen, S.; Akerstrom, T.; Zankari, A.; Dahl, B.; Pedersen, B.K. Exercise induces expression of leukaemia inhibitory factor in human skeletal muscle. *J. Physiol.* **2008**, *586*, 2195–2201. [CrossRef]
31. Donnikov, A.; Shkurnikov, M.Y.; Akimov, E.B.; Grebenyuk, E.S.; Khaustova, S.A.; Shahmatova, E.M.; Tonevitsky, A.G. Effect of a six-hour marathon ultra-race on the levels of IL-6, LIF, and SCF. *Bull. Exp. Biol. Med.* **2009**, *148*, 819–821. [CrossRef]
32. Hilton, D.J.; Nicola, N.A.; Waring, P.M.; Metcalf, D. Clearance and fate of leukemia-inhibitory factor (LIF) after injection into mice. *J. Cell Physiol.* **1991**, *148*, 430–439. [CrossRef]
33. Hashemi, M.S.; Ghaedi, K.; Salamian, A.; Karbalaie, K.; Emadi-Baygi, M.; Tanhaei, S.; Baharvand, H. FNDC5 knockdown significantly decreased neural differentiation rate of mouse embryonic stem cells. *Neuroscience* **2013**, *231*, 296–304. [CrossRef]
34. Moon, H.S.; Dincer, F.; Mantzoros, C.S. Pharmacological concentrations of irisin increase cell proliferation without influencing markers of neurite outgrowth and synaptogenesis in mouse H19-7 hippocampal cell lines. *Metab. Clin. Exp.* **2013**, *62*, 1131–1136. [CrossRef]

5. Li, D.J.; Li, Y.H.; Yuan, H.B.; Qu, L.F.; Wang, P. The novel exercise-induced hormone irisin protects against neuronal injury via activation of the Akt and ERK1/2 signaling pathways and contributes to the neuroprotection of physical exercise in cerebral ischemia. *Metab. Clin. Exp.* **2017**, *68*, 31–42. [CrossRef] [PubMed]
6. Fox, J.; Rioux, B.V.; Goulet, E.D.; Johanssen, N.M.; Swift, D.L.; Bouchard, D.R.; Loewen, H.; Sénéchal, M. Effect of an acute exercise bout on immediate post-exercise irisin concentration in adults: A meta-analysis. *Scand. J. Med. Sci. Sports* **2018**, *28*, 16–28. [CrossRef] [PubMed]
7. Pekkala, S.; Wiklund, P.K.; Hulmi, J.J.; Ahtiainen, J.P.; Horttanainen, M.; Pöllänen, E.; Mäkelä, K.A.; Kaiunalainen, H.; Häkkinen, K.; Nyman, K.; et al. Are skeletal muscle FNDC5 gene expression and irisin release regulated by exercise and related to health? *J. Physiol.* **2013**, *591 Pt 21*, 5393–5400. [CrossRef]
8. Tsuchiya, Y.; Ando, D.; Takamatsu, K.; Goto, K. Resistance exercise induces a greater irisin response than endurance exercise. *Metabolism* **2015**, *64*, 1042–1050. [CrossRef] [PubMed]
9. Huh, J.Y.; Panagiotou, G.; Mougios, V.; Brinkoetter, M.; Vamvini, M.T.; Schneider, B.E.; Mantzoros, C.S. FNDC5 and irisin in humans: I. Predictors of circulating concentrations in serum and plasma and II. mRNA expression and circulating concentrations in response to weight loss and exercise. *Metabolism* **2012**, *61*, 1725–1738. [CrossRef]
10. Daskalopoulou, S.S.; Cooke, A.B.; Gomez, Y.-H.; Mutter, A.F.; Filippaios, A.; Mesfum, E.T.; Mantzoros, C.S. Plasma irisin levels progressively increase in response to increasing exercise workloads in young, healthy, active subjects. *Eur. J. Endocrinol.* **2014**, *171*, 343–352. [CrossRef]
11. Huh, J.Y.; Siopi, A.; Mougios, V.; Park, K.H.; Mantzoros, C.S. Irisin in response to exercise in humans with and without metabolic syndrome. *J. Clin. Endocrinol. Metab.* **2015**, *100*, E453–E457. [CrossRef]
12. Wrann, C.D.; White, J.P.; Salogiannnis, J.; Laznik-Bogoslavski, D.; Wu, J.; Ma, D.; Lin, J.D.; Greenberg, M.E.; Spiegelman, B.M. Exercise induces hippocampal BDNF through a PGC-1α/FNDC5 pathway. *Cell Metab.* **2013**, *18*, 649–659. [CrossRef]

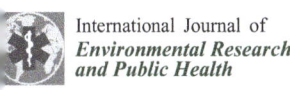

Article

The Role of Social Media in Sports Vision

Henrique Nascimento [1], Clara Martinez-Perez [1,2,*], Cristina Alvarez-Peregrina [3] and Miguel Ángel Sánchez-Tena [1,4]

1. ISEC LISBOA—Instituto Superior de Educação e Ciências, 1750-179 Lisboa, Portugal; henrique.nascimento@iseclisboa.pt (H.N.); masancheztena@ucm.es (M.Á.S.-T.)
2. Faculty of Sport Sciences, Universidad Europea de Madrid, 28670 Madrid, Spain
3. School of Biomedical and Health Science, Universidad Europea de Madrid, 28670 Madrid, Spain; cristina.alvarez@universidadeuropea.es
4. Department of Optometry and Vision, Faculty of Optics and Optometry, Universidad Complutense de Madrid, 28037 Madrid, Spain
* Correspondence: clara.perez@iseclisboa.pt

Abstract: Background: Sports vision is a relatively new specialty. The objective is to provide ophthalmological and optometric care services for the care of vision in the sports field. An increasing number of athletes and coaches are trying to improve visual skills and they seek information on social media. The current excess of information has made it increasingly difficult to identify high quality articles. For this reason, alternative metrics are useful tools to identify publications that draw attention to society. This research aims to study the influence of social networks on the importance of vision in sport. Methods: Altmetric Explorer was used to perform a search using "sport", "vision" and "eye" as keywords. The 100 outcomes with the most attention were analyzed and correlated with the number of citations in the Web of Science (WoS) using the Spearman correlation coefficient. Results: The 100 best Altmetric Attention Scores (AASs) were published in 67 journals and had a mean AAS value of 30.22 ± 62.37 The results were discussed mainly on Twitter, with a mean of 113.99 ± 43.86 tweets and retweets and a mean of 75.92 ± 79.92 readers in Mendeley. There was no correlation between AAS and WoS Cites for the top 100 outcomes and the correlation was low if we considered the total research results rather than the top 100. Conclusions: The citations are not related to the impact of scientific articles on social networks. Sports vision is a specialty with a growing interest in social media.

Keywords: sport vision; social media; social network analysis; Altmetric

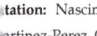

1. Introduction

Nowadays, sports and media share a symbiotic relationship in which both exert an inexhaustible and continuous influence. The media generates revenue through sport while sports and related contents are transmitted through the media in order to develop and expand [1]. This is associated with the fact that many people around the world, especially the younger generation, take part in debates on Facebook, tweet or like a picture on a daily basis [2]. In this regard, sports clubs use advanced and effective communication tools, creating a positive image through social media with the aim of reaching out to people [3].

On the other hand, competition in sport relies on athletes having a diverse set of physical and mental skills. Athletes and coaches are constantly looking for ways to improve these skills and given the demanding nature of sports with regard to perception, visual and motor skills are often the foci of sports training programs. Consequently, social media play an increasingly important role in showing ever-improving skills to action sports participants and in contributing to the creation of new links between corporations, action sports organizations and communities [4,5]. These new links have increased the visibility of the specialty of "sports vision" in the field of optometry. The aim of this specialty is to improve and preserve visual functions for better sporting performance. Thus, in the last

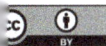

10 years, the number of publications on this subject has increased by 30% due to the great interest of both coaches and athletes in improving visual skills and performance on the playing field. Since 2011, the number of publications has increased significantly (1911–2010: 34.96% of publications; 2011–2020: 65.04% of publications). 2019 was the year with the highest number of publications [6–11].

For many years, the Journal Impact Factor (JIF) was the best tool to determine a journal's impact. Nowadays, social networks such as Mendeley or Twitter offer data (known as alternative metrics or Altmetrics), which allow the measurement of the impact of research in a broader way than by means of citations [12]. The term "Altmetrics" was coined by Jason Priem in 2010 to help researchers filter information and identify relevant sources. Originally, this term was used to refer to the metrics derived from social media activity and other alternative sources of information that transcend the scientific field [13]. However, it is now used with very different metrics and sources that combine with each other [14]. This is particularly important in research where several scholars have found limitations in traditional bibliometric measurements because the information displayed on social media is targeted at a large population [15,16].

Altmetric Explorer tracks the attention that research findings such as academic papers and datasets draw online. In other words, Altmetrics provides an overview of how research is shared and discussed online including by audience [17]. This is highly relevant to sports vision as more and more athletes, coaches, physical trainers and teams are seeking information about training techniques to improve their visual skills.

To date, many studies have analyzed the top Altmetric articles in various areas of health. However, the top Altmetric articles on the influence of vision in sport have not been analyzed. This research aims to study the influence of social networks on the importance of vision in sport.

2. Materials and Methods

2.1. Database

The search was conducted using Altmetric Explorer (Altmetric LLP, London, UK). The search was performed on 5 April 2021 using "sport", "vision" and "eye" as keywords. The search field for the first two keywords was Subject Area (applying filters for abstract, title and keywords) and for the third keyword, a query was used that included all fields. All publications resulting from this search were included in the study. The top 100 with the highest attention according to the Altmetric Attention Score (AAS) were analyzed by two researchers who excluded irrelevant results. For the selection of the most mentioned articles, the AAS provided by Altmetric.com was chosen. The data provided by Altmetric are the most comprehensive, covering the vast majority of social media activity associated with scientific articles. The AAS reflects a weighted total of the mentions of the article by the different online platforms. Thus, a news item is worth eight points, a tweet is worth one point and a Facebook post is worth a quarter point [18]. To perform the analysis, the number of articles with the highest AAS was established as the average of the most cited and most downloaded articles of each journal (after rounding the average number of each journal). The articles with an AAS mat were then identified by an Altmetric Explorer search (Altmetric LLP, London, UK).

2.2. Data Analysis

The Web of Science (WoS) was used to obtain the number of citations for each result, which was then compared with the AAS for the same search date.

The correlation between the number of citations on the WoS and the publication data obtained with the AAS was tested using the Spearman correlation coefficient with SPSS software (IBM, Armonk, NY, USA).

3. Results

The Altmetric Explorer search provided 157 research outputs out of 234 published according to the Web of Science (WoS). A total of 201 of these outputs were mentioned at least once, with a total of 2993 mentions. The first output was from 1995, with one mention in video databases. The years 2017 and 2020 had the highest number of outputs ($n = 26$) followed by 2018 ($n = 23$) and 2019 ($n = 21$). There was a low correlation between publication date and the AAS (Altmetric Attention Score) ($r = 0.145$; $p = 0.028$). Table 1 shows the mean and standard deviation of mentions since 2007 and the total number of mentions in any of the sources studied according to the year as that is when the first iPhone appeared and social networks began to have relevance.

Table 1. Mean and standard deviation of mentions by source and total number of mentions that Altmetric Explorer tracked by sport and vision according to year.

	Mean ± SD	2007	2008	2009	2010	2011	2012	2013	2014	2015	2016	2017	2018	2019	2020	2021
News	12.6 ± 17.3	0	0	0	9	3	5	15	7	8	63	38	23	13	5	0
Blog	2.4 ± 3.2	0	0	0	12	5	2	6	0	3	2	1	1	3	1	0
Policy *	0.4 ± 0.7	0	0	0	1	0	1	2	0	0	2	0	0	0	0	0
Patent **	1.3 ± 2.9	0	0	0	1	0	9	8	0	2	0	0	0	0	0	0
Twitter	162.3 ± 160.7	0	5	2	505	22	37	254	20	185	243	339	289	187	329	18
Peer review **	0.1 ± 0.3	0	0	0	0	0	0	1	0	1	0	0	0	0	0	0
Facebook	12.2 ± 13.5	0	0	0	10	3	17	27	5	33	23	41	18	3	3	0
Wikipedia	1.3 ± 1.5	0	0	1	1	2	3	3	0	5	0	0	0	2	2	0
Google †	1.3 ± 2.3	0	0	0	1	9	1	0	0	0	0	3	1	2	2	0	0
Reddit ***	0.1 ± 0.2	0	0	0	0	0	0	0	0	0	0	0	1	0	0	0
Video ††	0.1 ± 0.2	0	0	0	0	1	0	0	0	0	0	0	0	0	0	0
Total	194.1 ± 179.8	0	5	3	540	45	75	316	32	237	336	421	333	210	340	18

* not trackable since 2016; ** not trackable since 2015; *** not trackable since 2017; † not trackable since 1999; †† not trackable since 2011.

Twitter was the source with the most mentions with the USA (769 posts and 556 profiles), the UK (666 posts and 344 profiles) and Australia (220 posts and 169 profiles) as the three most active countries sharing information on this social network. A total of 769 posts and 556 profiles were not related to any country (Table 2).

Table 2. Mention of the journals on the different social media platforms.

Journal Title	News	Blog	Twitter	Facebook	Wikipedia	Google	Video
Optometry and Vision Science	41	2	107	32	0	0	1
JAMA Ophthalmology	75	6	84	26	0	7	0
Journal of the Neurological Sciences	0	0	122	5	2	0	0
Medicine & Science in Sports & Exercise	11	3	59	11	0	0	0
Journal of Science and Medicine in Sport	0	0	49	0	2	0	0
Journal of Pediatric Ophthalmology and Strabismus	1	0	19	1	5	1	0
Experimental Brain Research	0	0	37	1	0	0	0
Journal of Sports Sciences	1	0	64	4	1	0	0
European Journal of Sports Sciences	0	0	24	0	0	0	0
Frontiers in Psychology	0	0	227	1	0	0	0
Total	129	11	792	81	10	8	1

The research outputs from the top 100 AASs were published in 67 journals and had a mean AAS value of 30.22 ± 62.37 (range 3 to 426). The outputs were mainly discussed on Twitter with a mean of 13.99 ± 43.86 tweets and retweets (range 0 to 484). Supplementary Figure S1 shows the mentions on social networks of the publications with the most AASs as well as the number of readers in Mendeley.

Regarding the journals, *Optometry and Vision Science* was the journal with the highest number of articles in the top 100 with a total of five papers. *Journal of Science and Medicine in Sport*, *JAMA Ophthalmology* and *Journal of the Neurological Sciences* fell behind *Optometry and Vision Science* with three articles each among the top 100. Tables 3 and 4 show the characteristics of the ten journals with the highest AAS on vision and sport. Thus, during the years included in the study, 23 out of 51 items published had an AAS higher than 1 and, of these, five had an AAS higher than 5. *JAMA Ophthalmology* had the highest cumulative AAS. The journals with the highest attraction were *JAMA Ophthalmology* and *Medicine & Science in Sports & Exercise* with a mean AAS per published item of 131.3 and 75.5, respectively. *Optometry and Vision Science* drew online attention to 61.5% of its published articles and this journal published the highest number of items with an AAS above 5.

Table 3. Journals in the top 10 Altmetric Attention Score in sport vision research.

Journal Title	n	Number of Mentioned Outputs	Total Mentions	AAS	IF	Citations, WoS
Optometry and Vision Science	13	10	180	371	8.470	186
JAMA Ophthalmology	4	4	198	525	6.198	68
Journal of the Neurological Sciences	7	6	141	57	3.115	357
Medicine and Science in Sports & Exercise	2	2	84	151	4.029	25
Journal of Science and Medicine in Sport	4	3	49	28	3.607	26
Journal of Pediatric Ophthalmology and Strabismus	3	2	15	26	1.100	85
Experimental Brain Research	2	2	38	21	1.591	16
Journal of Sports Sciences	8	4	58	32	2.597	152
European Journal of Sports Sciences	3	3	24	12	2.781	11
Frontiers in Psychology	5	4	226	7	2.067	47
Total	51			1230		973

n: Number of published items; AAS: Altmetric Attention Score.

Table 4. AAS rank for each of the journals studied.

Journal Title	AAS/Article	n/AAS	n/AAS Range			
			1	2–5	6–10	>10
Optometry and Vision Science	28.5	8 (61.5%)	2	2	1	3
JAMA Ophthalmology	131.3	0 (0%)	0	0	0	0
Journal of the Neurological Sciences	8.1	3 (42.8%)	2	1	0	0
Medicine & Science in Sports & Exercise	75.5	0 (0%)	0	0	0	0
Journal of Science and Medicine in Sport	7.0	2 (50%)	1	1	0	0
Journal of Pediatric Ophthalmology and Strabismus	8.7	0 (0%)	0	0	0	0
Experimental Brain Research	10.5	0 (0%)	0	0	0	0
Journal of Sports Sciences	4.0	4 (50%)	2	1	1	0
European Journal of Sports Sciences	4.0	2 (66.7%)	1	1	0	0
Frontiers in Psychology	1.4	4 (80%)	3	1	0	0
Total		23	11	7	2	3

n: Number of published items; AAS: Altmetric Attention Score.

In terms of Field of Research (FoR) of the top 100 outputs, 75 were classified in division 11: Medical and Health Sciences and 23 of them in division 17: Psychology and Cognitive Sciences. The main area of the journals in which it was published was Medical and Health Sciences with 74 of the 100 outputs studied. Regarding the main areas of the reviews in which sports vision articles appeared, we found Neurosciences with 19 of the 100 outputs and Human Movement and Sports Science with 16 of the 100 outputs.

Table 5 shows the five outputs with the highest AAS as well as other traditional bibliometric parameters.

Table 5. Top five research outputs about sport vision according to the Altimetric Attention Score (AAS).

AAS	Title	Journal/ Collection Title	Publication Date (dd/mm/yyyy)	Mentions	Citations, WoS
426	Transitions between Central and Peripheral Vision Create Spatial/Temporal Distortions: A Hypothesis Concerning the Perceived Break of the Curveball	PLoS ONE	13/10/2010	601	37
379	Epidemiology of Sports-Related Eye Injuries in the United States	JAMA Ophthalmology	01/12/2016	189	16
167	Vision and Vestibular System Dysfunction Predicts Prolonged Concussion Recovery in Children	Clinical Journal of Sport Medicine	28/03/2018	247	37
162	What Do Football Players Look at? An Eye-Tracking Analysis of the Visual Fixations of Players in 11 v 11 Elite Football Match Play	Frontiers in Psychology	16/10/2020	239	0
154	Academic Difficulty and Vision Symptoms in Children with Concussion	Optometry and Vision Science	01/01/2018	124	19

When studying the correlation between the AAS and WoS Cites, no correlation was found between both values for the top 100 outputs ($r = 0.195$; $p > 0.05$). However, a low correlation was found when analyzing the total outputs ($r = 0.147$; $p = 0.024$).

4. Discussion

Visual skills are essential for most sports because visual information can account for up to 85–95% of the sensory information an athlete receives on the playing field. This is why sports vision is now a fundamental part of athlete development and daily training has the potential to enhance performance [19,20]. The study by Spera et al. [21] showed that athletes with a visual impairment had less chance of winning a competition. This is because the functions of the loss of vision affects movement coordination, balance and emotional state, which are important particularly for martial arts. Another study showed that good vision is important for the athlete and training will allow a quick response to different types of stimuli [22].

In recent years, a growing interest on the part of trainers and athletes has led to an increase in posts about this area of research on social media and how to try to improve visual skills for better results on the playing field. As a consequence, it has also become increasingly important to know how the population is receiving this information.

In this regard, altmetrics covers social media activity in the form of mentions on social media, academic activity in digital libraries, popularity indexes in reference managers, scholarly comments through scientific blogs and references on social media [23].

This study is relevant in terms of understanding the impact of sports vision research on society. Compared with other subject areas, sports vision seems to be a topic that currently receives little attention, with a mean AAS value of 30.22 in the top 100 research outputs. This may be due to the fact that the number of publications on sports vision has increased since 2011, which means that it is a new specialty in the field of optometry [6]. However, it is important to note that only 34 of the top 100 research outputs were published in optometry, ophthalmology or sports journals. The top two research outputs according to the AAS were published in *PLoS ONE* [24] and *JAMA Ophthalmology* [25], with 500 and 117 mentions and 37 and 16 citations on the WoS, respectively. In third position was the publication by Master et al. in 2018 in the *Clinical Journal of Sport Medicine* [26] with

111 mentions and 37 citations on the Web of Science. This difference may be due to the fact that this research area is multi-disciplinary and researchers in this field tend to be published in journals with a wide range of research topics.

Analyzing the five most relevant papers in terms of the AAS, the article by Saphiro et al. [24] entitled "Transitions between central and peripheral vision create spatial/temporal distortions: a hypothesis concerning the perceived break of the curveball" was first. It describes the perception of the ball in baseball. In terms of metrics, it could be observed that the largest number of mentions occurred on Twitter although it could also be found on other social networks. This could be explained by the fact that this is one of the most popular sports in the United States and the news was published in The Washington Post newspaper, which gave it a very high visibility. The article analyses the surprise at the explanation offered by science of the perception the batter has of the ball when he tries to hit it as the visual perception does not match the reality, thus worsening the outcome in batting. The relevance of this analysis should not be disregarded as it might make a certain team win matches and even championships if they can count on a good pitcher who is able to give enough spin to the ball so as to cause an erroneous visual perception. The news became popular and was echoed on Twitter where the hashtag "the curveball illusion" caught the attention of readers and helped in its dissemination. It was a blend of science, sport and perception.

In second position was the article by Haring et al. [25] entitled "Epidemiology of Sports-Related Eye Injuries in the United States", which provided an annual incidence of sports-related eye trauma broken down by age, sex, the mechanism of the injury and related activity as well as factors associated with short-term vision problems. As a result, they found that, in the United States, about 70% of eye injuries are sports-related. Again, baseball and basketball appear as the sports with the highest incidence of eye injuries. As these are the two major sports in the United States, they are more widespread and relevant. In relation to this article, the importance of eye protection plans in sport was highlighted. In this case, it was the magazine itself that first spread the article through Twitter. Scientific journals taking part in this type of dissemination is a relatively new practice, which highlights the inclusion of social networks in science outreach plans.

In position 3 and 5 of the most relevant papers were those on American football and the head concussions that occur in the practice of this sport. It is a sport with a high incidence of concussion during its practice. As can be seen in article [27], a total of 1302 concussions were analyzed between 2015 and 2019 in 1004 players, of which 80% of the cases refer to football within the National Football League (NFL) professional league in the United States. Again, this is another highly popular sport in this country.

These papers analyze the repercussions that this type of concussion can have on children's development.

In this instance, the tweets came from the medical area, from medical professionals with many followers disseminating this scientific knowledge and expressing their concern.

In fourth position we have to highlight the study by Aksum et al. [28] published in October 2020. Even if it did not have any citations on the WoS, it was one of the five papers that drew the most attention on social media. This indicated the importance of evaluating alternative metrics that give faster information than traditional metrics about the interest in a certain research project. The attraction of this paper was due to the fact that it analyses the importance of vision on the playing field in elite soccer players and, as mentioned above, a greater number of coaches and athletes are looking to improve their visual skills.

This article refers to soccer, a major sport in Europe and Asia as proven by the fact that most of the tweets came from Sweden and China.

With regard to the years, 2010 and 2017 were the years where publications drew the highest attraction with 540 and 421 mentions, respectively. In those years, the papers by Shapiro et al. [24] and Gallaway et al [29] are worth mentioning. However, when we compared altmetric studies with bibliometric studies, the year 2019 stood out due to the large number of publications and great progress in the research field [6].

This difference may be due to the fact that in 2010, three major multi-sport events took place, the Winter Olympic Games, the FIFA World Cup and the Commonwealth Games. Thus, in countries such as Spain, during that year, interest in sport increased as this country won the World Cup, Alberto Contador, a Spanish cyclist, won the Tour de France and Rafael Nadal, a Spanish tennis player, took over from Roger Federer as a prominent figure in the world of tennis. During 2017, a historic Super Bowl final took place and sprinter Usain Bolt ran his last international races. All this led to increased social interest in the world of sport. On the other hand, in terms of the number of scientific publications, 2019 was the most relevant year, most definitely due to the run up to the Tokyo 2020 Olympic Games. Unfortunately, it is not possible to confirm whether these publications really drew more attention because of the one-year suspension of the Olympic Games due to the pandemic.

In terms of sources, Twitter was the most widely used with the United States and the United Kingdom leading in profiles and tweets on sports vision research. This was consistent with the US being the country with the largest number of users (59,350,000 users) and both the UK and the US being English-speaking countries, which gives rise to a possible connection between the different research groups. At the same time, it was observed that the most prominent articles in this rank referred to three priority sports in the United States: basketball, baseball and American football.

However, if compared with other studies such as the one conducted by Kharmalki et al. [30], Instagram was found to entice a higher participation in the area of sport in general compared with Facebook and YouTube. This may be due to the fact that fans currently use Instagram more to interact with their sports team compared with Facebook, Twitter or YouTube as they prefer instant viewing. In addition, there is growing evidence that fans have moved away from the traditional way of consuming sports where there is only one-way communication and are more drawn to social networking sites where communication is instant and they are connected to a two-way communication network.

As a result, it is expected that in the near future, given the growing interest in the influence of vision on sports performance, public engagement on social media will increase. It should be noted that despite the growing interest in training visual skills to improve athletic performance, it is still unknown how visual training will improve performance on the field of play. Therefore, the increased interest in social networks about the influence of vision in sport will help to develop various training programs in the future to continue training the most relevant visual skills for sport in order to improve performance on the field of play. In addition, it is also hoped that sports vision techniques can be used to assess and rehabilitate sports-related concussions.

The number of publications has grown but it is yet to be seen how it will influence the interest shown on social media.

5. Conclusions

Social networks play an important role for sport vision.

This study offered a new insight into the use and impact of online research given the increase of open access publications. In addition, it showed that Twitter was the social media network with the highest number of mentions of scientific articles in the area of sports vision, with the United States being the country with the highest number of mentions.

The more powerful social networks are to publish the news, the more it can lead to a greater reach and credibility of the investigation.

In this sense, American football is the sport that presented the most interest on social media in which Twitter stood out followed by Facebook. The article with the greatest attraction was published in *PLoS ONE*. Therefore, it should be noted that the citations were not related to the impact on social networks of the scientific article as the most published journal on social media is *Optometry and Vision Science*.

Supplementary Materials: The following are available online at https://www.mdpi.com/article/10.3390/ijerph18105354/s1, Figure S1: Overview of attention for the output of the five articles with the highest AAS.

Author Contributions: Conceptualization, H.N.; C.M.-P.; C.A.-P. and M.Á.S.-T.; methodology, C.A.-P. and M.Á.S.-T.; software, C.M.-P.; C.A.-P.; validation, H.N.; C.M.-P.; C.A.-P. and M.Á.S.-T.; formal analysis, C.M.-P.; C.A.-P.; investigation, C.A.-P. and M.Á.S.-T.; resources, C.M.-P.; C.A.-P. data curation, C.A.-P. and M.Á.S.-T.; writing—original draft preparation, H.N.; C.M.-P.; writing—review and editing, H.N.; C.M.-P.; C.A.-P. and M.Á.S.-T.; visualization, H.N.; C.M.-P.; C.A.-P. and M.Á.S.-T.; supervision, C.A.-P. and M.Á.S.-T.; project administration, M.Á.S.-T.; funding acquisition. All authors have read and agreed to the published version of the manuscript.

Funding: This research received no external funding.

Institutional Review Board Statement: Not applicable.

Informed Consent Statement: Not applicable.

Conflicts of Interest: The authors declare no conflict of interest.

References

1. Kim, N.K.; Park, S.P. The Relationship between Media Sports Involvement Experiences and Sports Values and Sports Participation *Int. J. Appl. Eng. Res.* **2017**, *12*, 9768–9773.
2. Parganas, P.; Anagnostopoulos, C.; Chadwick, S. 'You'll never tweet alone': Managing sports brands through social media. *J. Brand Manag.* **2015**, *22*, 551–568. [CrossRef]
3. Nicholson, M.; Kerr, A.A.; Sherwood, M. *Sport and the Media: Managing the Nexus*; Routledge: New York, NY, USA, 2015.
4. Gilchrist, P.; Wheaton, B. New media technologies in lifestyle sport. In *Digital Media Sport: Technology, Power and Culture in the Network Society*; Hutchins, B., Rowe, D., Eds.; Routledge: New York, NY, USA, 2013.
5. Thorpe, H. *Transnational Migration and Mobilities in Action Sport Cultures*; Palgrave Macmillan: London, UK, 2014.
6. Nascimento, H.; Martinez-Perez, C.; Alvarez-Peregrina, C.; Sánchez-Tena, M.Á. Citations Network Analysis of Vision and Sport *Int. J. Environ. Public Health* **2020**, *17*, 7574. [CrossRef] [PubMed]
7. Appelbaum, L.G.; Erickson, G. Sports vision training: A review of the state-of-the-art in digital training techniques. *Int. Rev. Sport Exerc. Psychol.* **2016**, *11*, 1–30. [CrossRef]
8. Appelbaum, L.G.; Lu, Y.; Khanna, R.; Detwiler, K.R. The Effects of Sports Vision Training on Sensorimotor Abilities in Collegiate Softball Athletes. *Athl. Train Sports Health Care.* **2016**, *8*, 154–163. [CrossRef]
9. Clark, J.F.; Ellis, J.K.; Bench, J.; Khoury, J.; Graman, P. High-Performance vision training improves batting statistics for University of Cincinnati baseball players. *PLoS ONE* **2012**, *7*, e29109. [CrossRef]
10. Formenti, D.; Duca, M.; Trecroci, A.; Ansaldi, L.; Bonfanti, L.; Alberti, G.; Iodice, P. Perceptual vision training in non-sport-specific context: Effect onperformance skills and cognition in young females. *Sci. Rep.* **2019**, *9*, 18671. [CrossRef]
11. Schwab, S.; Memmert, D. The Impact of a Sports Vision Training Program in Youth Field Hockey Players. *J. Sports Sci. Med.* **2012**, *11*, 624–631. [PubMed]
12. Cronin, B.; Sugimoto, C.R. *Beyond Bibliometrics: Harnessing Multi-Dimensional Indicators of Performance*; MIT Press: Cambridge MA, USA, 2014.
13. Priem, J.; Taraborelli, D.; Groth, P.; Neylon, C. Altmetrics: A Manifesto. Available online: http://altmetrics.org/manifesto (accessed on 15 April 2021).
14. Moed, H.F.; Glänzel, W.; Schmoch, U. *Handbook of Quantitative Science and Technology Research*; Springer: Berlin, Germany, 2018.
15. Nederhof, A.J. Bibliometric monitoring of research performance in the Social Sciences and the Humanities: A Review. *Scientometrics* **2006**, *66*, 81–100. [CrossRef]
16. Hammarfelt, B. Using altmetrics for assessing research impact in the humanities. *Scientometrics* **2014**, *101*, 1419–1430. [CrossRef]
17. Maggio, L.; Meyer, H.; Artino, A. Beyond citation rates: Real-time impact analysis of health professions education research via altmetrics. *Acad. Med.* **2017**, *92*, 1449–1455. [CrossRef] [PubMed]
18. Trueger, N.S.; Thoma, B.; Hsu, C.H.; Sullivan, D.; Peters, L.; Lin, M. The Altmetric Score: A New Measure for Article-Level Dissemination and Impact. *Ann. Emerg. Med.* **2015**, *66*, 549–553. [CrossRef]
19. Knudson, D.; Kluka, D.A. The impact of vision and vision training on sport performance. *JPERD* **1997**, *68*, 17–24. [CrossRef]
20. Williams, A.M.; Ward, P.; Knowles, J.M.; Smeeton, N.J. Anticipation skill in a real-world task: Measurement, training, and transfer in tennis. *J. Exp. Psychol. Appl.* **2002**, *8*, 259–270. [CrossRef] [PubMed]
21. Spera, R.; Belviso, I.; Sirico, F.; Palermi, S.; Massa, B.; Mazzeo, F.; Montesano, P. Jump and balance test in judo athletes with or without visual impairments. *J. Hum. Sport Exercis.* **2019**, *14*, S937–S947. [CrossRef]
22. Sirico, F.; Romano, V.; Sacco, A.M.; Belviso, I.; Didonna, V.; Nurzynska, D.; Castaldo, C.; Palermi, S.; Sannino, G.; Della Valle E.; et al. Effect of Video Observation and Motor Imagery on Simple Reaction Time in Cadet Pilots. *J. Funct. Morphol. Kinesiol* **2020**, *5*, 89. [CrossRef] [PubMed]

3. Alonso Arévalo, J.; Cordón-Garcia, J.A.; Maltrás Barba, B. Altmetrics: Medición de la influencia de los medios en el impacto social de la investigación. *Cuad. Doc. Multimed.* **2016**, *27*. [CrossRef]
4. Shapiro, A.; Lu, Z.L.; Huang, C.B.; Knight, E.; Ennis, R. Transitions between central and peripheral vision create spatial/temporal distortions: A hypothesis concerning the perceived break of the curveball. *PLoS ONE* **2010**, *5*, e13296. [CrossRef]
5. Haring, R.S.; Sheffield, I.D.; Canner, J.K.; Schneider, E.B. Epidemiology of Sports-Related Eye Injuries in the United States. *JAMA Ophthalmol.* **2016**, *134*, 1382–1390. [CrossRef]
6. Master, C.L.; Master, S.R.; Wiebe, D.J.; Storey, E.P.; Lockyer, J.E.; Podolak, O.E.; Grady, M.F. Vision and Vestibular System Dysfunction Predicts Prolonged Concussion Recovery in Children. *Clin. J. Sport Med.* **2018**, *28*, 139–145. [CrossRef]
7. Mack, C.D.; Solomon, G.; Covassin, T.; Theodore, N.; Cárdenas, J.; Sills, A. Epidemiology of Concussion in the National Football League, 2015–2019. *Sports Health* **2021**, 19417381211011446. [CrossRef]
8. Aksum, K.M.; Magnaguagno, L.; Bjørndal, C.T.; Jordet, G. What Do Football Players Look at? An Eye-Tracking Analysis of the Visual Fixations of Players in 11 v 11 Elite Football Match Play. *Front. Psychol.* **2020**, *11*, 562995. [CrossRef] [PubMed]
9. Gallaway, M.; Scheiman, M.; Mitchell, G.L. Vision Therapy for Post-Concussion Vision Disorders. *Optom. Vis. Sci.* **2017**, *94*, 68–73. [CrossRef] [PubMed]
10. Kharmalki, G.W.; Raizada, S. Social Media Marketing in Sports: The Rise of Fan Engagement through Instagram. *Soc. Mark. Sports* **2020**, *23*, SP231721. [CrossRef]

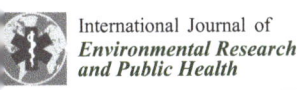

Article

Effects of Ultratrail Running on Neuromuscular Function, Muscle Damage and Hydration Status. Differences According to Training Level

Francisco Pradas [1,2], David Falcón [1,2], Carlos Peñarrubia-Lozano [1,2], Víctor Toro-Román [3,*], Luis Carrasco [4] and Carlos Castellar [1,2]

1 ENFYRED Research Group, Faculty of Health and Sports Sciences, University of Zaragoza, 22001 Huesca, Spain; franprad@unizar.es (F.P.); dfalcon@unizar.es (D.F.); carlospl@unizar.es (C.P.-L.); castella@unizar.es (C.C.)
2 Department of Corporal Expression, Faculty of Health and Sports Sciences, University of Zaragoza, 22001 Huesca, Spain
3 School of Sport Sciences, University of Extremadura, Avenida de la Universidad s/n, 10003 Cáceres, Spain
4 BIOFANEX Research Group, Department of Physical Education and Sport, Faculty of Education Sciences, University of Seville, 41004 Seville, Spain; lcarrasco@us.es
* Correspondence: vtoro@unex.es; Tel.: +34-927-257-460 (ext. 57833)

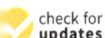

Citation: Pradas, F.; Falcón, D.; Peñarrubia-Lozano, C.; Toro-Román, V.; Carrasco, L.; Castellar, C. Effects of Ultratrail Running on Neuromuscular Function, Muscle Damage and Hydration Status. Differences According to Training Level. *Int. J. Environ. Res. Public Health* **2021**, *18*, 5119. https://doi.org/10.3390/ijerph18105119

Academic Editor: Paul B. Tchounwou

Received: 15 April 2021
Accepted: 9 May 2021
Published: 12 May 2021

Publisher's Note: MDPI stays neutral with regard to jurisdictional claims in published maps and institutional affiliations.

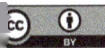

Copyright: © 2021 by the authors. Licensee MDPI, Basel, Switzerland. This article is an open access article distributed under the terms and conditions of the Creative Commons Attribution (CC BY) license (https://creativecommons.org/licenses/by/4.0/).

Abstract: The status of trail running races has exponentially grown in recent years. The present study aimed to: (a) evaluate the acute response of ultratrail racing in terms of neuromuscular function, muscle damage and hydration status; (b) analyze if responses could differ according to training levels. Twenty runners participated in the present study. The participants were divided into amateur training level ($n = 10$; 43.30 ± 4.52 years) or high level competitors ($n = 10$; 41.40 ± 6.18). Neuromuscular response (squat jump, countermovement jump and Abalakov jump), muscle damage (alanine aminotransferase, bilirubin, creatine kinase and leukocytes) and hydration status (sodium and creatinine) were evaluated before and after the Guara Somontano Ultratrail Race (108 km distance, with an accumulated slope of 5800 m). The height and power achieved by vertical jumps were lower after the race ($p < 0.001$). The post-race muscle damage and creatinine parameters increased in both groups ($p < 0.001$). The high-level group obtained lower percentages of change in squat jump and countermovement jump than the amateur-level group ($p < 0.05$). However, the increase in creatinine was greater for the high-level group ($p < 0.05$). Ultratrail racing reduces neuromuscular function and increases muscle damage. High-level runners showed less neuromuscular fatigue compared to amateur ones.

Keywords: trail running; jump; neuromuscular; hydration

1. Introduction

Ultratrail is a form of very long-distance mountain racing included in trail running. Given its extreme characteristics, this kind of racing can be considered very taxing, or even dangerous, for our organism [1]. Ultratrail racing is performed on routes with adverse orography. Its distance exceeds that of marathons [2,3], and ranges between 80 km and 300 km [4]. The fact that ultratrail runners face unstable environmental and weather conditions for long periods of time, and constant changes in the topography of land and altitude [4], with considerable positive and negative slopes [5], is also emphasized.

Despite trail running races being extremely hard, the organization of the sport has exponentially grown worldwide in recent times [6–8], and Spain is no exception [9]. The marked demand expected today of such races has drawn more participants, to the extent that the number of runners in races must be limited, which has led to some runners becoming professionals with enhanced ultratrail race performance [10].

Ultratrail races are multifactorial events that include physiological, neuromuscular, biomechanical and psychological variables [2]. Depending on exertion while running these races, research works indicate that according to ventilator thresholds (VT), in physiological terms these races place mean training intensities at 85.7% for zone I (<VT1), 13.9% for zone II (VT1–VT2) and 0.4% for zone III (>VT2) [11]. Cardiac responses during races lasting between 14 and 7 h present intensities of 64% [12] and 82% [13] of maximum heart rate (HR_{max}), respectively. Different research works have analyzed lactate kinetics during such races, and have obtained results that are below the onset of blood lactate accumulation (OBLA) [14,15]. Finally, as regards the psychophysiological component, values between 13 and 14 points have been obtained on the rate perceived exertion (RPE) scale [16].

In ultratrail endurance races, optimum performance might depend on high maximal oxygen consumption (VO_{2max}) levels, high VO_{2max} fraction utilization percentages and low oxygen transport cost [2]. Along these lines, it has been demonstrated that maximum aerobic power can be a limiting factor to running on positive slopes [17], which are usual for ultratrail routes. When considering the types of routes that ultratrail races are organized along, it would appear that adapting to exertions, in which eccentric-type activations predominate, could be important for facing the ascents and constant loads that come into play when running on irregular sloping surfaces. The eccentric capacity to maintain maximum racing speed would be a determining factor in zones with negative slopes [18].

The increasing numbers of both participants and ultratrail races have favored different research studies being performed in an attempt to analyze the impact that this racing has on health. Indeed, ultratrail races have been associated with a negative energy balance [13], muscle harm and inflammation [19,20], neuromuscular fatigue [21,22], cardiac dysfunctions, myocardial damage [13] and dehydration [1].

The relationship between hydration status and performance has been described [23,24] Hydration status is directly related to physical performance [25]. Previous studies have reported the consequences of dehydration at the physical level, which can negatively affect sports performance [26,27]. A small decrement in hydration status impaired physiologic function and performance during a trail running race [28]. In addition, dehydration status could negatively affect the neuromuscular response [29].

Bearing in mind the marked physical stress that the organism is submitted to while running an ultratrail race, it can be stated that running such races in an unplanned and uncontrolled manner can have very negative consequences for the health of the people practicing this sport [1]. Indeed, knowing the limits of the organism's physiological responses while practicing long intense exercise is necessary to avoid resorting to urgent medical assistance [30]. However, the impact of an ultratrail race could differ from one individual to another because they have distinct training levels. This means that more studies need to be conducted to elucidate this statement [31,32]. The impacts of such races could be very different depending on the participants' training levels, owing to their distinct physiological profiles [33]. Hence, the objectives of the present study were to (a) evaluate the acute responses to an ultratrail race in terms of neuromuscular function muscle damage and hydration status; (b) analyze if responses could differ according to training levels.

2. Materials and Methods

2.1. Participants

Twenty runners participated in this quasiexperimental study, and were divided into an amateur-level group ($n = 10$) and a high-level group ($n = 10$) according to their training levels [34]. The high-level group was made up of runners who trained for a minimum of 8 h/week and achieved positive accumulated slopes of more than 50,000 m in the 12 months before the test. The amateur group was formed by those runners who did not meet any of the set requirements. The study was conducted on a population of 176 male participants who completed the race. The minimum sample size was 20 participants (confidence level = 95%; margin of error = 21%). The characteristics of the participants in each group are found in Table 1.

Table 1. Characteristics of our participants.

Parameters	Amateur Level (n = 10)	High Level (n = 10)	p
Age (years)	43.30 ± 4.52	41.40 ± 6.18	0.443
Height (m)	1.77 ± 0.06	1.76 ± 0.06	0.780
Experience (year)	5.80 ± 2.52	4.60 ± 1.26	0.196
Weekly training (h)	6.50 ± 0.70	11.05 ± 2.94	<0.001
Annual slopes (m)	33,716.7 ± 4427.7	56,426.6 ± 8184.6	0.001

All the participants were informed about the study purpose and signed a consent form before enrolling. The protocol was reviewed and approved by the Ethical Committee of Clinical Research of Aragon (Spain) following the guidelines of the Helsinki Declaration of Ethics, updated at the World Medical Assembly in Fortaleza (2013) for research involving human subjects. A code was assigned to each participant to collect and treat samples in order to maintain their anonymity.

In order to participate in this study, the participants had to meet the following inclusion criteria: (a) male; (b) finished the race route; (c) had no injuries after a race in at least the 2 months prior to the test; (d) not on a special diet or any pharmacological treatment; (e) no cardiovascular or metabolic diseases.

2.2. Procedures

This study was carried out while organizing the Guara Somontano UltraTrail Race (GSUR) (Figure 1), which took place in the town of Alquézar (Huesca, Spain). The total race distance was 108 km, with 5800 meters of positive accumulated slope. The maximum permitted time to finish it in was 24 h. During this race the mean temperature was 14 ± 4.4 °C and relative humidity was 57 ± 16.1% (Figure 1).

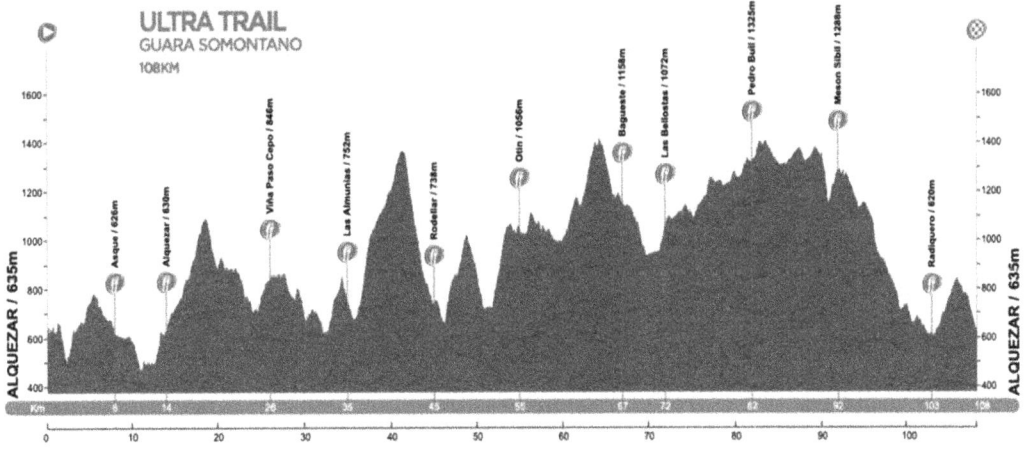

Figure 1. Race profile (taken from the organization's website).

The week before competition, the participants underwent body composition and physical performance evaluations. In parallel to these evaluations, the runners completed an open *ad hoc* survey with supplementary information about their experience, and the characteristics of their training over the past year (h/week and accumulated slope). To determine hydration during races, the volumes of liquids drunk by racers were calculated at both supply points and throughout the race according to individual drinking frequency.

Volunteers recorded the amounts of water ingested at each supply point using two 250 cc bottles as a reference. At each refreshment point, two 250 cc bottles were given to each participant.

2.3. Anthropometric Measurements

The participants' morphological characteristics were evaluated in the morning and always under the same conditions. Body height was measured to the nearest 0.1 cm using a wall-mounted stadiometer (Seca 220, Seca, Hamburg, Germany). Body weight was measured to the nearest 0.01 kg on calibrated electronic digital scales (Seca 769, Seca, Hamburg, Germany), barefooted. A Holtain© 610ND (Holtain, Crymych, Wales, UK) skin fold compass, accurate to ±0.2 mm and a tape (Seca 212, Seca, Hamburg, Germany) with an accuracy of ±1 mm were employed to take anthropometric assessments. The obtained anthropometric measurements were height, weight, six skin folds (abdominal, suprailiac, subscapular, tricipital, thigh and leg) and perimeters (arm and leg in a relaxed 90° position). The equations of Yushaz were used to calculate the percentage of fat [35] and the equation according to Lee to determine the percentage of muscle [36]. All the measurements were taken by the same operator, who was skilled in kinanthropometric techniques, and in accordance with the International Society for the Advancement of Kinanthropometry recommendations [37]. Body weight was recorded 2 h before and immediately after the race finished.

2.4. Physical Performance Evaluation

In order to determine the corresponding physical performance values, a progressive and maximum laboratory test was done on a treadmill (Pulsar, h/p/cosmos®, Nussdorf, Germany). The test was run on a 1% slope and began at a speed of 8 km/h, which increased 1 km/h every minute. Before the test began, the participants warmed up for 5 min on the treadmill operating at a speed of 6 $km.h^{-1}$. Respired gases were collected with an Oxycon Pro analyzer (Erich Jaeger GmbH, Hoechberg, Germany). A pulsometer (Vantage M, Polar, Finland) was used to evaluate the maximal heart rate.

2.5. Neuromuscular Function

Neuromuscular function was evaluated by different jumping tests: squat jump (SJ), countermovement jump (CMJ) and Abalakov jump (ABK) [38,39]. The former tests were chosen to measure the neuromuscular function of leg extensor muscles, because they can perform jumps with a high degree of reliability [40,41]. A jump mat system (Chronojump Boscosystems, Barcelona, Spain) was employed to measure the height and time during jumps. Three attempts were made for all jump types; there was a 30-s rest between jumps. The best jump was selected to be later analyzed. Evaluations were done 2 h before the race began and then immediately after the race finished (approximately 1 to 5 min after the race). The protocols of each jump test were applied by following the original protocol proposed by Bosco et al. [39].

In order to perform SJ, the participants started in a squatting position with knees bent at 90° and arms on hips to avoid influencing the jump. A goniometer was used to verify the knee angle. The participants had to remain in this squatting position for 3 s before performing SJ. For CMJ, the subjects started from an upright standing position with hands on hips to avoid any arm movement. Then as a single sequence, they made a swift downward movement, followed immediately by a rapid vertical movement to jump as high as possible. Finally, during the ABK test, the participants had to begin by squatting and flexing their knees 90°, followed by swinging their arms to help them to jump as high as possible.

2.6. Blood Samples

Twenty milliliters of venous blood (antecubital vein) was withdrawn from each participant in both the pre- and post-race evaluations (90 min before and 10 min after finishing the race). Blood samples were collected in two 5-mL Vacutainer tubes (Vacutainer, beliver industrial state, plymouth PL6 7BP, United Kingdom) without anticoagulant for serum isolation and in two 5-mL tubes containing ethylenediaminetetraacetic acid (EDTA) as an anticoagulant. Once collected, blood samples were coagulated for 25–30 min at room temperature and then centrifuged at 2500 rpm for 10 min to remove the clots. Serum samples were aliquoted into Eppendorf tubes (Eppendorf AG, Hamburg, Germany), previously washed with diluted nitric acid, and conserved at −80 °C until the biochemical analysis.

2.7. Determining Muscle Damage Markers and Hydration Status

A 2-mL blood sample was used to determine leukocytes (leu) with an analyzer model Coulter model AcT diff. The rest, a 3-mL blood sample, was employed to determine creatinine (Cr), alanine aminotransferase (ALT), creatine kinase (CK), sodium (Na) and bilirubin (BIL) by spectrophotometric techniques. Complete biochemistry was processed in the laboratory of the San Jorge University Hospital by a Chemistry Analyzer model Advia 1650 (Bayer, Germany).

2.8. Statistical Analysis

Data were processed with IBM SPSS 25.0 Statistics for Macintosh (IBM Corp., Armonk, NY, USA). A descriptive analysis was performed to show the means and standard deviations. The variables' normality distribution was analyzed by the Shapiro–Wilk test and the homogeneity of variances by the Levene test. The Student's t-test was applied to determine differences in the participants' characteristics and the percentages of change (pre-race vs. post-race). A two-way ANOVA (group effect + race effect) was used to show differences between the studied variables. Effect size was calculated for the two-way ANOVA using partial eta-squared (η^2) as a low effect (0.01–0.06), moderate effect (0.06–0.14) and high effect (>0.14) [42]. The $p < 0.05$ differences were considered statistically significant.

3. Results

Table 2 shows the characteristics of the participants in both groups. Significant differences existed in weekly training hours, annual slope achieved while training, times recorded during the GSUR test, maximum speed and percentage of fat ($p < 0.05$).

Table 2. Body composition, physical tests and result during GSUR.

Parameters	Amateur Level (n = 10)	High Level (n = 10)	p
Time during the race (h)	19.87 ± 1.84	15.31 ± 0.81	<0.001
VO$_{2max}$ (L/min)	4.11 ± 0.37	4.46 ± 0.45	0.079
HR$_{max}$ (bpm)	179.50 ± 7.20	177.29 ± 6.76	0.605
Maximum speed (km/h)	15.00 ± 0.81	16.40 ± 0.96	0.003
Fat mass (%)	10.72 ± 2.28	8.83 ± 1.45	0.040
Muscle mass (%)	43.40 ± 3.65	45.07 ± 2.93	0.276
Water intake (L)	9.64 ± 3.08	11.17 ± 3.79	0.337

VO$_{2max}$: maximal oxygen consumption; HR$_{max}$: maximum heart rate.

Tables 3 and 4 indicate the changes in neuromuscular function, muscle damage and dehydration before and after the race, as well as intergroup differences. For these differences, we observed significant differences for ALT and bilirubin ($p < 0.05$). For the effect that racing had, we found significant differences in SJ, CMJ, ABK, CK, ALT, BIL, leu and Cr ($p < 0.001$). Finally, we observed significant differences in bilirubin when the group x race interaction was analyzed ($p < 0.05$).

Table 3. Neuromuscular function before and after the race according to training level.

Parameters	Time	Amateur Level (n = 10)	High Level (n = 10)	Group Effect	η^2	Race Effect	η^2	Group x Race	η^2
SJ (cm)	Pre	25.50 ± 4.38	27.12 ± 5.29	0.102	0.072	<0.001	0.470	0.597	0.008
	Post	16.74 ± 3.91	19.87 ± 4.31						
CMJ (cm)	Pre	29.86 ± 5.08	31.14 ± 6.33	0.182	0.049	<0.001	0.430	0.554	0.010
	Post	20.11 ± 5.01	23.39 ± 4.64						
ABK (cm)	Pre	34.08 ± 6.44	36.66 ± 8.93	0.189	0.047	<0.001	0.360	0.922	0.000
	Post	24.52 ± 4.88	27.51 ± 5.25						
SJ (W)	Pre	810.80 ± 78.87	821.20 ± 91.68	0.638	0.006	<0.001	0.327	0.906	0.000
	Post	684.80 ± 71.57	702.20 ± 120.62						
CMJ (W)	Pre	876.90 ± 84.09	866.00 ± 107.53	0.659	0.005	<0.001	0.290	0.420	0.018
	Post	740.10 ± 71.11	777.20 ± 103.15						
ABK (W)	Pre	935.30 ± 79.98	950.20 ± 106.14	0.663	0.005	<0.001	0.333	0.949	0.000
	Post	811.80 ± 95.25	822.90 ± 90.97						

CMJ: countermovement jump; SJ: squat jump; ABK: Abalakov jump; η^2: eta-squared.

Table 4. Weight, muscle harm parameters and hydration status before and after the race according to training level.

Parameters	Time	Amateur Level (n = 10)	High Level (n = 10)	Group Effect	η^2	Race Effect	η^2	Group x Race	η^2
Weight (kg)	Pre	76.01 ± 10.84	75.23 ± 6.87	0.640	0.006	0.474	0.014	0.846	0.001
	Post	74.52 ± 10.21	73.58 ± 8.56						
CK (U/L)	Pre	164.30 ± 69.39	193.60 ± 42.11	0.074	0.086	<0.001	0.817	0.091	0.077
	Post	3251.60 ± 1011.89	4261.50 ± 1469.60						
ALT (U/L)	Pre	18.60 ± 2.50	23.50 ± 3.92	0.017	0.147	<0.001	0.537	0.904	0.000
	Post	31.70 ± 9.67	37.10 ± 7.46						
BIL (mg/dL)	Pre	0.597 ± 0.148	0.600 ± 0.156	0.028	0.128	<0.001	0.698	0.024	0.133
	Post	1.219 ± 0.205	0.967 ± 0.169						
Leu ($\times 10^3/\mu L$)	Pre	5.93 ± 1.00	5.99 ± 0.93	0.589	0.008	<0.001	0.843	0.650	0.006
	Post	15.04 ± 2.29	15.72 ± 3.35						
Cr (mg/dL)	Pre	0.900 ± 0.137	0.855 ± 0.101	0.380	0.021	<0.001	0.634	0.081	0.082
	Post	1.202 ± 0.239	1.335 ± 0.107						
Na (mmol/L)	Pre	140.10 ± 2.33	140.70 ± 1.76	0.194	0.046	0.432	0.017	0.599	0.008
	Post	140.30 ± 2.11	141.70 ± 3.12						

CK: creatinine kinase; ALT: alanine aminotransferase; BIL: bilirubin; Leu: leukocytes; Cr: creatinine; Na: sodium; η^2: eta-squared.

Figures 2 and 3 depict the percentages of change (pre vs. post) of the previously studied parameters. Figure 2 illustrates the significant differences in the height of both SJ and CMJ, and loss in the high-level group was lower ($p < 0.05$). Figure 3 shows differences in creatinine ($p < 0.05$), for which a more marked increase was observed in the high-level group.

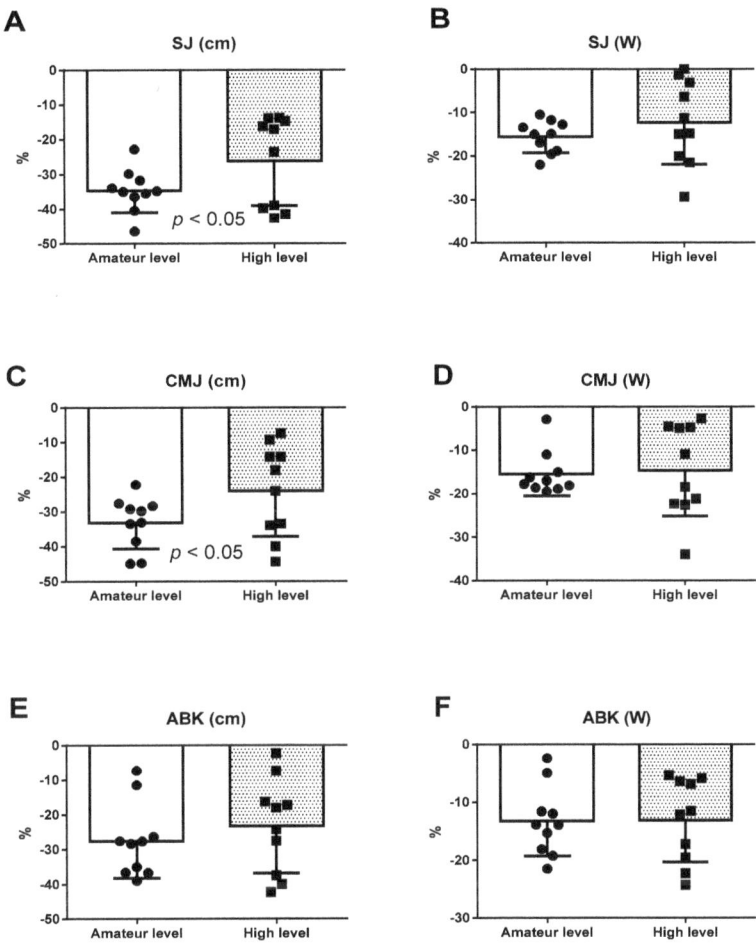

Figure 2. (**A**) Percentage of change in height for SJ; (**B**) percentage of change in power for SJ; (**C**) percentage of change in height for CMJ; (**D**) percentage of change in power for CMJ; (**E**) percentage of change in height for ABK; (**F**) percentage of change in power for ABK; black circle: values of amateur levels participants; black square: values of high levels participants; SJ: squat jump; CMJ: countermovement jump; SJ: squat jump; ABK: Abalakov jump.

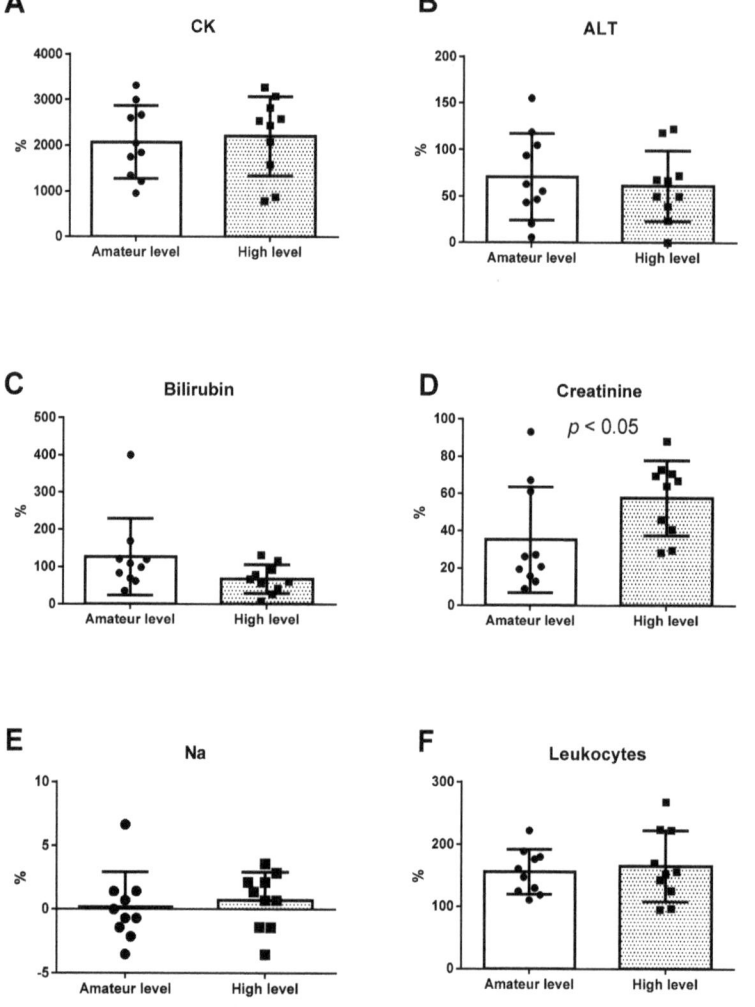

Figure 3. (**A**) Percentage of change in CK; (**B**) percentage of change in ALT; (**C**) percentage of change in bilirubin; (**D**) percentage of change in creatinine; (**E**) percentage of change in Na; (**F**) percentage of change in leukocytes; black circle: values of amateur levels participants; black square: values of high levels participants; CK: creatinine kinase; ALT: alanine aminotransferase; Na: sodium.

4. Discussion

The present study's objectives were to: (a) evaluate the acute responses of running an ultratrail race in terms of neuromuscular function, muscle damage and hydration status; (b) analyze if responses could differ according to training level. The GSUR reduced the power and height of the SJ, CMJ and ABK jumps for all the participants. The muscle damage and dehydration markers increased in both groups. However, the percentages of loss in the SJ and CMJ heights were lower in the high-level group than in the amateur-level group ($p < 0.05$). The percentage of increase in creatinine levels was higher in the high-level group ($p < 0.05$). Research concerning the study of trail running has increased in recent years [43–46]

In general, the responses observed during the GSUR were similar to those reported in other races [12,13,47,48]. Likewise, the study participants presented similar characteristic to runners, as reported by former studies [22,49]. According to similar studies, ultratrail racing could have a distinct impact, particularly for neuromuscular and creatinine parameters, depending on training level [31,32].

For the neuromuscular function parameters, significant reductions in the height and power of all jumps were noted after the race (Table 3). These results fall in line with those previously reported by other authors. For instance, Martínez-Navarro et al. [50] observed lower SJ heights after races covering 65 km and 107 km. Balducci et al. [51] reported a 20% loss in CMJ after a 75 km race, as Gatterer et al. did [52]. However, Rousanoglou et al. [53] observed no significant differences in CMJ height after a mountain marathon race until 5 after min after finishing the race. Apart from ultratrail races being long-distance runs, they involve marked slopes, which implies engaging a high eccentric force component [47] that can cause high levels of muscle damage and fatigue which, in turn, have been associated with excitation–relaxation coupling failure [54,55]. Excitation–contraction coupling failure results in a lower free calcium level in the cytosol, and thus, in less muscle power [55,56]. Hence, ultratrail endurance mountain racing events strongly impact peripheral fatigue by diminishing muscle function and performance [22,56]. The lower jump heights after racing were expected due to functional alterations and the reduced capacity to produce maximum power induced by racing characteristics [13,53]. On this matter, Millet et al. [22], Giandolini et al. [54] and Saugy et al. [21] respectively observed how voluntary maximum knee extensor contraction diminished (35%, 35% and 13%), as did foot flexor contraction (39%, 28% and 10%), after mountain races. In these circumstances, it is not surprising that jump tests are often employed to evaluate neuromuscular fatigue in muscle groups [57–59], especially fatigue induced by ultradistance tests. In fact, after repeatedly applying jump tests after a 90-kilometer race, Chambers et al. [60] reported significant drops in SJ and CMJ heights, which remained for 18 consecutive days after the competition.

Our study also observed how fatigue affected the amateur-level group runners to a greater extent because the reductions in the SJ (Figure 2A) and CMJ (Figure 2C) heights were significantly more marked in this group. These results fall in line with what El-Ashker et al. indicated [61], who found that the subjects with a higher level of training presented better neuromuscular function with fatigue. Nonetheless, these intergroup differences were not noted for either the ABK jump (Figure 2E) or developed power (W) in all jumps (Figure 2B,D,F). These results coincide partly with those from the meta-analysis carried out by Claudino et al. [62] because the achieved CMJ height seemed to better define the degree of the neuromuscular fatigue of knee extensors than other jumps and kinetic parameters, which showed a higher coefficient of variation, such as developed power.

For muscle and liver damage and inflammation, the present study observed higher CK, ALT and bilirubin concentrations after racing. The obtained results fall in line with those reported for mountain races covering different distances: 43 km [63], 54 km [13], 217 km [48], 280 km [64] and 330 km [65]. The CK and liver enzyme levels, among others, were the most widespread markers to indicate skeletal muscle damage [66]. According to data on jump tests, lower jump heights could be related to high CK and ALT levels in blood [67]. This relation suggests that continuous eccentric actions performed on negative slopes might damage muscle fibers, which leads to the release of muscle proteins in the bloodstream, such as CK [13,68]. The fact that ALT rose could be related to both muscle damage caused by eccentric contractions and liver cell lesions [69]. However, it is known that ALT concentrations are higher in the liver and kidneys, and lower in skeletal muscle [70]. It is also known that the degree of liver lesion is proportional to workload [71]. Likewise, a rise in bilirubin levels after a race has been found by others studies [72–74]. Increased bilirubin can be caused by hemolysis produced mainly by mechanical factors and the effect of free radicals [75]. The percentage increase in bilirubin in the amateur level group could have been due to the lower amount of antioxidants in this group compared to the high-level group [75]. As an adaptation, regular physical training increases the levels of antioxidants in the body, increasing the efficiency of the antioxidant system [76,77]. The radicals produced during exercise could increase hemolysis and bilirubin levels.

The rising levels of leukocytes observed in the present study fall in line with previous studies [64,78,79]. Leukocytosis caused by running could be due to increased inflammation caused by muscle damage [80,81]. Acute physical exercise can lead to more cardiac output, vascular vasodilatation and blood flow, which exert stronger mechanical forces on the endothelium which, in turn, leads to leukocytes separating from the endothelium and entering circulation [82]. Moreover, catecholamines and cortisol are secreted during exercise, which could also contribute to increase leukocytes [81,83].

No differences were observed in the plasma Na concentration for hydration status. Creatinine levels rose after racing ($p < 0.001$) and the percentage of change was higher for the high-level group ($p < 0.05$). These differences are probably related to strong kidney and muscle impacts. After ultratrail races, runners generally suffer dehydration and body weight loss [1,84]. Drinking plenty of liquids during races is recommended to avoid dehydration [1]. Different hydration strategies are used during ultratrail races to avoid dehydration [85]. The problems of dehydration regarding metabolic and neuromuscular performance were previously outlined [25,28]. Acute kidney lesions are often reported after endurance races, with a prevalence of up to 80% during ultratrail running, but most do not pose serious health problems, and kidney function normally recovers completely after a few days [86,87]. The present study found no significant differences between drinking liquids while racing, unlike some other studies [88]. This could be related to no differences being found in Na concentrations. Plasma Na concentration is the most frequently used parameter to evaluate dehydration status [89]. Former studies reported increased Na after trail races [90,91]. The fact that our study found high creatinine concentrations in runners coincides with previous studies [87,92]. These changes would probably have a multifactorial basis, to which both dehydration and a lower exercise-related glomerular filtration rate would contribute [93]. The fact that serum creatinine concentration positively correlates with lean muscle mass and varies with training type has been demonstrated [88,94].

The study has its limitations: (a) its sample size was small; (b) food intake while racing was not controlled, which could have affected the muscle and neuromuscular damage markers, as other studies have reported [56,95]; (c) only the male gender was studied; (d) it did not evaluate the same markers while the race was underway or in post-race hours to evaluate evolution. As each ultratrail race is unique, these results cannot be completely extrapolated to other races.

5. Conclusions

Ultratrail racing lowers neuromuscular function and increases muscle damage/inflammation. High-level runners suffer less neuromuscular fatigue than amateur-level runners. However, the creatinine levels in the high-level group increased more in metabolic terms.

It is worth knowing the impacts of trail racing in order to schedule and adapt training sessions according to race demands. According to the obtained results, training programs and racing strategies must include muscle damage prevention to reduce ultratrail runners muscle fatigue.

Author Contributions: Conceptualization, F.P., L.C. and C.C.; methodology, F.P.; C.C. and D.F. formal analysis, V.T.-R. and C.P.-L.; writing—original draft preparation, F.P., V.T.-R. and L.C.; writing—review and editing, D.F., C.P.-L. and C.C. All authors have read and agreed to the published version of the manuscript.

Funding: The present research was funded by a research grant from the Instituto de Estudios Altoaragoneses of the Diputación Provincial de Huesca (Spain) and with public funds from the Dirección General de Investigación e Innovación del Gobierno de Aragón to the ENFYRED research group.

Institutional Review Board Statement: The study was conducted according to the guidelines of the Declaration of Helsinki, and approved by the Ethics Committee of the Department of Health and Consumption of the Government of Aragon (protocol code 16/2017; date: 29/09/2017).

Informed Consent Statement: Informed consent was obtained from all subjects involved in the study.

Data Availability Statement: Information about the UTGS race is available at http://utgs.es/ (accessed on 11 May 2021).

Acknowledgments: We thank all the runners who participated in this research work and the Centro de Medicina del Deporte del Gobierno de Aragón for its invaluable help and collaboration.

Conflicts of Interest: The authors declare no conflict of interest.

References

1. Knechtle, B.; Nikolaidis, P.T. Physiology and Pathophysiology in Ultra-Marathon Running. *Front. Physiol.* **2018**, *9*, 634. [CrossRef] [PubMed]
2. Garbisu-Hualde, A.; Santos-Concejero, J. What are the Limiting Factors During an Ultra-Marathon? A Systematic Review of the Scientific Literature. *J. Hum. Kinet.* **2020**, *72*, 129–139. [CrossRef]
3. Millet, G.P.; Millet, G.Y. Ultramarathon is an outstanding model for the study of adaptive responses to extreme load and stress. *BMC Med.* **2012**, *10*, 77. [CrossRef]
4. Rochat, N.; Gesbert, V.; Seifert, L.; Hauw, D. Enacting Phenomenological Gestalts in Ultra-Trail Running: An Inductive Analysis of Trail Runners' Courses of Experience. *Front. Psychol.* **2018**, *9*, 2038. [CrossRef] [PubMed]
5. Vernillo, G.; Savoldelli, A.; Zignoli, A.; Trabucchi, P.; Pellegrini, B.; Millet, G.P.; Schena, F. Influence of the world's most challenging mountain ultra-marathon on energy cost and running mechanics. *Graefe's Arch. Clin. Exp. Ophthalmol.* **2014**, *114*, 929–939. [CrossRef] [PubMed]
6. Hoffman, M.D.; Ong, J.C.; Wang, G. Historical Analysis of Participation in 161 km Ultramarathons in North America. *Int. J. Hist. Sport* **2010**, *27*, 1877–1891. [CrossRef]
7. Perić, M.; Slavić, N. Event sport tourism business models: The case of trail running. *Sport Bus. Manag. Int. J.* **2019**, *9*, 164–184. [CrossRef]
8. Peter, L.; Rust, C.; Knechtle, B.; Rosemann, T.; Lepers, R. Sex differences in 24 hour ultra-marathon performance—A retrospective data analysis from 1977 to 2012. *Clinics* **2014**, *69*, 38–46. [CrossRef]
9. Urbaneja, J.S.; Torbidoni, E.I.F. El Trail running in Spain. Origin, evolution and current situation. *Retos Nuevas Tend. Educ. Física Deport. Recreación* **2018**, *33*, 123–128.
10. Scheer, V. Participation Trends of Ultra Endurance Events. *Sports Med. Arthrosc. Rev.* **2019**, *27*, 3–7. [CrossRef]
11. Fornasiero, A.; Savoldelli, A.; Fruet, D.; Boccia, G.; Pellegrini, B.; Schena, F. Physiological intensity profile, exercise load and performance predictors of a 65 km mountain ultra-marathon. *J. Sports Sci.* **2017**, *36*, 1287–1295. [CrossRef]
12. Clemente-Suárez, V.J. Psychophysiological response and energy balance during a 14 h ultraendurance mountain running event. *Appl. Physiol. Nutr. Metab.* **2015**, *40*, 269–273. [CrossRef]
13. Ramos-Campo, D.J.; Ávila-Gandía, V.; Alacid, F.; Soto-Méndez, F.; Alcaraz, P.E.; López-Román, F.J.; Rubio-Arias, J. Ángel Muscle damage, physiological changes, and energy balance in ultra-endurance mountain-event athletes. *Appl. Physiol. Nutr. Metab.* **2016**, *41*, 872–878. [CrossRef]
14. Linderman, J.K.; Laubach, L.L. Energy balance during 24 hours of treadmill running. *J. Exerc. Physiol. Online* **2004**, *7*, 37–44.
15. Clemente, V.J. Modificaciones de parámetros bioquímicos después de una maratón de montaña. *Eur. J. Hum. Mov.* **2011**, *27*, 75–83.
16. Jeukendrup, A.E.; Moseley, L.; Mainwaring, G.I.; Samuels, S.; Perry, S.; Mann, C.H. Exogenous carbohydrate oxidation during ultraendurance exercise. *J. Appl. Physiol.* **2006**, *100*, 1134–1141. [CrossRef]
17. Townshend, A.D.; Worringham, C.J.; Stewart, I.B. Spontaneous Pacing during Overground Hill Running. *Med. Sci. Sports Exerc.* **2010**, *42*, 160–169. [CrossRef] [PubMed]
18. Born, D.-P.; Stöggl, T.; Swarén, M.; Björklund, G. Near-Infrared Spectroscopy: More Accurate Than Heart Rate for Monitoring Intensity in Running in Hilly Terrain. *Int. J. Sports Physiol. Perform.* **2017**, *12*, 440–447. [CrossRef] [PubMed]
19. Rojas-Valverde, D.; Sánchez-Ureña, B.; Pino-Ortega, J.; Gómez-Carmona, C.; Gutiérrez-Vargas, R.; Timón, R.; Olcina, G. External Workload Indicators of Muscle and Kidney Mechanical Injury in Endurance Trail Running. *Int. J. Environ. Res. Public Health* **2019**, *16*, 3909. [CrossRef]
20. Carmona, G.; Roca, E.; Guerrero, M.; Cussó, R.; Irurtia, A.; Nescolarde, L.; Brotons, D.; Bedini, J.L.; Cadefau, J.A. Sarcomere Disruptions of Slow Fiber Resulting From Mountain Ultramarathon. *Int. J. Sports Physiol. Perform.* **2015**, *10*, 1041–1047. [CrossRef] [PubMed]
21. Saugy, J.; Place, N.; Millet, G.Y.; Degache, F.; Schena, F.; Millet, G.P. Alterations of Neuromuscular Function after the World's Most Challenging Mountain Ultra-Marathon. *PLoS ONE* **2013**, *8*, e65596. [CrossRef] [PubMed]
22. Millet, G.Y.; Tomazin, K.; Verges, S.; Vincent, C.; Bonnefoy, R.; Boisson, R.-C.; Gergelé, L.; Féasson, L.; Martin, V. Neuromuscular Consequences of an Extreme Mountain Ultra-Marathon. *PLoS ONE* **2011**, *6*, e17059. [CrossRef]

23. Judelson, D.A.; Maresh, C.M.; Farrell, M.J.; Yamamoto, L.M.; Armstrong, L.E.; Kraemer, W.J.; Volek, J.S.; Spiering, B.A.; Casa, D.J.; Anderson, J.M. Effect of Hydration State on Strength, Power, and Resistance Exercise Performance. *Med. Sci. Sports Exerc.* **2007** *39*, 1817–1824. [CrossRef] [PubMed]
24. Murray, B. Hydration and Physical Performance. *J. Am. Coll. Nutr.* **2007**, *26*, 542S–548S. [CrossRef]
25. Campa, F.; Piras, A.; Raffi, M.; Trofè, A.; Perazzolo, M.; Mascherini, G.; Toselli, S. The Effects of Dehydration on Metabolic and Neuromuscular Functionality during Cycling. *Int. J. Environ. Res. Public Health* **2020**, *17*, 1161. [CrossRef]
26. Castro Sepúlveda, M.; Cerda Kohler, H.; Pérez Luco, C.; Monsalves, M.; Andrade, D.C.; Hermann, Z.F.; Báez San Martín, E.; Ramírez Campillo, R. Hydration status after exercise affect resting metabolic rate and heart rate variability. *Nutr. Hosp.* **2014**, *17*, 1273–1277.
27. Barley, O.R.; Chapman, D.W.; Blazevich, A.J.; Abbiss, C.R. Acute Dehydration Impairs Endurance Without Modulating Neuromuscular Function. *Front. Physiol.* **2018**, *9*, 1562. [CrossRef] [PubMed]
28. Casa, D.J.; Stearns, R.L.; Lopez, R.M.; Ganio, M.S.; McDermott, B.P.; Yeargin, S.W.; Yamamoto, L.M.; Mazerolle, S.M.; Roti, M.W.; Armstrong, L.E.; et al. Influence of Hydration on Physiological Function and Performance During Trail Running in the Heat. *J. Athl. Train.* **2010**, *45*, 147–156. [CrossRef] [PubMed]
29. Judelson, D.A.; Maresh, C.M.; Anderson, J.M.; Armstrong, L.E.; Casa, D.J.; Kraemer, W.J.; Volek, J.S. Hydration and Muscular Performance. *Sports Med.* **2007**, *37*, 907–921. [CrossRef] [PubMed]
30. Rojas-Valverde, D.; Sánchez-Ureña, B.; Crowe, J.; Timón, R.; Olcina, G.J. Exertional rhabdomyolysis and acute kidney injury in endurance sports: A systematic review. *Eur. J. Sport Sci.* **2021**, *21*, 261–274. [CrossRef] [PubMed]
31. Collado Andrés, C.; Hernando, B.; Hernando, C.; Martínez-Cadenas, C. ¿ Qué repercusión a nivel fisiológico puede tener realizar una carrera de ultratrail? *Ágora Salut.* **2020**, *7*, 57–66. [CrossRef]
32. Khodaee, M.; Spittler, J.; VanBaak, K.; Changstrom, B.; Hill, J. Effects of Running an Ultramarathon on Cardiac, Hematologic, and Metabolic Biomarkers. *Int. J. Sports Med.* **2015**, *36*, 867–871. [CrossRef] [PubMed]
33. Oliveira-Rosado, J.; Duarte, J.P.; Sousa-E-Silva, P.; Costa, D.C.; Martinho, D.V.; Sarmento, H.; Valente-Dos-Santos, J.; Rama, L.M.; Tavares, Ó.M.; Conde, J.; et al. Physiological profile of adult male long-distance trail runners: Variations according to competitive level (national or regional). *Einstein (São Paulo)* **2020**, *18*, eAO5256. [CrossRef] [PubMed]
34. Hohl, R.; de Rezende, F.N.; Millet, G.Y.; da Mota, G.R.; Marocolo, M. Blood cardiac biomarkers responses are associated with 24 h ultramarathon performance. *Heliyon* **2019**, *5*, e01913. [CrossRef] [PubMed]
35. Porta, J.; Galiano, D.; Tejedo, A.; González, J.M. Valoración de la composición corporal. Utopías y realidades. In *Manual de Cineantropometría*; Esparza Ros, F., Ed.; Ágora para la Educación Física y el Deporte: Madrid, Spain, 1993; pp. 113–170.
36. Lee, R.C.; Wang, Z.; Heo, M.; Ross, R.; Janssen, I.; Heymsfield, S.B. Total-body skeletal muscle mass: Development and cross-validation of anthropometric prediction models. *Am. J. Clin. Nutr.* **2000**, *72*, 796–803. [CrossRef] [PubMed]
37. Stewart, A.; Marfell-Jones, M. *International Society for Advancement of Kinanthropometry International Standards for Anthropometric Assessment*; International Society for the Advancement of Kinanthropometry: Lower Hutt, New Zealand, 2011; ISBN 0620362073 9780620362078.
38. Komi, P.V.; Bosco, C. Utilization of stored elastic energy in leg extensor muscles by men and women. *Med. Sci. Sports* **1978**, *10*, 261–265. [PubMed]
39. Bosco, C.; Luhtanen, P.; Komi, P.V. A simple method for measurement of mechanical power in jumping. *Eur. J. Appl. Physiol. Occup. Physiol.* **1983**, *50*, 273–282. [CrossRef] [PubMed]
40. Rodríguez-Rosell, D.; Mora-Custodio, R.; Franco-Márquez, F.; Yáñez-García, J.M.; González-Badillo, J.J. Traditional vs. Sport Specific Vertical Jump Tests: Reliability, Validity, and Relationship With the Legs Strength and Sprint Performance in Adult and Teen Soccer and Basketball Players. *J. Strength Cond. Res.* **2017**, *31*, 196–206. [CrossRef] [PubMed]
41. Bosco, C.; Ito, A.; Komi, P.V.; Luhtanen, P.; Rahkila, P.; Rusko, H.; Viitasalo, J.T. Neuromuscular function and mechanical efficiency of human leg extensor muscles during jumping exercises. *Acta Physiol. Scand.* **1982**, *114*, 543–550. [CrossRef] [PubMed]
42. Hopkins, W.G.; Marshall, S.W.; Batterham, A.M.; Hanin, J. Progressive Statistics for Studies in Sports Medicine and Exercise Science. *Med. Sci. Sports Exerc.* **2009**, *41*, 3–12. [CrossRef]
43. Méndez-Alonso, D.; Prieto-Saborit, J.; Bahamonde, J.; Jiménez-Arberás, E. Influence of Psychological Factors on the Success of the Ultra-Trail Runner. *Int. J. Environ. Res. Public Health* **2021**, *18*, 2704. [CrossRef]
44. Suter, D.; Sousa, C.V.; Hill, L.; Scheer, V.; Nikolaidis, P.T.; Knechtle, B. Even Pacing Is Associated with Faster Finishing Times in Ultramarathon Distance Trail Running—The "Ultra-Trail du Mont Blanc" 2008–2019. *Int. J. Environ. Res. Public Health* **2020**, *17*, 7074. [CrossRef] [PubMed]
45. Robert, M.; Stauffer, E.; Nader, E.; Skinner, S.; Boisson, C.; Cibiel, A.; Feasson, L.; Renoux, C.; Robach, P.; Joly, P.; et al. Impact of Trail Running Races on Blood Viscosity and Its Determinants: Effects of Distance. *Int. J. Mol. Sci.* **2020**, *21*, 8531. [CrossRef] [PubMed]
46. Matos, S.; Clemente, F.M.; Silva, R.; Pereira, J.; Carral, J.M.C. Performance and Training Load Profiles in Recreational Male Trail Runners: Analyzing Their Interactions during Competitions. *Int. J. Environ. Res. Public Health* **2020**, *17*, 8902. [CrossRef]
47. Abos, A.; Gonzalez, L.G.; Solana, A.A.; Serrano, J.S.; Sanz, M. RICYDE. Revista internacional de ciencias del deporte. *RICYDE Rev. Int. Cienc. Deport.* **2016**, *10*, 43–56. [CrossRef]

8. Belli, T.; Macedo, D.V.; De Araújo, G.G.; Dos Reis, I.G.M.; Scariot, P.P.M.; Lazarim, F.L.; Nunes, L.A.S.; Brenzikofer, R.; Gobatto, C.A. Mountain Ultramarathon Induces Early Increases of Muscle Damage, Inflammation, and Risk for Acute Renal Injury. *Front. Physiol.* **2018**, *9*, 1368. [CrossRef] [PubMed]
9. Zanchi, D.; Viallon, M.; Le Goff, C.; Millet, G.P.; Giardini, G.; Croisille, P.; Haller, S. Extreme Mountain Ultra-Marathon Leads to Acute but Transient Increase in Cerebral Water Diffusivity and Plasma Biomarkers Levels Changes. *Front. Physiol.* **2017**, *7*, 664. [CrossRef]
10. Martínez-Navarro, I.; Sanchez-Gómez, J.M.; Aparicio, I.; Priego-Quesada, J.I.; Pérez-Soriano, P.; Collado, E.; Hernando, B.; Hernando, C. Effect of mountain ultramarathon distance competition on biochemical variables, respiratory and lower-limb fatigue. *PLoS ONE* **2020**, *15*, e0238846. [CrossRef] [PubMed]
11. Balducci, P.; Clémençon, M.; Trama, R.; Blache, Y.; Hautier, C. Performance factors in a mountain ultramarathon. *Int. J. Sports Med.* **2017**, *38*, 819–826. [CrossRef]
12. Gatterer, H.; Schenk, K.; Wille, M.; Raschner, C.; Faulhaber, M.; Ferrari, M.; Burtscher, M. Race Performance and Exercise Intensity of Male Amateur Mountain Runners During a Multistage Mountain Marathon Competition Are Not Dependent on Muscle Strength Loss or Cardiorespiratory Fitness. *J. Strength Cond. Res.* **2013**, *27*, 2149–2156. [CrossRef] [PubMed]
13. Rousanoglou, E.N.; Noutsos, K.; Pappas, A.; Bogdanis, G.; Vagenas, G.; Bayios, I.A.; Boudolos, K.D. Alterations of Vertical Jump Mechanics after a Half-Marathon Mountain Running Race. *J. Sports Sci. Med.* **2016**, *15*, 277–286. [PubMed]
14. Giandolini, M.; Gimenez, P.; Temesi, J.; Arnal, P.J.; Martin, V.; Rupp, T.; Morin, J.-B.; Samozino, P.; Millet, G.Y. Effect of the Fatigue Induced by a 110-km Ultramarathon on Tibial Impact Acceleration and Lower Leg Kinematics. *PLoS ONE* **2016**, *11*, e0151687. [CrossRef]
15. Fitts, R.H. Cellular mechanisms of muscle fatigue. *Physiol. Rev.* **1994**, *74*, 49–94. [CrossRef] [PubMed]
16. Urdampilleta, A.; Arribalzaga, S.; Viribay, A.; Castañeda-Babarro, A.; Seco-Calvo, J.; Mielgo-Ayuso, J. Effects of 120 vs. 60 and 90 g/h Carbohydrate Intake during a Trail Marathon on Neuromuscular Function and High Intensity Run Capacity Recovery. *Nutrients* **2020**, *12*, 2094. [CrossRef] [PubMed]
17. Wu, P.P.-Y.; Sterkenburg, N.; Everett, K.; Chapman, D.W.; White, N.; Mengersen, K. Predicting fatigue using countermovement jump force-time signatures: PCA can distinguish neuromuscular versus metabolic fatigue. *PLoS ONE* **2019**, *14*, e0219295. [CrossRef] [PubMed]
18. Jiménez-Reyes, P.; Pareja-Blanco, F.; Cuadrado-Peñafiel, V.; Ortega-Becerra, M.; Párraga, J.; González-Badillo, J.J. Jump height loss as an indicator of fatigue during sprint training. *J. Sports Sci.* **2017**, *37*, 1029–1037. [CrossRef] [PubMed]
19. Watkins, C.M.; Barillas, S.R.; Wong, M.A.; Archer, D.C.; Dobbs, I.J.; Lockie, R.G.; Coburn, J.W.; Tran, T.T.; Brown, L.E. Determination of Vertical Jump as a Measure of Neuromuscular Readiness and Fatigue. *J. Strength Cond. Res.* **2017**, *31*, 3305–3310. [CrossRef]
20. Chambers, C.; Noakes, T.D.; Lambert, E.V.; Lambert, M.I. Time course of recovery of vertical jump height and heart rate versus running speed after a 90-km foot race. *J. Sports Sci.* **1998**, *16*, 645–651. [CrossRef]
21. El-Ashker, S.; Chaabene, H.; Prieske, O.; Abdelkafy, A.; Ahmed, M.A.; Muaidi, Q.I.; Granacher, U. Effects of Neuromuscular Fatigue on Eccentric Strength and Electromechanical Delay of the Knee Flexors: The Role of Training Status. *Front. Physiol.* **2019**, *10*, 782. [CrossRef]
22. Claudino, J.G.; Cronin, J.; Mezêncio, B.; McMaster, D.T.; McGuigan, M.; Tricoli, V.; Amadio, A.C.; Serrão, J.C. The countermovement jump to monitor neuromuscular status: A meta-analysis. *J. Sci. Med. Sport* **2017**, *20*, 397–402. [CrossRef]
23. Da Ponte, A.; Giovanelli, N.; Antonutto, G.; Nigris, D.; Curcio, F.; Cortese, P.; Lazzer, S. Changes in cardiac and muscle biomarkers following an uphill-only marathon. *Res. Sports Med.* **2017**, *26*, 100–111. [CrossRef] [PubMed]
24. Kłapcińska, B.; Waśkiewicz, Z.; Chrapusta, S.J.; Sadowska-Krępa, E.; Czuba, M.; Langfort, J. Metabolic responses to a 48-h ultra-marathon run in middle-aged male amateur runners. *Graefe's Arch. Clin. Exp. Ophthalmol.* **2013**, *113*, 2781–2793. [CrossRef] [PubMed]
25. Mrakic-Sposta, S.; Gussoni, M.; Moretti, S.; Pratali, L.; Giardini, G.; Tacchini, P.; Dellanoce, C.; Tonacci, A.; Mastorci, F.; Borghini, A.; et al. Effects of Mountain Ultra-Marathon Running on ROS Production and Oxidative Damage by Micro-Invasive Analytic Techniques. *PLoS ONE* **2015**, *10*, e0141780. [CrossRef] [PubMed]
26. Skenderi, K.P.; Kavouras, S.A.; Anastasiou, C.A.; Yiannakouris, N.; Matalas, A.-L. Exertional Rhabdomyolysis during a 246-km Continuous Running Race. *Med. Sci. Sports Exerc.* **2006**, *38*, 1054–1057. [CrossRef]
27. Del Coso, J.; Salinero, J.J.; Abián-Vicen, J.; González-Millán, C.; Garde, S.; Vega, P.; Pérez-González, B. Influence of body mass loss and myoglobinuria on the development of muscle fatigue after a marathon in a warm environment. *Appl. Physiol. Nutr. Metab.* **2013**, *38*, 286–291. [CrossRef]
28. Friden, J.; Sjöström, M.; Ekblom, B. Myofibrillar damage following intense eccentric exercise in man. *Int. J. Sports Med.* **1983**, *4*, 170–176. [CrossRef]
29. Nagel, D.; Seiler, D.; Franz, H.; Jung, K. Ultra-Long-Distance Running and the Liver*. *Int. J. Sports Med.* **1990**, *11*, 441–445. [CrossRef]
30. Prati, D.; Taioli, E.; Zanella, A.; Della Torre, E.; Butelli, S.; Del Vecchio, E.; Vianello, L.; Zanuso, F.; Mozzi, F.; Milani, S.; et al. Updated Definitions of Healthy Ranges for Serum Alanine Aminotransferase Levels. *Ann. Intern. Med.* **2002**, *137*, 1–10. [CrossRef]
31. Wu, H.-J.; Chen, K.-T.; Shee, B.-W.; Chang, H.-C.; Huang, Y.-J.; Yang, R.-S. Effects of 24 h ultra-marathon on biochemical and hematological parameters. *World J. Gastroenterol.* **2004**, *10*, 2711–2714. [CrossRef]

72. De Paz, J.A.; Villa, J.G.; López, P.; González-Gallego, J. Effects of long-distance running on serum bilirubin. *Med. Sci. Sports Exerc.* **1995**, *27*, 1590–1594. [CrossRef]
73. Shin, K.; Jee, H.; Lee, Y.; Kim, T.K.; Kim, H.S.; Park, Y.; Kim, Y. Effects of an extreme endurance ultra-marathon on musculoskeletal and hematologic functions. *Gazz. Medica Ital. Arch. Sci. Med.* **2014**, *173*, 283–289.
74. Jastrzębski, Z.; Żychowska, M.; Jastrzębska, M.; Prusik, K.; Prusik, K.; Kortas, J.; Ratkowski, W.; Konieczna, A.; Radzimiński, Ł. Changes in blood morphology and chosen biochemical parameters in ultra-marathon runners during a 100-km run in relation to the age and speed of runners. *Int. J. Occup. Med. Environ. Health* **2016**, *29*, 801–814. [CrossRef] [PubMed]
75. Witek, K.; Ścisłowska, J.; Turowski, D.; Lerczak, K.; Lewandowska-Pachecka, S.; Pokrywka, A. Total bilirubin in athletes, determination of reference range. *Biol. Sport* **2017**, *1*, 45–48. [CrossRef]
76. Mena, P.; Maynar, M.; Gutiérrez, J.M.; Maynar, J.; Timon, J.; Campillo, J.E. Erythrocyte Free Radical Scavenger Enzymes in Bicycle Professional Racers. Adaptation to Training. *Int. J. Sports Med.* **1991**, *12*, 563–566. [CrossRef]
77. Powers, S.K.; Deminice, R.; Ozdemir, M.; Yoshihara, T.; Bomkamp, M.P.; Hyatt, H. Exercise-induced oxidative stress: Friend or foe? *J. Sport Health Sci.* **2020**, *9*, 415–425. [CrossRef]
78. Žákovská, A.; Knechtle, B.; Chlíbková, D.; Miličková, M.; Rosemann, T.; Nikolaidis, P.T. The Effect of a 100-km Ultra-Marathon under Freezing Conditions on Selected Immunological and Hematological Parameters. *Front. Physiol.* **2017**, *8*, 638. [CrossRef]
79. Rowlands, D.S.; Pearce, E.; Aboud, A.; Gillen, J.B.; Gibala, M.J.; Donato, S.; Waddington, J.M.; Green, J.G.; Tarnopolsky, M.A. Oxidative stress, inflammation, and muscle soreness in an 894-km relay trail run. *Graefe's Arch. Clin. Exp. Ophthalmol.* **2012**, *112*, 1839–1848. [CrossRef]
80. Wells, C.L.; Stern, J.R.; Hecht, L.H. Hematological changes following a marathon race in male and female runners. *Graefe's Arch. Clin. Exp. Ophthalmol.* **1982**, *48*, 41–49. [CrossRef]
81. Tossige-Gomes, R.; Ottone, V.; Oliveira, P.; Viana, D.; Araújo, T.; Gripp, F.; Rocha-Vieira, E. Leukocytosis, muscle damage and increased lymphocyte proliferative response after an adventure sprint race. *Braz. J. Med. Biol. Res.* **2014**, *47*, 492–498. [CrossRef]
82. Simpson, R.J.; Kunz, H.; Agha, N.; Graff, R. Exercise and the Regulation of Immune Functions. *Prog. Mol. Biol. Transl. Sci.* **2015**, *135*, 355–380. [CrossRef] [PubMed]
83. Foster, N.K.; Martyn, J.B.; Rangno, R.E.; Hogg, J.C.; Pardy, R.L. Leukocytosis of exercise: Role of cardiac output and catecholamines. *J. Appl. Physiol.* **1986**, *61*, 2218–2223. [CrossRef] [PubMed]
84. Newmark, S.R.; Toppo, F.R.; Adams, G. Fluid and electrolyte replacement in the ultramarathon runner. *Am. J. Sports Med.* **1991**, *19*, 389–391. [CrossRef] [PubMed]
85. Bouscaren, N.; Faricier, R.; Millet, G.; Racinais, S. Heat Acclimatization, Cooling Strategies, and Hydration during an Ultra-Trail in Warm and Humid Conditions. *Nutrients* **2021**, *13*, 1085. [CrossRef] [PubMed]
86. Lipman, G.S.; Krabak, B.J.; Waite, B.L.; Logan, S.B.; Menon, A.; Chan, G.K. A Prospective Cohort Study of Acute Kidney Injury in Multi-stage Ultramarathon Runners: The Biochemistry in Endurance Runner Study (BIERS). *Res. Sports Med.* **2014**, *22*, 185–192. [CrossRef] [PubMed]
87. Kao, W.-F.; Hou, S.-K.; Chiu, Y.-H.; Chou, S.-L.; Kuo, F.-C.; Wang, S.-H.; Chen, J.-J. Effects of 100-km Ultramarathon on Acute Kidney Injury. *Clin. J. Sport Med.* **2015**, *25*, 49–54. [CrossRef] [PubMed]
88. Reid, S.A.; King, M.J. Serum Biochemistry and Morbidity Among Runners Presenting for Medical Care After an Australian Mountain Ultramarathon. *Clin. J. Sport Med.* **2007**, *17*, 307–310. [CrossRef] [PubMed]
89. Chlíbková, D.; Rosemann, T.; Posch, L.; Matoušek, R.; Knechtle, B. Pre- and Post-Race Hydration Status in Hyponatremic and Non-Hyponatremic Ultra-Endurance Athletes. *Chin. J. Physiol.* **2016**, *59*, 173–183. [CrossRef]
90. Cejka, C.; Knechtle, B.; Knechtle, P.; Rüst, C.A.; Rosemann, T. An increased fluid intake leads to feet swelling in 100-km ultra-marathoners—An observational field study. *J. Int. Soc. Sports Nutr.* **2012**, *9*, 11. [CrossRef]
91. Burge, J.; Knechtle, B.; Knechtle, P.; Gnädinger, M.; Rüst, C.A.; Rosemann, T. Maintained Serum Sodium in Male Ultra-Marathoners—The Role of Fluid Intake, Vasopressin, and Aldosterone in Fluid and Electrolyte Regulation. *Horm. Metab. Res.* **2012**, *44*, 711. [CrossRef]
92. Hoffman, M.D.; Stuempfle, K.J.; Fogard, K.; Hew-Butler, T.; Winger, J.; Weiss, R.H. Urine dipstick analysis for identification of runners susceptible to acute kidney injury following an ultramarathon. *J. Sports Sci.* **2013**, *31*, 20–31. [CrossRef]
93. Noakes, T.D.; Carter, J.W. Biochemical parameters in athletes before and after having run 160 kilometres. *South. Afr. Med. J.* **1976**, *50*, 1562–1566.
94. Schutte, J.E.; Longhurst, J.C.; Gaffney, F.A.; Bastian, B.C.; Blomqvist, C.G. Total plasma creatinine: An accurate measure of total striated muscle mass. *J. Appl. Physiol.* **1981**, *51*, 762–766. [CrossRef] [PubMed]
95. Viribay, A.; Arribalzaga, S.; Mielgo-Ayuso, J.; Castañeda-Babarro, A.; Seco-Calvo, J.; Urdampilleta, A. Effects of 120 g/h of Carbohydrates Intake during a Mountain Marathon on Exercise-Induced Muscle Damage in Elite Runners. *Nutrients* **2020**, *12*, 1367. [CrossRef] [PubMed]

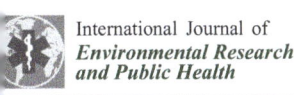

Article

Analysis of Game Performance Indicators during 2015–2019 World Padel Tour Seasons and Their Influence on Match Outcome

Adrián Escudero-Tena [1], Bernardino Javier Sánchez-Alcaraz [2,*], Javier García-Rubio [1] and Sergio J. Ibáñez [1]

1. Training Optimization and Sport Performance Research Group (GOERD), Sport Science Faculty, University of Extremadura, 10005 Caceres, Spain; adescuder@alumnos.unex.es (A.E.-T.); jagaru@unex.es (J.G.-R.); sibanez@unex.es (S.J.I.)
2. Department of Physical Activity and Sport, Faculty of Sport Sciences, University of Murcia, C/ Argentina, s/n, 30700 Murcia, Spain
* Correspondence: bjavier.sanchez@um.es; Tel.: +34-6-2694-3147

Abstract: A better understanding of the demands of in-game competition demands may improve coaching strategies, training designs, and injury prevention programs. However, there is limited information regarding performance analysis in professional padel. This study aimed to analyse performance indicators and their influence on match outcomes regarding sex, tournament round, and set number. The sample contained 1070 sets from 532 matches of the 2016 to 2019 World Padel Tour seasons. Variables including sex, round, game result, stroke effectiveness, and break points were registered through systematic observation. A non-parametric approach was applied to evaluate differences between sex, match outcome, and tournament round. The results showed significant differences between winners and losers regarding sex in break points (male $d = 2.13$, $p = 0.00$; female $d = 2.22$, $p = 0.00$), smash winners (male $d = 0.85$, $p = 0.00$; female $d = 0.69$, $p = 0.00$), groundstroke winners (male $d = 1.01$, $p = 0.00$; female $d = 1.18$, $p = 0.00$), volley winners (male $d = 1.08$, $p = 0.00$; female $d = 0.91$, $p = 0.00$), and errors (male $d = 0.76$, $p = 0.00$; female $d = 0.65$, $p = 0.00$). Furthermore, differences in shot effectiveness between winners and errors increased in the last set of the match and in the last round of the tournament ($p < 0.05$). Therefore, shot effectiveness seems to be a key factor in professional padel that distinguishes between winning and losing players. Such knowledge may have implications in the design of appropriate game strategies and specific training sessions to improve performance and to prevent sport injuries.

Keywords: racket sports; performance analysis; technical indicators; tactical indicators; paddle tennis

Citation: Escudero-Tena, A.; Sánchez-Alcaraz, B.J.; García-Rubio, J.; Ibáñez, S.J. Analysis of Game Performance Indicators during 2015–2019 World Padel Tour Seasons and Their Influence on Match Outcome. *Int. J. Environ. Res. Public Health* **2021**, *18*, 4904. https://doi.org/10.3390/ijerph18094904

Academic Editor: Paul B. Tchounwou

Received: 29 March 2021
Accepted: 29 April 2021
Published: 4 May 2021

Publisher's Note: MDPI stays neutral with regard to jurisdictional claims in published maps and institutional affiliations.

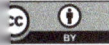

Copyright: © 2021 by the authors. Licensee MDPI, Basel, Switzerland. This article is an open access article distributed under the terms and conditions of the Creative Commons Attribution (CC BY) license (https://creativecommons.org/licenses/by/4.0/).

1. Introduction

Padel is a recent sport [1], which is practised in pairs (two vs. two) on a 20 × 10 m court surrounded by walls or glass and metal fences, which allow the bouncing of the ball, and is scored like tennis [2]. In recent years, there has been an enormous growth in the number of players and courts, as it is now practised in more than 40 countries around the world [3,4]. Furthermore, a professional padel circuit has been developed (World Padel Tour), with tournaments in several countries. Padel practice has significant advantages compared with other racket sports, which renders it a powerful tool for health promotion, namely: high technical skills are not required to start practicing, the long duration of rallies increases player enjoyment, it can be played outdoors, and its equipment is inexpensive [2,5,6]. Because padel is played largely in recreational environments [3], the sport seems to play an important role in promoting physical habits.

Investigations in padel have increased in the last few years [7], and have mainly focused on describing match activity and detecting effective performance indicators [8] in four fundamental aspects: temporal structure [9–11], players' movements and distance covered on the court [12–14], design and validation of observation instruments [15,16] and game actions, such as technical or tactical parameters [8,17–19]. These researchers have sought to identify performance indicators that describe and explain effective players behaviours during the competition [11] with the aim to provide objective information on real game situations [20]. For example, occupying offensive positions close to the net seems to be a determinant to winning the point in padel [14,21]. These investigations have shown that more than 80% of the padel winning points are completed from the attack position, using different strokes such as volleys (20–25%), the tray, and the smash (12–18%) [12,22,23].

However, these results may be especially relevant when analysed according to the result of the match, since they would show the strokes that are most used to win a padel match. The results of some studies indicated that the winning pairs perform a significantly higher percentage of smashes and volleys and a lower number of ground strokes, walls strokes, and lobs than the losing pairs [24]. Moreover, padel players' performance was characterised by the ratio between winning shots and errors [25]. Considering the effectiveness of the strokes, the winning pairs achieved a higher percentage of winners (5.6%) and a lower percentage of errors (7.5%) than the losing pairs [18] in areas close to the net [23,26]. However, studies about winners and error distribution in failed to distinguish between the different padel strokes [26].

Previous researchers have found sex-related differences during competition [22,27,28]. Higher values in play time, total time, as well as in the number and type of strokes have been observed in women than in men [27]. Hence, different performance profiles of padel could exist respective of sex [28]. However, information about performance indicators regarding sex or tournament round is still limited. This information is vital for planning specific and effective training sessions [6], designing players' tactics for better performance and developing sport injury prevention programs [18]. Therefore, the aim of this study was to analyse different performance stroke indicators in a large sample of professional padel matches (four World Padel Tour seasons) and their influence on match outcome with regard to sex, tournament round, and set number.

2. Materials and Methods

2.1. Sample and Variables

The sample contained 1070 sets from 532 matches corresponding to the tournaments in which World Padel Tour provided statistics during the 2016 to 2019 seasons. Sets were classified according to tournament round and sex: quarter finals (men: $n = 375$; women $n = 171$), semi-finals (men: $n = 174$; women: $n = 172$), and finals (men: $n = 83$; women $n = 95$). Sets decided with a tie-break (7-6) were excluded. The matches were played following the official game regulations [2]. The ethics board of the local university reviewed and approved the study. The following variables were analysed: sex (male and female matches), round (quarter-finals, semi-finals, and finals), game result (winning and losing pair), stroke effectiveness (smash winners, volley winners, total number of winners, and total number of errors), number of break points and break points won.

- Sex: male and female matches.
- Tournament round: quarter-finals, semi-finals, and finals.
- Set number: first set, second set, and third set.
- Match outcome: Winning and losing pair.
- Performance variables (N):
    ○ Stroke effectiveness: total smashes, smash winners, volley winners, total winners, and total errors.
    ○ Break points: break points and break points won.

2.2. Procedure

The matches were downloaded from the official channel of the World Padel Tour (https://www.youtube.com/user/WorldPadelTourAJPP (accessed on 1 July 2020). Sup plementary Material Table S1 shows the links to each video. Lince video analysis software (Observesport, 1.0, Barcelona, Spain) was used to collect and register the data [29]. One observer, specialising in padel (over 5 years' experience), was specifically trained to perform the analysis of the recordings. The observer was specifically trained in the use of the observational instrument over two weeks. The training focused on the clear identification of the performance variables (smash winners, volley winners, total number of winners, and total number of errors). Once the observer finished the training process, they analysed a total of 107 sets to calculate inter-rater reliability. These results were compared with the official match statistics. Consistency of records was analysed using the free-marginal multirater kappa [30] and the weighted kappa [31]. The score obtained was $k = 0.93$, indicating a very good strength of agreement with scores over 0.92 [32].

2.3. Data Analysis

Performance statistics of the matches were entered onto a spreadsheet (Microsoft Excel, Redmon, USA) for processing purposes. From the spreadsheet, the data were exported to the IBM SPSS 25.0 statistical package for Macintosh (IBM Corp: Armonk, NY, USA) for analysis. Performance variables were categorised game-by-game [33]. Then, a descriptive exploration of the data obtained was carried out and mean (M) and standard deviation (SD) were calculated. Subsequently, the Kolmogorov–Smirnov tests were performed for the study of normality and the Levene test for the homogeneity of variances. We compared the statistics on the performance variables according to match outcome, sex, and tournament round using the Mann–Whitney U-test. The effect size was calculated from Cohen's d [34]. The Cohen's d effect size was interpreted as small (0.20–0.50), medium (0.50–0.80), or large (>0.80) [35]. A significance level of $p < 0.05$ was established.

3. Results

Table 1 shows performance differences between winning and losing players according to players' sex. Winning pairs showed significantly higher values in break points won, break points, smash winners, smashes, volley winners, and total winners, and significantly lower values in errors in both men and women. Furthermore, the effect size was large in break points won, break points, winners, and volley winners for both male and female players.

Table 1. Performance differences between winning and losing players according to players' sex.

Performance Variables (N)	Men					Women				
	Winning Pair	Loser Pair				Winning Pair	Losing Pair	Total		
	M	M	U	p	d	M	M	U	p	d
Break points won	0.22	0.04	31,409.50	0.00 *	2.13	0.26	0.06	13,543.50	0.00 *	2.22
Break points	0.46	0.20	84,491.50	0.00 *	1.15	0.55	0.28	43,021.00	0.00 *	1.08
Errors	0.77	1.04	117,438.00	0.00 *	0.76	0.94	1.21	61,342.00	0.00 *	0.65
Smash winners	1.01	0.73	108,996.00	0.00 *	0.85	0.67	0.44	59,784.50	0.00 *	0.69
Smashes	1.56	1.40	35,024.00	0.00 *	0.29	1.07	0.91	23,729.00	0.00 *	0.27
Winners	1.51	1.09	20,040.50	0.00 *	1.01	1.75	1.21	11,512.00	0.00 *	1.18
Volley winners	0.91	0.60	26,356.50	0.00 *	1.08	0.96	0.65	10,472.00	0.00 *	0.91

Note: M = Mean; * = $p < 0.05$: d = effect size.

Table 2 shows performance differences between winning and losing players according to players' sex and tournament round. All performance variables, except smashes in the semi-final round, showed statistical differences between winning and losing pairs in the three rounds analysed for both male and female players. Furthermore, these differences decreased in the most of the performance variables from quarter-finals to finals, especially in the female category. However, the effect size in male smash winners and female volley winners increased from the quarter-finals to the finals.

Table 2. Performance differences between winning and losing players according to players' sex and tournament round.

Performance Variables (N)	Men											
	Quarter-Finals				Semi-Finals				Finals			
	Winning Pair	Losing Pair			Winning Pair	Losing Pair			Winning Pair	Losing Pair		
	M	M	p	d	M	M	p	d	M	M	p	d
Break points won	0.22	0.05	0.00 *	2.10	0.22	0.05	0.00 *	2.29	0.21	0.04	0.00 *	1.97
Break points	0.47	0.29	0.00 *	1.24	0.45	0.22	0.00 *	1.00	0.47	0.20	0.00 *	1.07
Errors	0.77	1.04	0.00 *	0.80	0.79	1.03	0.00 *	0.67	0.76	1.05	0.00 *	0.77
Smash winners	1.00	0.73	0.00 *	0.80	1.01	0.72	0.00 *	0.91	1.07	0.75	0.00 *	0.95
Smashes	1.57	1.40	0.00 *	0.30	1.46	1.39	0.24	0.18	1.72	1.45	0.04 *	0.45
Winners	1.50	1.08	0.00 *	1.11	1.52	1.11	0.00 *	1.02	1.50	1.14	0.00 *	0.67
Volley winners	0.92	0.60	0.00 *	1.08	0.91	0.58	0.00 *	1.16	0.83	0.62	0.00 *	0.83

Performance Variables (N)	Women											
	Quarter-Finals				Semi-Finals				Finals			
	Winning Pair	Losing Pair			Winning Pair	Losing Pair			Winning Pair	Losing Pair		
	M	M	p	d	M	M	p	d	M	M	p	d
Break points won	0.28	0.07	0.00 *	2.32	0.25	0.06	0.00 *	2.18	0.26	0.07	0.00 *	2.10
Break points	0.56	0.25	0.00 *	1.35	0.54	0.29	0.00 *	0.97	0.53	0.31	0.00 *	0.84
Errors	0.92	1.23	0.00 *	0.78	0.95	1.19	0.00 *	0.56	0.96	1.22	0.00 *	0.60
Smash winners	0.63	0.39	0.00 *	0.78	0.70	0.47	0.00 *	0.64	0.68	0.46	0.00 *	0.63
Smashes	1.03	0.85	0.04 *	0.31	1.06	0.98	0.43	0.11	1.18	0.90	0.01 *	0.50
Winners	1.78	1.16	0.00 *	1.33	1.69	1.19	0.00 *	1.15	1.79	1.32	0.00 *	0.93
Volley winners	0.96	0.67	0.00 *	0.90	0.96	0.65	0.00 *	0.86	0.95	0.62	0.00 *	0.94

Note: M = Mean; * = $p < 0.05$; d = effect size.

Table 3 shows performance differences between winning and losing players according to player sex and set number. All performance variables, except smashes in the second and third sets and female volley winners in the third set, showed statistical differences between winning and losing pairs in the three sets analysed for both male and female players. Furthermore, differences in break points won, break points, and winners decreased during the match because the effect size is lower from the first to third sets, for both the male and female categories. Effect size also decreased from the first to third sets in the female category for volley and smash winners. However, the effect size increased from the first to third sets in errors for male and female players, and also in male volley and smash winners.

Table 3. Performance differences between winning and losing players according to players' sex and set number.

Performance Variables (N)	Men											
	First Set				Second Set				Third Set			
	Winning Pair	Losing Pair			Winning Pair	Losing Pair			Winning Pair	Losing Pair		
	M	M	p	d	M	M	p	d	M	M	p	d
Break points won	0.23	0.04	0.00 *	2.18	0.22	0.05	0.00 *	2.11	0.20	0.05	0.00 *	2.02
Break points	0.47	0.19	0.00 *	1.23	0.46	0.21	0.00 *	1.11	0.43	0.21	0.00 *	0.98
Errors	0.78	1.04	0.00 *	0.76	0.77	1.04	0.00 *	0.73	0.74	1.03	0.00 *	0.84
Smash winners	0.99	0.69	0.00 *	0.90	1.03	0.77	0.00 *	0.78	1.02	0.73	0.00 *	0.91
Smashes	1.53	1.32	0.00 *	0.40	1.62	1.51	0.17	0.17	1.46	1.31	0.13	0.35
Winners	1.52	1.06	0.00 *	1.14	1.50	1.10	0.00 *	0.95	1.48	1.18	0.00 *	0.81
Volley winners	0.90	0.58	0.00 *	1.10	0.92	0.62	0.00 *	1.02	0.89	0.55	0.00 *	1.14

Table 3. Cont.

Performance Variables (N)	Women											
	First Set				Second Set				Third Set			
	Winning Pair	Losing Pair			Winning Pair	Losing Pair			Winning Pair	Losing Pair		
	M	M	p	d	M	M	p	d	M	M	p	d
Break points won	0.26	0.06	0.00 *	2.26	0.27	0.07	0.00 *	2.18	0.26	0.06	0.00 *	2.10
Break points	0.54	0.27	0.00 *	1.08	0.54	0.27	0.00 *	0.97	0.76	0.32	0.00 *	0.84
Errors	0.97	1.24	0.00 *	0.66	0.92	1.18	0.00 *	0.56	0.88	1.23	0.00 *	0.60
Smash winners	0.66	0.41	0.00 *	0.75	0.67	0.46	0.00 *	0.64	0.68	0.48	0.00 *	0.63
Smashes	1.06	0.84	0.00 *	0.41	1.06	0.97	0.40	0.11	1.15	0.93	0.27	0.50
Winners	1.69	1.17	0.00 *	1.14	1.81	1.21	0.00 *	1.15	1.74	1.32	0.00 *	0.93
Volley winners	1.02	0.62	0.00 *	1.26	0.91	0.68	0.00 *	0.86	0.88	0.67	0.09	0.94

Note: M = Mean; * = $p < 0.05$; d = effect size.

4. Discussion

The aim of this study was to analyse different performance stroke indicators in a large sample of matches (four World Padel Tour seasons) and their influence on match outcomes regarding sex, tournament round, and set number. This study highlighted the differences between winners and losers in some performance indicators for players. Several investigations have analysed these parameters, but mainly in the male category and not in a large sample of matches and tournaments [23,36]. This is also the first study to classify these performance variables according to tournament round and set number. The main results showed that the winning pairs demonstrated a significantly higher number of break points won, break points, smash winners, smashes, winners, and volley winners, and a significantly lower number of errors in both men and women; these results are similar to those of other studies that analysed the strokes that are most used to win a padel match [23]. Considering that smash and volley shots are performed in offensive positions, these results confirm the data already provided by similar studies, which suggest that winning players perform a significantly higher percentage of shots in positions close to the net [8,18]. More specifically, winning players performed more attack strokes in 85% of the points in a padel match [37], and the winning shots were performed with flat and topspin smashes [25].

One of the main contributions of this study is that winning pairs showed a significantly higher number of break points played and break points won, confirming that padel players must be effective when they are returning and trying to move to the offensive position during the first shots of the rally [18]. An investigation of padel has illustrated the advantage of serving by comparing points won by servers and receiving players after different numbers of shots within rallies, which lasted until shot 7 in women and shot 12 in men [19]. Therefore, coaches should consider designing exercises during training seasons including the return of serves to the server and defensive shots, such as deep lobs to the corners of the court [7,38,39], as well as strategies to win the point when players are not serving [40]. Interestingly, our findings showed a significantly lower number of errors for winning pairs, in both the male and female categories. Similar results were reported by previous studies that quantified the number of errors in professional male players, indicating that 40% of the errors are made during the first 4 s of the rally [6]. Decision-making might account for these differences by a winning players' shot selection when hitting the ball, varying directions, and height and enhancing scoring options [8,25]. Considering these results, it seems that an effective game style when players are in the return-of-serve situation will increase the chance of executing more break points and less errors, so the possibilities to win the padel match in male and female categories would rise.

In regard to the tournament round and set number, all performance variables, except smashes, showed statistical differences between winning and loser pairs in the three rounds and sets analysed, for both male and female players. However, the differences in stroke effectiveness and break point variables between winning and losing pairs decreased during the tournament (from the quarter-finals to the finals), especially in the female category, and during the match (from the first to third set). These data confirm that there is a significantly increased equality of the scores in the last rounds of the tournament, and when the players play a third set in a match. This is remarkable considering that 30% of the matches in professional padel are decided in a third set [41]. Thus, the results of this investigation imply special attention should be paid to conditioning sessions to incorporate decider sets and matches to better replicate game-like conditions, as it is well-understood that high cardiorespiratory capacity and muscular endurance in players delays fatigue and aids in recovery [42].

The current study adds novel insights into notational analysis in padel, considering for the first time, a large sample of tournaments and seasons. However, some limitations to the study should be noted. First, the number of performance indicators analysed is low. Future research should consider studying other variables such as court zones, shot directions, or players' hand-dominance and game side, due to their relation to padel match outcomes [8,24,25]. Second, we analysed only three tournament rounds; future studies should consider including qualifying rounds. Finally, although these data constitute a useful guide for training designs and injury prevention programs, notational analysis studies should explore game dynamics in padel through shot-by-shot analysis.

5. Conclusions

This study presented new contributions on performance indicators in professional padel. Shot effectiveness seemed to be a key factor in professional padel that distinguished between winning and losing players. The data showed that winning pairs demonstrated a significantly higher number of break points won, total break points, smash winners, total smashes, total winners, volley winners, and a significantly lower number of errors, in both men and women. Moreover, the match equality increased during the tournament (from the quarter-finals to the finals), and during the match (from the first to third set). This knowledge may have implications in the design of appropriate game strategies and specific training sessions to improve performance and to prevent sport injuries. The findings of this study suggest that coaches should consider training volleys and smash winners, returns of serve, and defensive shots such as lobs to enhance winning options. As a practical application, sex differences should be considered when coaches prescribe sessions based on stroke volume, due to women performing more volleys and men more smashes.

Supplementary Materials: The following are available online at https://www.mdpi.com/article/10.3390/ijerph18094904/s1. Table S1: links to each video.

Author Contributions: Conceptualization, A.E.-T., B.J.S.-A., and S.J.I.; methodology, A.E.-T., B.J.S.-A and S.J.I.; formal analysis, A.E.-T., J.G.-R., and S.J.I.; investigation, A.E.-T., J.G.-R. and S.J.I.; data collection, A.E.-T.; writing—original draft preparation, A.E.-T.; writing—review and editing, B.J.S.-A J.G.-R., and S.J.I.; funding acquisition, S.J.I. All authors have read and agreed to the published version of the manuscript.

Funding: This work was partially subsidized by the Aid to Research Groups (GR18170) from the Regional Government of Extremadura (Department of Economy and Infrastructure), with the contribution of the European Union through FEDER.

Institutional Review Board Statement: The study was conducted according to the guidelines of the Declaration of Helsinki, and approved by the Ethics Committee of University of Extremadura (67/2017).

Conflicts of Interest: The authors declare no conflict of interest.

References

1. Sánchez-Alcaraz, B.J. History of padel [Historia del pádel]. *Mater. Hist. Deport.* **2013**, *11*, 57–60.
2. International Padel Federation. *Rules of Padel*; FIP: Lausanne, Switzerland, 2020.
3. Courel-Ibáñez, J.; Sánchez-Alcaraz, B.J.; García, S.; Echegaray, M. Evolution of padel in spain according to practitioners' gender and age [Evolución del pádel en España en función del género y edad de los practicantes]. *Cult. Cienc. Deport.* **2017**, *12*, 39–46 [CrossRef]

4. International Padel Federation. *List of IPF Associated Countries*; FIP: Lausanne, Switzerland, 2020.
5. Courel-Ibáñez, J.; Sánchez-Alcaraz, B.J.; Muñoz, D.; Grijota, F.J.; Chaparro, R.; Díaz, J. Gender reasons for practicing paddle tennis [Motivos de género para la práctica de pádel]. *Apunt. Educ. Fis. Deport.* **2018**, *133*, 116–125. [CrossRef]
6. Courel-Ibáñez, J.; Sánchez-Alcaraz, B.J.; Cañas, J. Game performance and length of rally in professional padel player. *J. Hum. Kinet.* **2017**, *55*, 161–169. [CrossRef] [PubMed]
7. Sánchez-Alcaraz, B.J.; Courel-Ibáñez, J.; Cañas, J. Temporal structure, court movements and game actions in padel: A systematic review [Estructura temporal, movimientos en pista y acciones de juego en pádel: Revisión sistemática]. *Retos Nuevas Tend. Deport. Educ. Física Recreación* **2018**, *33*, 221–225.
8. Courel-Ibáñez, J.; Sánchez-Alcaraz, B.J.; Muñoz, D. Exploring game dynamics in padel: Implications for assessment and training. *J. Strength Cond. Res.* **2019**, *33*, 1971–1977. [CrossRef]
9. García-Benítez, S.; Courel-Ibáñez, J.; Pérez-Bilbao, T.; Felipe, J.L. Game responses during young padel match play: Age and sex comparisons. *J. Strength Cond. Res.* **2018**, *32*, 1144–1149. [CrossRef]
10. Sañudo, B.; De Hoyo, M.; Carrasco, L. Structural characteristics and physiological demands of the paddle competition [Demandas fisiológicas y características estructurales de la competición en pádel masculino]. *Apunt. Educ. Física Deportes* **2008**, *94*, 23–28.
11. Courel-Ibáñez, J.; Sánchez-Alcaraz, B.J. Effect of situational variables on points in elite padel players [Efecto de las variables situacionales sobre los puntos en jugadores de pádel de élite]. *Apunt. Educ. Física Deportes* **2017**, *127*, 68–74. [CrossRef]
12. Priego Quesada, J.I.; Olaso Melis, J.; Llana Belloch, S.; Pérez Soriano, P.; González García, J.C.; Sanchís Almenara, M. Padel: A quantitative study of the shots and movements in the high-performance. *J. Hum. Sport Exerc.* **2013**, *8*, 925–931. [CrossRef]
13. Ramón-Llín, J.; Guzmán, J.; Llana, S.; Vuckovic, G.; Muñoz, D.; Sánchez-Alcaraz Martínez, B.J. Analysis of distance covered in padel based on level of play and number of points per match. *Retos* **2021**. [CrossRef]
14. Ramón-Llin, J.; Guzmán, J.F.; Belloch, S.L.; Vučković, G.; James, N. Comparison of distance covered in paddle in the serve team according to performance level. *J. Hum. Sport Exerc.* **2013**, *8*, 738–742. [CrossRef]
15. Díaz, J.; Muñoz, D.; Muñoz, J.; Ibañez, S.J. Design and validation of an observational instrument for final actions in padel. *Rev. Int. Med. Cienc. Act. Física Deporte* **2021**, *21*, 197–210.
16. Fernández de Ossó, A.; Leon, J.A. Technical and tactical assessment tool for padel. *Rev. Int. Med. Cienc. Act. Física Deporte* **2017**, *17*, 693–714.
17. Muñoz, D.; Sánchez-Alcaraz, B.J.; Courel-Ibáñez, J.; Diaz, J.; Julian, A.; Munoz, J. Differences in winning the net zone in padel between professional and advance players. *J. Sport Health Res.* **2017**, *9*, 223–231.
18. Courel-Ibáñez, J.; Sánchez-Alcaraz, J.B.; Cañas, J. Effectiveness at the net as a predictor of final match outcome in professional padel players. *Int. J. Perform. Anal. Sport* **2015**, *15*, 632–640. [CrossRef]
19. Sánchez-Alcaraz, B.J.; Muñoz, D.; Pradas, F.; Ramón-Llin, J.; Cañas, J.; Sánchez-Pay, A. Analysis of Serve and Serve-Return Strategies in Elite Male and Female Padel. *Appl. Sci.* **2020**, *10*, 6693. [CrossRef]
20. McGarry, T.; O'Donoghue, P.; Sampaio, J. *Routledge Handbook of Sports Performance Analysis*; Routledge: London, UK, 2013.
21. Carrasco, L.; Romero, S.; Sañudo, B.; de Hoyo, M. Game analysis and energy requirements of paddle tennis competition. *Sci. Sports* **2011**, *26*, 338–344. [CrossRef]
22. García-Benítez, S.; Pérez-Bilbao, T.; Echegaray, M.; Felipe, J.L. The influence of gender on temporal structure and match activity patterns of professional padel tournaments. *Cult. Cienc. Deport.* **2016**, *33*, 241–247. [CrossRef]
23. Ramón-llin, J.; Guzmán, J.; Martínez-Gallego, R.; Muñoz, D.; Sánchez-Pay, A.; Sánchez-Alcaraz, B.J. Stroke Analysis in Padel According to Match Outcome and Game Side on Court. *Int. J. Environ. Res. Public Health* **2020**, *17*, 7838. [CrossRef] [PubMed]
24. Courel-Ibáñez, J.; Sánchez-Alcaraz, B.J. The role of hand dominance in padel: Performance profiles of professional players. *Motricidade* **2018**, *14*, 33–41. [CrossRef]
25. Sánchez-Alcaraz, B.J.; Perez-Puche, D.T.; Pradas, F.; Ramón-Llin, J.; Sánchez-Pay, A.; Muñoz, D. Analysis of Performance Parameters of the Smash in Male and Female Professional Padel. *Int. J. Environ. Res. Public Health* **2020**, *17*, 7027. [CrossRef]
26. Sánchez-Alcaraz, B.J. Game actions and temporal structure diferences between male and female professional paddle players [Diferencias en las acciones de juego y la estructura temporal entre el pádel masculino y femenino profesional]. *Acción Mot.* **2014**, *12*, 17–22.
27. Torres-Luque, G.; Ramirez, A.; Cabello-Manrique, D.; Nikolaidis, P.T.; Alvero-Cruz, J.R. Match analysis of elite players during paddle tennis competition. *Int. J. Perform. Anal. Sport* **2015**, *15*, 1135–1144. [CrossRef]
28. Lupo, C.; Condello, G.; Courel-Ibáñez, J.; Gallo, C.; Conte, D.; Tessitore, A. Effect of gender and match outcome on professional padel competition. *Ricyde Rev. Int. Ciencias Deport.* **2018**, *14*, 29–41. [CrossRef]
29. Gabin, B.; Camerino, O.; Anguera, M.T.; Castañer, M. Lince: Multiplatform Sport Analysis Software. *Procedia Soc. Behav. Sci.* **2012**, *46*, 4692–4694. [CrossRef]
30. Randolph, J.J. Free-marginal multirater kappa: An alternative to Fleiss' fixed-marginal multirater kappa. In Proceedings of the Joensuu University Learning and Instruction Symposium, Joensuu, Finland, 14–15 October 2005.
31. Robinson, G.; O'Donoghue, P.G. A weighted kappa statistic for reliability testing in performance analysis of sport. *Int. J. Perform. Anal. Sport* **2007**, *7*, 12–19. [CrossRef]
32. Altman, D.G. *Practical Statistics for Medical Research*; Chapman and Hall: London, UK, 1991.
33. Hughes, M.D.; Barnett, T. What is performance analysis? In *Basics of Performance Analysis*; Hughes, M.D., Ed.; Centre for Performance Analysis, UWIC: Cardiff, UK, 2007.

34. Cohen, J. Statistical Power Analysis for the Behavioural Science. In *Statistical Power Anaylsis for the Behavioral Sciences*, 2nd ed.; Lawrence Erlbaum: Hillsdale, MI, USA, 1988; ISBN 0805802835.
35. Cohen, J. Quantitative methods in psychology: A power primer. *Psychol. Bull.* **1992**, *112*, 155–159. [CrossRef]
36. Sánchez-Alcaraz, B.J.; Courel-Ibáñez, J.; Muñoz, D.; Infantes-Córdoba, P.; de Zumarán, F.S.; Sánchez-Pay, A. Análisis de las acciones de ataque en el pádel masculino profesional. *Apunts* **2020**, 29–34. [CrossRef]
37. Sánchez-Alcaraz, B.J.; Courel-Ibáñez, J.; Muñoz, D.; Infantes, P.; Sáez de Zuramán, F. Analysis of the attack actions in professional padel. *Apunt. Educ. Física Deportes* **2020**, in press.
38. Escudero-Tena, A.; Fernández-Cortes, J.; García-Rubio, J.; Ibáñez, S.J. Use and efficacy of the lob to achieve the offensive position in women's professional padel. Analysis of the 2018 wpt finals. *Int. J. Environ. Res. Public Health* **2020**, *17*, 4061. [CrossRef]
39. Muñoz, D.; Courel-Ibáñez, J.; Sánchez-Alcaraz, B.J.; Díaz, J.; Grijota, F.J.; Munoz, J. Analysis of the use and effectiveness of lobs to recover the net in the context of padel [Análisis del uso y eficacia del globo para recuperar la red en función del contexto de juego en pádel]. *Retos Nuevas Tend. Deport. Educ. Física Recreación* **2017**, *31*, 19–22.
40. Ramón-Llin, J.; Guzmán, J.F.; Llana, S.; Martínez-Gallego, R.; James, N.; Vučković, G. The effect of the return of serve on the server pair's movement parameters and rally outcome in padel using cluster analysis. *Front. Psychol.* **2019**, *10*, 1–8. [CrossRef] [PubMed]
41. Sánchez-Alcaraz Martínez, B.J.; Siquier-Coll, J.; Toro-Román, V.; Sánchez-Pay, A.; Muñoz, D. Analysis of the parameters related to score in world padel tour 2019: Differences by gender, round and tournament type. *Retos* **2021**. [CrossRef]
42. Courel-Ibáñez, J.; Herrera-Gálvez, J.J. Fitness testing in padel: Performance differences according to players' competitive level. *Sci. Sports* **2020**, *35*, e11–e19. [CrossRef]

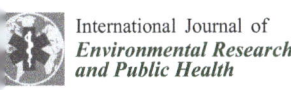

Article

Associations between Inter-Limb Asymmetries in Jump and Change of Direction Speed Tests and Physical Performance in Adolescent Female Soccer Players

Elena Pardos-Mainer [1], Chris Bishop [2], Oliver Gonzalo-Skok [3], Hadi Nobari [4,5,6,7], Jorge Pérez-Gómez [5] and Demetrio Lozano [1,*]

1. Health Sciences Faculty, Universidad San Jorge, Autov A23 km 299, 50830 Villanueva de Gállego, 50830 Zaragoza, Spain; epardos@usj.es
2. Faculty of Science and Technology, London Sports Institute, London NW4 4BT, UK; C.Bishop@mdx.ac.uk
3. Head of Return to Play, Sevilla Futbol Club, 41005 Sevilla, Spain; oligons@hotmail.com
4. Department of Physical Education and Sports, University of Granada, 18010 Granada, Spain; hadi.nobari1@gmail.com
5. HEME Research Group, Faculty of Sport Sciences, University of Extremadura, 10003 Cáceres, Spain; jorgepg100@gmail.com
6. Department of Exercise Physiology, Faculty of Sport Sciences, University of Isfahan, Isfahan 81746-7344, Iran
7. Sports Scientist, Sepahan Football Club, Isfahan 81887-78273, Iran
* Correspondence: dlozano@usj.es; Tel.: +34-607-417-795

Citation: Pardos-Mainer, E.; Bishop, C.; Gonzalo-Skok, O.; Nobari, H.; Pérez-Gómez, J.; Lozano, D. Associations between Inter-Limb Asymmetries in Jump and Change of Direction Speed Tests and Physical Performance in Adolescent Female Soccer Players. *Int. J. Environ. Res. Public Health* 2021, *18*, 3474. https://doi.org/10.3390/ijerph18073474

Received: 23 February 2021
Accepted: 25 March 2021
Published: 27 March 2021

Publisher's Note: MDPI stays neutral with regard to jurisdictional claims in published maps and institutional affiliations.

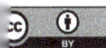

Copyright: © 2021 by the authors. Licensee MDPI, Basel, Switzerland. This article is an open access article distributed under the terms and conditions of the Creative Commons Attribution (CC BY) license (https://creativecommons.org/licenses/by/4.0/).

Abstract: The association between asymmetries in jump and change of direction (COD) with physical performance in several sports show inconclusive results. The purposes of this study were to: (1) measure inter-limb asymmetries in three distinct groups in adolescent female soccer players and, (2) to determine the association between inter-limb asymmetries and physical performance in different age groups. Fifty-four players were distributed in three age groups: U-18, U-16 and U-14. All of them performed a series of jumps, sprints and change of direction speed tests. Asymmetries were assessed as the percentage difference between limbs, with the equation: 100/Max value (right and left) * in value (right and left) * −1 + 100. Mean inter-limb asymmetries were 2.91%, 4.82% and 11.6% for 180° COD, single leg hop and single leg countermovement jump tests respectively, but higher percentages of asymmetries were observed in many players individually. U-18 and U-16 showed significant differences on 180° left COD compared to U-14. Effect size (ES): 0.80 and 0.74, respectively; U-18 presented differences on single left leg hop test compared to U-14, ES: −0.72; U-16 also showed differences on 40 m speed compared to U-14, ES 0.87 (All $p < 0.05$). Jumping and COD physical tests show asymmetries in adolescent female soccer players, but these asymmetries do not interfere with physical performance. The largest asymmetry was observed in the single leg countermovement jump, and no asymmetries between groups were found. Due to the high variability in the direction of asymmetries, it is recommended to consider players' individual asymmetries for designing specific training programs.

Keywords: athletic performance; youth sports; females; football

1. Introduction

Women's football has witnessed a notable increase in popularity during the last decade [1], particularly at the youth level, where a ~4% increase in participation has been observed in the last 5 years [1]. Such impact has resulted in both increased demands during competition and training, as well as greater skill levels during matches [2]. Given these changes to the youth female game, a better understanding of the physical demands players face face across different age categories seems warranted.

In soccer, many high-intensity actions are performed unilaterally such as: jumping, sprinting, changing direction and kicking [3,4]. Given the prevalence of these actions occurring on one side, and the associated positional differences in soccer, inter-limb asymmetries should be expected in athletes who compete in this sport. Inter-limb asymmetries have been a reference on researches in latest years, it means to the concept of comparing the performance or function between limbs [5]. Literature has showed the requirement to investigate the connection between asymmetry and measures of physical performance [6–8], as the prevalence of asymmetry alone provides us with limited information as to the impact on athletic performance. Previous research in team sport athletes has shown that asymmetry may simply be a by-product of competing in a single sport over time [9]. Furthermore, the existing evidence base is still unclear as to whether asymmetry is consistently a problem for team sport athletes.

Only three studies have investigated the relationship between inter-limb asymmetries and measures of physical performance in female soccer players [6,10,11]. Bishop et al. [10] showed jump height asymmetry of 9.2% in the unilateral drop jump, which showed significant associations with linear sprint (r = 0.52–0.58) and change of direction (COD) speed (r = 0.52–0.66) tests in adult female soccer players. Otherwise, no relationships were found between countermovement jump (CMJ) asymmetry and linear or COD speed. Similarly, Bishop et al. [6], found jump height asymmetry of 12.5% from the unilateral CMJ was associated with reduced speed performance (r = 0.49–0.59) in academy youth female soccer players. In contrast, Loturco et al. [11] showed jump height asymmetry of 9.8% and 10.6% from the unilateral squat jump and CMJ respectively, with no association with speed and power performance in professional female soccer players. Thus, with this conflicting evidence and lack of studies in female soccer players, it is not obvious if the differences in results are linked to the level (i.e., youth vs. professional), or motor activities performed (i.e., unilateral vs. bilateral horizontal or vertical jumps, straight running vs. COD). Thus more researches are necessary to establish a correlation between inter-limb asymmetry and physical performance, specifically in adolescent female soccer players.

Inter-limb asymmetries has also been associated with injury risk [12,13], highlighting the important to analyse the effect of exercise-induced fatigue during training or sport practice due to inter-limb asymmetries on the risk of injuries [12,14]. Some studies have observed that greater inter-limb asymmetries and lower physical fitness showed a higher predisposition to injury [15]. It is known that athletic performance is influenced by players fatigue and it could be accentuated by asymmetries [7–16]. A reduced athletic performance was found with only 5% differences inter-lib asymmetries [7], however, other studies did not find a relationship between asymmetries and deterioration on physical performance [17]. So the influence of asymmetries on fatigue and the negative effects on exercise performance required more investigations.

Furthermore, there is an insufficiency of literature researching how side to side differences interact with physical performance between different chronological age groups. Read et al. [18] and Kellis et al. [19] examined different chronological age groups in youth male soccer players. Read et al. [18] showed that single-leg countermovement jump landing force asymmetry was significantly higher for circa and post-peak height velocity (PHV) ($p < 0.001$; d = 0.41–0.43) compared with those who were pre-PHV; whereas Kellis et al. [19] founded that asymmetry, during diverse strength parameters using a isokinetic dynamometry, was not affected by age. On the other hand, Bishop et al. [7] recently observed elite male soccer players (under (U-16 to U-23) and they founded that jump height of single leg CMJ was related with slower sprint and COD speed times (r = 0.54–0.87). However, these studies have been executed in youth male soccer players, and to the authors' knowledge, no comparable data is available in adolescent female soccer players. Consequently, obtained results have not demonstrate conclusive findings when we try to determine the relation between inter-limb asymmetries and measures of physical performance, particularly in adolescent female soccer players.

Therefore, the objectives of this study were: (1) to measure inter-limb asymmetries in three distinct age groups in adolescent female soccer players, and (2) to determine the association between inter-limb asymmetries and measures of physical performance in different age groups.

2. Materials and Methods

2.1. Participants

Fifty-four adolescent female soccer players from three different teams of the same Spanish the club academy squad (Iberdrola Women's First Division) participated in this study. They were distributed in three age groups: U-18 (n = 18; age: 16.9 ± 0.5 years; height 161.8 ± 9.2 cm; mass 57.7 ± 9.3 kg), U-16 (n = 21; age: 14.9 ± 0.5 years; height 159.8 ± 5.3 cm; mass 53.6 ± 8.1 kg) and U-14 (n = 15; age: 13.7 ± 0.6 years; height 154.1 ± 7.9 cm; mass 48.9 ± 7.9 kg). A priori power analysis identified that when aiming to assess differences between three independent groups at a statistical power of 0.8, with an alpha level of 0.05 and effect size of 0.8, 21 players were required for each group. Thus, the present study is under-powered. However, it is worth noting that the present group were adolescent female and studies using such samples are likely to be under-powered given the limited number of athletes associated with this specific population. All the players have more than 4 years of training experience in soccer. The physical training sessions, in all teams, consisted of training exercises for coordination, agility, speed and injury prevention that allow maintaining the level of physical condition. Participants were healthy and without any disease or injury that could interfere with the study results. Informed consents were obtained from all players involved in this investigation. In accordance with the Declaration of Helsinki, the informed consents of all the players were obtained and the study was approved by the Ethical Committee for Clinical Research of the Government of Aragon (CP19/039, CEICA, Zaragoza, Spain).

2.2. Procedures

To ensure the standardized distribution of the groups, all the players followed the same protocols during the two sessions of physical tests. Do not participate in any strenuous exercise 24 h in advance. Do not take the last meal 3 h before the tests. Don't drink caffeinated beverages. The tests were performed at the same time of the day (6 p.m. to 8 p.m.). The first session was used to familiarize all participants with the jump, sprint and COD speed test. The second session, separated by 72 h, the tests were carried out in a random and balanced order, for the correct data collection. The order of the tests was jump, sprint and COD speed test. These tests were performed by the same group of investigators, and were carried out on days with stable environmental conditions measured by a wet bulb globe temperature monitor (~22 °C and ~20% humidity), days that did not comply with these environmental conditions were discarded, in an artificial grass soccer field where every team had their training sessions. All participants completed a rise, activate, mobilize and potentiate (RAMP) system warm-up protocol [20]. A 3-min rest period was provided after the last practice trial and the start of data collection. Three attempts per test were allowed with 3 min of passive recovery between repetitions. Players wore athletic shoes (for jump tests) and soccer boots (for linear sprint and COD test).

2.3. Single Leg Countermovement Jump Test

To calculate the vertical jump capacity, a single leg CMJ was used the Optojump tool (Optojump, Microgate, Bolzano, Italy). All subjects were instructed to perform a maximum vertical jump with their hands on their hips and to land in a vertical position with their knees bent, controlled and balanced, and held in the landing position for 2–3 s. Three attempts were made and the best jump was selected for analysis.

2.4. Single Leg Hop Test

To calculate single leg hop was used a standard measuring tape (30 m M13; Stanley, New Britain, CT, USA). Each subject started behind the starting line and jumped as far as possible (horizontal distance), landing on the same leg, controlled and balanced, and held in the landing position for 2–3 s [21]. Three attempts were made and the best jump was selected for analysis.

2.5. 40-m Sprint Test

To calculate the running speed, it was recorded with photoelectric cells (Microgate). The sprint time of 40 m, and the partial times of 10, 20 and 30 m were measured. Subjects like previous studies started with the front foot 0.5 m before the start [22]. The photoelectric cells were mounted on tripods 0.75 m above the ground and 3 m apart [23]. The test was prepared, and the player chose the moment of departure. The time began to count when the player cut the first photocell. Subjects were given verbal encouragement during each sprint. Three attempts were made and the best time was selected for analysis.

2.6. 180° Change of Direction Speed Test

To calculate the 10-m sprint test with a 180° COD, it was recorded with photoelectric cells (Microgate). The 180° COD is a modification of the 505 test [24], with good test-retest reliability [25]. Subjects started with the front foot 0.5 m before the start. and a test was carried out at a maximum speed of 10 m. plus 5 m, turn 180° on the right or left foot and 5 m to the finish line. The photoelectric cells were mounted on tripods 0.75 m above the ground and 3 m apart [23]. The test was prepared, and the player chose the moment of departure. The time began to count when the player cut the first photocell. Subjects were given verbal encouragement during each repetition. Three attempts were made and the best time was selected for analysis.

2.7. Statistical Analysis

All data were recorded as mean and standard deviation (SD). Normality was analyzed with the Shapiro-Wilk test and none of the variables had a normal distribution. Within-session reliability of test measures was computed using a two-way random intraclass correlation coefficient (ICC) with absolute agreement and 95% confidence intervals, and the coefficient of variation (CV). The interpretation of the ICC values was excellent (>0.90), good (0.75–0.90), moderate (0.5–0.75) and bad (<0.50) [26] and as an acceptable criterion of responsibility a CV lower than 10% [27].

Noting that asymmetries may favour either side depending on which limb scores larger [4]. The consistency of the asymmetries was calculated with the Kappa coefficient and they were interpreted as poor ($\leq$0), mild (0.01–0.20), regular (0.21–0.40), moderate (0.41–0.60), substantial (0.61–0, 80), almost perfect (0.81–0.99) and perfect [28]. SPSS statistical software (Version 19.0; SPSS Inc, Chicago, IL, USA) was used.

Inter-limb asymmetries were quantified as the percentage difference between the two limbs using the following equation [29].

$$100/\text{Max value (right and left)} * \text{Min value (right and left)} * -1 + 100$$

A one-way analysis of variance was conducted to determine systematic bias between age groups for mean test scores and asymmetry values, with statistical significance set at $p < 0.05$ identified via Bonferroni post-hoc analysis. The relationships between inter-limb asymmetry scores and test scores were analysed using Spearman's ρ correlations To determine the magnitude of differences between the groups for each variable, effect sizes (ES) were calculated using standardized mean difference corrected as Hedges'g [30] These were interpreted in line with Hopkins et al. [31] where trivial (<0.2), small (>0.2–0.6), moderate (>0.6–1.2), large (>1.2–2.0), very large (>2.0–4.0) and near perfect (>4.0).

3. Results

Table 1 shows the reliability within the session and shows high reliability except for COD of 180° (ICC: 0.85–0.87) and linear velocity of 10 m (ICC: 0.83), while acceptable CV was obtained for all tests (<10%).

Table 1. Mean test scores ± standard deviation (SD) and reliability for all players.

Test	Mean ± SD	% Asymmetry	CV (%)	ICC (95% CI)
SLCMJ$_R$ (cm)	11.4 ± 2.79	11.6 ± 7.54	4.3	0.95 (0.88; 0.98)
SLCMJ$_L$ (cm)	11.3 ± 3.05		5.8	0.95 (0.87; 0.98)
SLH$_R$ (cm)	120.9 ± 15.9	4.82 ± 3.87	2.8	0.96 (0.89; 0.98)
SLH$_L$ (cm)	121.1 ± 12.6		2	0.93 (0.82; 0.97)
180° COD$_R$ (s)	3 ± 0.14	2.91 ± 2.10	1.4	0.87 (0.69; 0.95)
180° COD$_L$ (s)	3.01 ± 0.16		1.4	0.85 (0.65; 0.94)
10 m (s)	2.08 ± 0.10	-	1.8	0.83 (0.62; 0.93)
20 m (s)	3.61 ± 0.17	-	1.1	0.94 (0.84; 0.97)
30 m (s)	5.10 ± 0.24	-	0.6	0.98 (0.95; 0.99)
40 m (s)	6.64 ± 0.34	-	0.6	0.98 (0.96; 0.99)

Note: SLCMJ: Single leg countermovement jump; SLH: Single leg hop test; 180° COD: 5 + 5 sprint test with a 180° change of direction; L: Left; R: Right; CV: Coefficient of variation; ICC: Intraclass correlation coefficient; CI: Confidence intervals.

Mean test scores and ES for each group are presented in Table 2. The U-18 group performed significantly better jumps and faster times than the U-14 in single leg hop test left and 180° COD left. The U-16 group were significantly faster than the U-14 over 40-m and 180° COD left. No other significant differences between groups were found.

Table 2. Mean data ± standard deviation for each age group and effect sizes between groups.

Test	U-18	U-16	U-14	ES U-18 vs. U-16	ES U-18 vs. U-14	ES U-16 vs. U-14
SLCMJ$_R$ (cm)	11.9 ± 2.6	11.7 ± 3.08	10.4 ± 2.34	−0.07 (trivial)	−0.57 (small)	−0.51 (small)
SLCMJ$_L$ (cm)	11.9 ± 3.2	11.8 ± 2.86	10.1 ± 2.77	0.02 (trivial)	−0.66 (moderate)	−0.76 (moderate)
As CMJ (%)	10.9 ± 5.96	11.6 ± 8.47	12.1 ± 8.34	0.09 (trivial)	0.16 (trivial)	0.05 (trivial)
SLH$_R$ (cm)	123.1 ± 12.6	123.6 ± 18.6	113.7 ± 10.2	0.11 (trivial)	−0.63 (moderate)	−0.74 (moderate)
SLH$_L$ (cm)	124.1 ± 3.6 *	123.1 ± 13.5	114.5 ± 8.95	0.04 (trivial)	−0.72 (moderate)	−0.90 (moderate)
As SLH (%)	3.68 ± 3.01	5.11 ± 4.19	5.77 ± 4.19	0.04 (trivial)	0.57 (small)	0.15 (trivial)
180° COD$_R$ (s)	2.96 ± 0.14	2.99 ± 0.14	3.07 ± 0.13	−0.03 (trivial)	0.40 (small)	0.90 (moderate)
180° COD$_L$ (s)	2.95 ± 0.14 *	2.98 ± 0.13 **	3.12 ± 0.15	−0.01 (trivial)	0.80 (moderate)	0.74 (moderate)
As COD (%)	2.57 ± 1.77	2.91 ± 2.31	3.32 ± 2.20	0.16 (trivial)	0.37 (small)	0.17 (trivial)
10 m (s)	2.05 ± 0.10	2.08 ± 0.10	2.12 ± 0.10	−0.29 (small)	0.23 (small)	0.69 (moderate)
20 m (s)	3.57 ± 0.17	3.63 ± 0.17	3.66 ± 0.14	−0.32 (small)	0.72 (moderate)	1.13 (moderate)
30 m (s)	5.04 ± 0.25	5.12 ± 025	5.16 ± 0.20	−0.32 (small)	0.60 (moderate)	0.48 (small)
40 m (s)	6.53 ±0.34	6.62 ± 0.34 **	6.84 ± 0.26	−0.27 (small)	1.03 (moderate)	0.87 (moderate)

Note: SLCMJ: Single leg countermovement jump; SLH: Single leg hop test; 180° COD: 5 + 5 sprint test with a 180° change of direction; L: Left; R: Right; ES: Effect size. U-18: Under 18; U-16: Under 16; U-14: Under 14. * Significant difference ($p < 0.05$) between U-18 and U-14 players. ** Significant difference ($p < 0.05$) between U-16 and U-14 players.

When comparing ES, trivial to moderate differences were evident between all group comparisons. Table 3 shows the levels of agreement for the asymmetry scores (Kappa coefficient).

The results showed substantial levels of agreement of U-16 between single leg CMJ and single leg hop test (0.45). The rest of the groups show poor to fair levels (range: −0.31 to 0.24) for all comparisons. Owing to the variable nature in both the magnitude and direction of asymmetry, individual inter-limb differences are presented for jump and COD speed tests in U-14 (Figure 1), U-16 (Figure 2) and U-18 (Figure 3) female soccer player.

Table 3. Kappa coefficients and descriptive levels of concordance of asymmetries between the jumping speed and COD tests.

Test Comparison	Kappa Coefficient	Descriptor
Under-14:		
SLCMJ- SLH	0.13	Slight
SLCMJ-180° COD	−0.13	Poor
SLH-180° COD	−0.31	Poor
Under-16:		
SLCMJ- SLH	0.45	Moderate
SLCMJ-180° COD	−0.03	Poor
SLH-180° COD	−0.03	Poor
Under-18:		
SLCMJ- SLH	−0.16	Poor
SLCMJ-180° COD	0.24	Fair
SLH-180° COD	0.10	Fair

Note: SLCMJ: Single leg countermovement jump; SLH: Single leg hop test; 180° COD: 5 + 5 sprint test with a 180° change of direction.

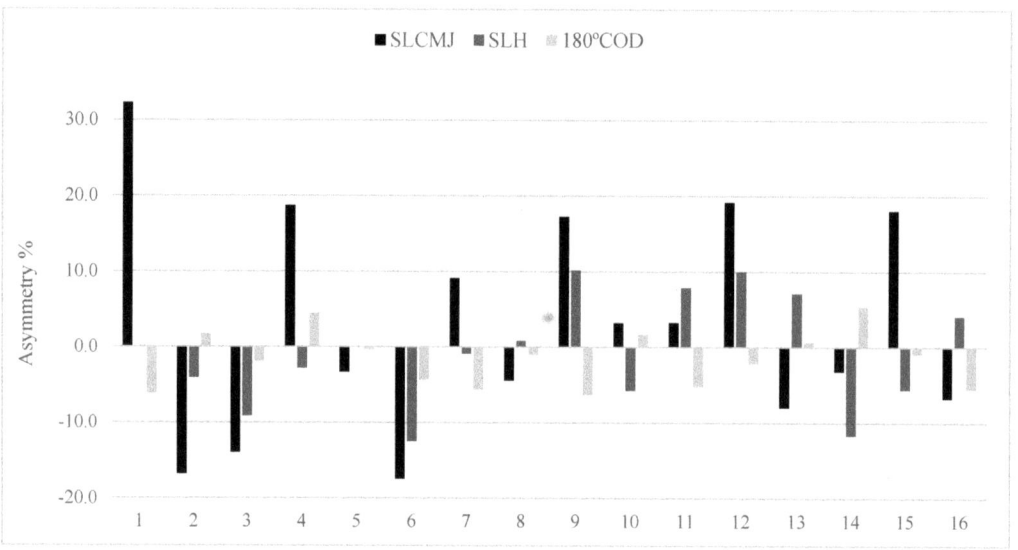

Figure 1. Data about individual asymmetry for single leg countermovement jump (SLCMJ), single leg hop (SLH) and 180° change of direction (180° COD) in the U-14 group. N.B: above 0 indicates right leg dominance and below 0 indicates left leg dominance.

Table 4 shows Spearman's ρ correlations between vertical and horizontal inter-limb asymmetry scores and tests data. No significant relationships were present between single leg CMJ and single leg hop inter-limb asymmetry scores and sprint or COD speed performance. Spearman's ρ correlations between COD speed inter-limb asymmetry scores and tests are shown in Table 5. No significant relationships were found between COD speed inter-limb asymmetry scores and sprint or jump performance.

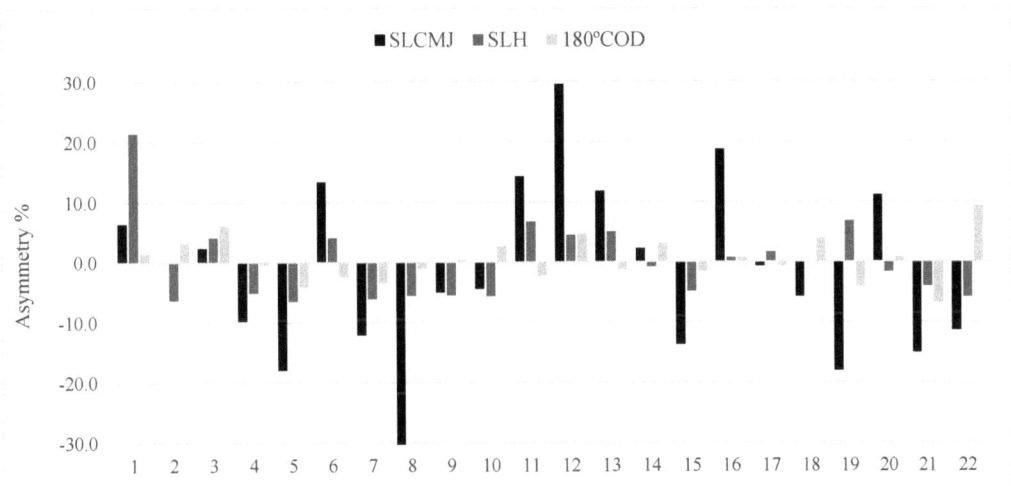

Figure 2. Data about individual asymmetry for single leg countermovement jump (SLCMJ), single leg hop (SLH) and 180° change of direction (180° COD) in the U-16 group. N.B: above 0 indicates right leg dominance and below 0 indicates left leg dominance.

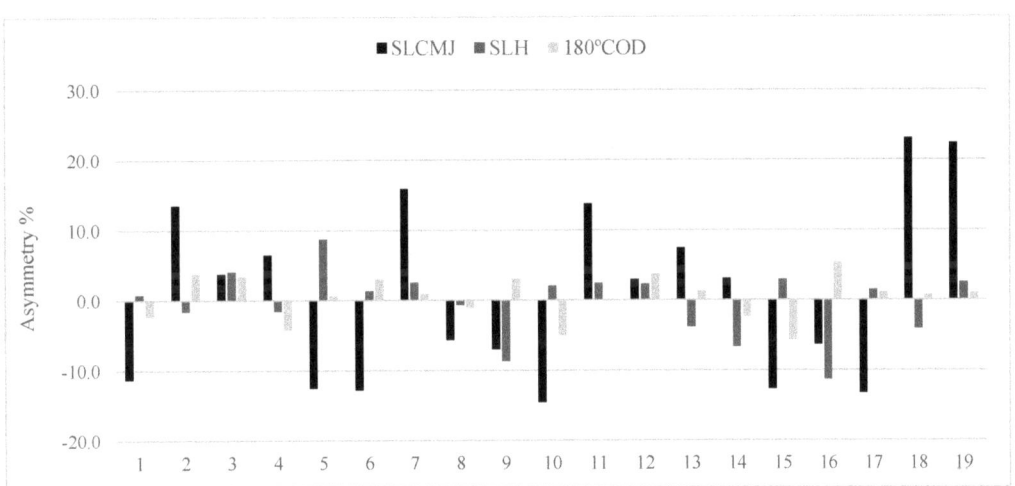

Figure 3. Data about individual asymmetry for single leg countermovement jump (SLCMJ), single leg hop (SLH) and 180° change of direction (180° COD) in the U-18 group. N.B: above 0 indicates right leg dominance and below 0 indicates left leg dominance.

Table 4. Spearman's ρ correlation between vertical and horizontal jump height asymmetry and test across age groups.

Test	Asymmetry SLCMJ			Asymmetry SLH		
	U-14	U-16	U-18	U-14	U-16	U-18
180° COD $_R$ (s)	−0.11	−0.16	−0.26	0.44	−0.06	0.50
180° COD $_L$ (s)	0.11	0.06	−0.36	0.35	−0.01	0.25
10 m (s)	−0.25	−0.05	−0.06	−0.06	−0.32	0.25
20 m (s)	−0.17	0.05	0.00	0.07	−0.34	0.25
30 m (s)	−0.21	0.07	0.09	0.04	−0.33	0.26
40 m (s)	0.10	0.10	0.12	−0.06	−0.33	0.22

Note: SLCMJ: Single leg countermovement jump; SLH: Single leg hop test; 180° COD: 5 + 5 sprint test with a 180° change of direction; L: Left; R: Right; U-18: Under 18; U-16: Under 16; U-14: Under 14.

Table 5. Spearman's ρ correlation between change of direction (COD) speed asymmetry and test across age groups.

Test	Asymmetry COD Speed		
	U-14	U-16	U-18
SLCMJ$_R$ (cm)	−0.01	−0.27	−0.32
SLCMJ$_L$ (cm)	−0.01	−0.01	−0.14
SLH$_R$ (cm)	−0.16	−0.49	−0.16
SLH$_L$ (cm)	−0.48	−0.39	−0.09
10 m (s)	0.48	0.24	0.35
20 m (s)	0.51	0.25	0.25
30 m (s)	0.45	0.26	0.16
40 m (s)	0.49	0.26	0.12

Note: SLCMJ: Single leg countermovement jump; SLH: Single leg hop test; 180° COD: 5 + 5 sprint test with a 180° change of direction; L: Left; R: Right; U-18: Under 18; U-16: Under 16; U-14: Under 14.

4. Discussion

The objectives of this study were to establish inter-limb asymmetry scores from the single leg CMJ, single leg hop test and 180° COD speed in adolescent female soccer players across different age groups, and to determine the relationship between these asymmetries and measures of physical performance. Outcomes demonstrated different magnitudes of asymmetry between tests. Vertical jump test showed larger asymmetry scores when comparing to horizontal jump test and COD speed test. There were no meaningful relationships between asymmetry scores and independent measures of physical performance. Moreover, asymmetries rarely favored the same side between jump and COD speed tests, highlighting the task-specific nature of inter-limb differences.

The totally of tests showed an exceptional relative reliability and an acceptable variability, and this can indicate that the results can be understood with confidence for next analysis [32]. The experience and the regular strength and conditioning training performed during the season may provide to the acceptable reliability of the data [33]. In relation to the asymmetry scores reported in the present study, the COD speed test (2.9%) showed a lower magnitude of asymmetry in comparison to the single leg CMJ test (11.6%), this is in contract with previous research [10,34]. Asymmetry is highly task-specific and although some tests produce larger asymmetry values, the inherent variability in asymmetry scores is still large for all tests, as shown by the varying magnitude of asymmetry at an individual level (see Figures 1–3). For this reason, it is advisable that researchers, coaches and practitioners calculate not only result measures (e.g., jump height and reactive strength index) but also test variability [10]. This will enable practitioners to determine when asymmetries are 'real (i.e., greater than the test error) or within the measured noise of the test [8].

An outstanding point to take into account from these results is that vertical jump (single leg CMJ: 11.6%) showed greater asymmetries than horizontal jump (single leg hop test: 4.8%), and this is in agreement with previous research [6,35]. In the same line

Bishop et al. [6] showed asymmetries of 12.5% and 6.8% in single leg CMJ and single leg hop test respectively, in elite youth female soccer players. It is possible that vertical jump may be more sensitive at identifying asymmetries because in these cases the study population are adolescent players. Children exercise horizontal hopping activities (e.g., hopscotch and somersault) from an early age [36,37]. These horizontal movement patterns are performed more than unilateral vertical tasks [6]. This can clarify the reason why inter-limb differences are not as horizontal jump, notwithstanding, more researches are still necessary to completely support this theory.

No significant differences between groups were during the asymmetry of CMJ, single leg hop and COD tests (Table 2). Intuitively, given the physical maturity of older athletes in comparison with younger, it seems logical to assume that these players would be able to be better asymmetry scores. In addition, there is a tendency for females' athletic performance to reach a plateau around the age of 13 years (puberty) [38], for this reason may be better asymmetry parameters in the older female groups in our study. This is supported in previous research by several studies which showed that older players outperformed younger players on jump and COD speed asymmetries [6,13,39–41].

The Kappa coefficient (Table 3) was calculated for the purpose of determining how usually asymmetries favoured the same side between tests. Results showed poor to fair levels of agreement for the side consistency of asymmetry between jumps and COD speed (Kappa range = −0.31 to 0.45). Simply put, if an asymmetry was favoured on the left limb during one of the jump tests, it was unlikely that the same side performed superiorly during the COD speed test. Previous research showed very low levels of agreement (<0.2) between different tests, indicating that asymmetries for these metrics favoured the imbalance [4,42]. In contrast, a comparison between both jumps in U-16 players showed moderate levels of agreement (Kappa: 0.45), corroborating that these asymmetries were more frequently present on the same side. The noticeably better levels of agreement between single leg CMJ and single leg hop test shows that these two tests shared some similarities in limb dominance, regardless of whether the focus was maximal jump height or distance. These results are partly in accordance with Bishop et al. [39] who showed a substantial level of agreement (Kappa: 0.61) between the squat jump and CMJ, in youth female soccer players. Consequently, these results demonstrate the variable nature of magnitude and direction of asymmetry and emphasize the require for more individual approach to data analysis [4] (Figures 1–3).

In Table 1 we have observed that inter-limb asymmetry metrics vary depend on the test used, and for this reason it is evident that not all female players react similarly to the same test referring to asymmetry. In this regard, group mean asymmetry scores ranged from 2.91 to 11.6%; however, many individual asymmetry values exceeded these percentages, mainly in vertical jump test (Figures 1–3). Literature has shown that asymmetries of >10% may decrease jump height [43] and increase COD speed times [44] indicating that the reduction of these differences may be favourable. Moreover, the direction of asymmetry to favour the left limb was observed in our results (i.e., non-dominant kicking limb) [10], in this case, 31–68% female players presented asymmetry on the left side for jump and COD speed tests. For these reasons, the individual information seems to be important to design a precise training program, with a view to reduce inter-limb asymmetries and therefore, to improve athletic performance and to decrease potential risk of injury [8,45]. In addition, other interesting methods for evaluating asymmetries could be used such us the Functional Movement Screen, ankle dorsiflexion or Y Balance test [40,46]. However, the problem to evaluate asymmetry from these tests, is that it is subjective interpretation of human movement quality [47]. Asymmetry is already a very noisy and variable concept, so to include subjective data could add more error to the equation.

There are no relevant relation between asymmetry results, emphasizing the independent nature of jumping, sprinting and COD speed test in adolescent female soccer players (Tables 3 and 4). This finding is supported by preceding studies [10,11], which do not observe any correlation between different asymmetry results in female soccer players.

Moreover, Bishop et al. [48] observed in a recent literature that comparing asymmetry scores over multiple tests levels of agreement were often poor (i.e., Kappa Coefficients < 0). Put simply, this indicates that the direction of asymmetry is rarely the same between tasks and provides further evidence of the task-specific nature of measuring side-to-side differences [49]. This highlights that if profiling asymmetry is deemed necessary, practitioners should do so using a variety of tests and not expect the same outcome between them. Furthermore, despite previous research in a comparable sample also showing no significant associations between asymmetry and independent measures of performance [11], the variable nature of asymmetry is undoubtedly a key factor in the lack of significant relationships with independent measures of athletic performance.

In this regard, it has been suggested to locate possible bilateral differences and imbalances between limbs is necessary to performed more than one type of exercise [42,50]. In addition, inter-limb asymmetries can also influence performance (e.g., greater symmetrical team-sports players look like they are faster than their asymmetrical counterparts) [35]. In this respect, strength and plyometric training are two of the most often used strategies to enhance soccer performance and high-intensity actions, just like decreasing asymmetries [40,41,51]. Therefore, adolescent female soccer players should make strength and plyometric exercises to improve performance and also, to reduce asymmetries.

In spite of the utility of these findings, the present study has several restrictions which must be recognized. Adolescent female soccer players have specific characteristics (e.g. anthropometry) and, so our outcomes cannot be extrapolated to other sports. Information on participation in other sports was not collected in the current sample. There were no differences in playing position due to the limited number of players presented in every single playing role. Consequently, we strongly recommend that future studies be conducted with the wider statistical population, collecting information about participation in other sports and considering more players for each playing positions. In addition, practitioners working in soccer may wish to consider defining limbs as 'dominant' and 'non-dominant' in respect to the preferred kicking limb; not as right and left, as in the present study. However, it is worth noting that this method does not always guarantee that the dominant limb will be the superior performing limb [10,52]. With that in mind, if limbs are defined within the context of dominance, close attention to the raw test scores (not just asymmetry) is required, so that the weaker or under-performing limb can be accurately identified. With this information, practitioners can accurately determine whether targeted training interventions are required.

5. Conclusions

In conclusion, jumping and COD physical tests show asymmetries in adolescent female soccer players, but these asymmetries do not interfere with their physical performance. The largest asymmetry was observed in the single leg countermovement jump, and no asymmetries between groups (U-18, U-16 and U-14) were found. Finally, the direction of asymmetry appears highly variable, so the individual analysis of asymmetries should be consider to perform more precise training interventions on an individual level.

Author Contributions: For research articles with several authors, a short paragraph specifying their individual contributions must be provided. The following statements should be used "Conceptualization, E.P.-M. and C.B.; methodology, E.P.-M. and C.B.; software, E.P.-M. and C.B.; validation, E.P.-M. C.B., O.G.-S., J.P.-G., and D.L.; formal analysis, E.P.-M. and C.B.; investigation, E.P.-M., O.G.-S., and C.B.; resources, E.P.-M., D.L. and C.B.; data curation, E.P.-M., J.P.-G. and C.B.; writing—original draft preparation, E.P.-M. and C.B.; writing—review and editing, O.G.-S., H.N., J.P.-G., and D.L. visualization, E.P.-M., and D.L.; supervision, E.P.-M., H.N. and D.L.; project administration, E.P.-M. and D.L. All authors have read and agreed to the published version of the manuscript.

Funding: This research received no external funding.

Institutional Review Board Statement: The study was conducted according to the Declaration of Helsinki and was approved by the Ethics Committee of Clinical Research from the Government of Aragón (CP19/039, CEICA, Spain).

Informed Consent Statement: Informed consent was obtained from all subjects involved in the study.

Data Availability Statement: The datasets generated and analyzed for this study can be requested by correspondence authors in epardos@usj.es and dlozano@usj.es.

Conflicts of Interest: The authors declare no conflict of interest.

References

1. FIFA. Women's Football Survey. 2014. Available online: https://img.fifa.com/image/upload/emtgxvp0ibnebltlvi3b.pdf (accessed on 18 August 2020).
2. Čović, N.; Jelešković, E.; Alić, H.; Rađo, I.; Kafedžić, E.; Sporiš, G.; McMaster, D.T.; Milanović, Z. Reliability, Validity and Usefulness of 30–15 Intermittent Fitness Test in Female Soccer Players. *Front. Physiol.* **2016**, *7*, 510. [CrossRef] [PubMed]
3. Gonzalo-Skok, O.; Tous-Fajardo, J.; Suarez-Arrones, L.; Arjol-Serrano, J.L.; Casajús, J.A.; Mendez-Villanueva, A. Single-Leg Power Output and Between-Limbs Imbalances in Team-Sport Players: Unilateral Versus Bilateral Combined Resistance Training. *Int. J. Sports Physiol. Perform.* **2017**, *12*, 106–114. [CrossRef] [PubMed]
4. Bishop, C.; Lake, J.; Loturco, I.; Papadopoulos, K.; Turner, A.; Read, P. Interlimb Asymmetries: The Need for an Individual Approach to Data Analysis. *J. Strength Cond. Res.* **2021**, *35*, 695–701. [CrossRef] [PubMed]
5. Keeley, D.W.; Plummer, H.A.; Oliver, G.D. Predicting Asymmetrical Lower Extremity Strength Deficits in College-Aged Men and Women Using Common Horizontal and Vertical Power Field Tests: A Possible Screening Mechanism. *J. Strength Cond. Res.* **2011**, *25*, 1632–1637. [CrossRef]
6. Bishop, C.; Read, P.; McCubbine, J.; Turner, A. Vertical and Horizontal Asymmetries Are Related to Slower Sprinting and Jump Performance in Elite Youth Female Soccer Players. *J. Strength Cond. Res.* **2021**, *35*, 56–63. [CrossRef] [PubMed]
7. Bishop, C.; Brashill, C.; Abbott, W.; Read, P.; Lake, J.; Turner, A. Jumping Asymmetries Are Associated with Speed, Change of Direction Speed, and Jump Performance in Elite Academy Soccer Players. *J. Strength Cond. Res.* **2019**. [CrossRef]
8. Bishop, C.; Turner, A.; Read, P. Effects of inter-limb asymmetries on physical and sports performance: A systematic review. *J. Sports Sci.* **2018**, *36*, 1135–1144. [CrossRef] [PubMed]
9. Hart, N.H.; Nimphius, S.; Weber, J.; Spiteri, T.; Rantalainen, T.; Dobbin, M.; Newton, R.U. Musculoskeletal Asymmetry in Football Athletes: A Product of Limb Function over Time. *Med. Sci. Sports Exerc.* **2016**, *48*, 1379–1387. [CrossRef] [PubMed]
10. Bishop, C.; Turner, A.; Maloney, S.; Lake, J.; LoTurco, I.; Bromley, T.; Read, P. Drop Jump Asymmetry is Associated with Reduced Sprint and Change-of-Direction Speed Performance in Adult Female Soccer Players. *Sports* **2019**, *7*, 29. [CrossRef]
11. LoTurco, I.; Pereira, L.A.; Kobal, R.; Abad, C.C.C.; Rosseti, M.; Carpes, F.P.; Bishop, C. Do asymmetry scores influence speed and power performance in elite female soccer players? *Biol. Sport* **2019**, *36*, 209–216. [CrossRef] [PubMed]
12. Heil, J.; Loffing, F.; Büsch, D. The Influence of Exercise-Induced Fatigue on Inter-Limb Asymmetries: A Systematic Review. *Sports Med. Open* **2020**, *6*, 1–16. [CrossRef] [PubMed]
13. Raya-González, J.; Clemente, F.M.; Castillo, D. Analyzing the Magnitude of Interlimb Asymmetries in Young Female Soccer Players: A Preliminary Study. *Int. J. Environ. Res. Public Health* **2021**, *18*, 475. [CrossRef] [PubMed]
14. Bishop, C.; McAuley, W.; Read, P.; Gonzalo-Skok, O.; Lake, J.; Turner, A. Acute Effect of Repeated Sprints on Interlimb Asymmetries During Unilateral Jumping. *J. Strength Cond. Res.* **2019**. [CrossRef] [PubMed]
15. Fort-Vanmeerhaeghe, A.; Milà-Villarroel, R.; Pujol-Marzo, M.; Arboix-Alió, J.; Bishop, C. Higher Vertical Jumping Asymmetries and Lower Physical Performance are Indicators of Increased Injury Incidence in Youth Team-Sport Athletes. *J. Strength Cond. Res.* **2020**. [CrossRef] [PubMed]
16. Fort-Vanmeerhaeghe, A.; Bishop, C.; Buscà, B.; Aguilera-Castells, J.; Vicens-Bordas, J.; Gonzalo-Skok, O. Inter-limb asymmetries are associated with decrements in physical performance in youth elite team sports athletes. *PLoS ONE* **2020**, *15*, e0229440. [CrossRef]
17. Maloney, S.J. The Relationship Between Asymmetry and Athletic Performance: A Critical Review. *J. Strength Cond. Res.* **2019**, *33*, 2579–2593. [CrossRef]
18. Read, P.J.; Oliver, J.L.; Myer, G.D.; De Ste Croix, M.B.; Lloyd, R.S. The Effects of Maturation on Measures of Asymmetry During Neuromuscular Control Tests in Elite Male Youth Soccer Players. *Pediatr. Exerc. Sci.* **2018**, *30*, 168–175. [CrossRef]
19. Kellis, S.; Gerodimos, V.; Kellis, E.; Manou, V. Bilateral isokinetic concentric and eccentric strength profiles of the knee extensors and flexors in young soccer players. *Isokinet. Exerc. Sci.* **2001**, *9*, 31–39. [CrossRef]
20. Jeffreys, I. Warm up Revisited—The "Ramp" Method of Optimising Performance Preparation. Available online: https://www.uksca.org.uk/assets/pdfs/UkscaIqPdfs/ramp-warmups-more-than-simply-shortterm-preparation-636825390373342631.pdf (accessed on 27 March 2021).
21. Munro, A.G.; Herrington, L.C. Between-Session Reliability of Four Hop Tests and the Agility T-Test. *J. Strength Cond. Res.* **2011**, *25*, 1470–1477. [CrossRef]

22. Nobari, H.; Silva, A.F.; Clemente, F.M.; Siahkouhian, M.; García-Gordillo, M. Ángel; Adsuar, J.C.; Pérez-Gómez, J. Analysis of Fitness Status Variations of Under-16 Soccer Players Over a Season and Their Relationships with Maturational Status and Training Load. *Front. Physiol.* **2021**, *11*, 597697. [CrossRef]
23. Nobari, H.; Polito, L.F.T.; Clemente, F.M.; Pérez-Gómez, J.; Ahmadi, M.; Garcia-Gordillo, M.A.; Silva, A.F.; Adsuar, J.C. Relationships Between Training Workload Parameters with Variations in Anaerobic Power and Change of Direction Status in Elite Youth Soccer Players. *Int. J. Environ. Res. Public Health* **2020**, *17*, 7934. [CrossRef] [PubMed]
24. Draper, J.A. The 505 test: A test for agility in horizontal plane. *Aust. J. Sci. Med. Sport* **1985**, *17*, 15–18.
25. Pardos-Mainer, E.; Casajús, J.A.; Gonzalo-Skok, O. Reliability and sensitivity of jumping, linear sprinting and change of direction ability tests in adolescent female football players. *Sci. Med. Footb.* **2018**, *3*, 183–190. [CrossRef]
26. Koo, T.K.; Li, M.Y. A Guideline of Selecting and Reporting Intraclass Correlation Coefficients for Reliability Research. *J. Chiropr. Med.* **2016**, *15*, 155–163. [CrossRef] [PubMed]
27. Cormack, S.J.; Newton, R.U.; McGuigan, M.R.; Doyle, T.L. Reliability of Measures Obtained During Single and Repeated Countermovement Jumps. *Int. J. Sports Physiol. Perform.* **2008**, *3*, 131–144. [CrossRef] [PubMed]
28. Viera, A.J.; Garrett, J.M. Understanding interobserver agreement: The kappa statistic. *Fam. Med.* **2005**, *37*, 360–363. [PubMed]
29. Bishop, C.; Read, P.; Lake, J.; Chavda, S.; Turner, A. Interlimb Asymmetries: Understanding How to Calculate Differences FROM Bilateral and Unilateral Tests. *Strength Cond. J.* **2018**, *40*, 1–6. [CrossRef]
30. Lakens, D. Calculating and reporting effect sizes to facilitate cumulative science: A practical primer for t-tests and ANOVAs. *Front. Psychol.* **2013**, *4*, 863. [CrossRef]
31. Hopkins, W.G.; Marshall, S.W.; Batterham, A.M.; Hanin, J. Progressive Statistics for Studies in Sports Medicine and Exercise Science. *Med. Sci. Sports Exerc.* **2009**, *41*, 3–13. [CrossRef]
32. Turner, A.; Brazier, J.; Bishop, C.; Chavda, S.; Cree, J.; Read, P. Data Analysis for Strength and Conditioning Coaches: Using excel to analyse reliability, differences, and relationships. *Strength Cond. J.* **2015**, *37*, 76–83. [CrossRef]
33. Bishop, C.; Berney, J.; Lake, J.; Loturco, I.; Blagrove, R.; Turner, A.; Read, P. Bilateral deficit during jumping tasks: Relationship with speed and change of direction speed performance. *J. Strength Cond. Res.* **2019**. [CrossRef] [PubMed]
34. Madruga-Parera, M.; Bishop, C.; Fort-Vanmeerhaeghe, A.; Beltran-Valls, M.R.; Skok, O.G.; Romero-Rodríguez, D. Interlimb Asymmetries in Youth Tennis Players: Relationships with Performance. *J. Strength Cond. Res.* **2020**, *34*, 2815–2823. [CrossRef] [PubMed]
35. Lockie, R.G.; Callaghan, S.J.; Berry, S.P.; Cooke, E.R.A.; Jordan, C.A.; Luczo, T.M.; Jeffriess, M.D. Relationship Between Unilateral Jumping Ability and Asymmetry on Multidirectional Speed in Team-Sport Athletes. *J. Strength Cond. Res.* **2014**, *28*, 3557–3566. [CrossRef]
36. Ridgers, N.D.; Stratton, G.; Fairclough, S.J.; Twisk, J.W.R. Children's physical activity levels during school recess: A quasi-experimental intervention study. *Int. J. Behav. Nutr. Phys. Act.* **2007**, *4*, 1–9. [CrossRef]
37. Wake, M.; Lycett, K.; Clifford, S.A.; Sabin, M.A.; Gunn, J.; Gibbons, K.; Hutton, C.; McCallum, Z.; Arnup, S.J.; Wittert, G. Shared care obesity management in 3-10 year old children: 12 month outcomes of HopSCOTCH randomised trial. *BMJ* **2013**, *346*, f3092. [CrossRef]
38. Rogol, A.D.; Clark, P.A.; Roemmich, J.N. Growth and pubertal development in children and adolescents: Effects of diet and physical activity. *Am. J. Clin. Nutr.* **2000**, *72*, 521S–528S. [CrossRef]
39. Bishop, C.; Pereira, L.A.; Reis, V.P.; Read, P.; Turner, A.N.; LoTurco, I. Comparing the magnitude and direction of asymmetry during the squat, countermovement and drop jump tests in elite youth female soccer players. *J. Sports Sci.* **2020**, *38*, 1296–1303 [CrossRef] [PubMed]
40. Pardos-Mainer, E.; Casajús, J.A.; Gonzalo-Skok, O. Adolescent female soccer players' soccer-specific warm-up effects on performance and inter-limb asymmetries. *Biol. Sport* **2019**, *36*, 199–207. [CrossRef]
41. Pardos-Mainer, E.; Casajús, J.A.; Bishop, C.; Gonzalo-Skok, O. Effects of Combined Strength and Power Training on Physical Performance and Interlimb Asymmetries in Adolescent Female Soccer Players. *Int. J. Sports Physiol. Perform.* **2020**, *15*, 1–9 [CrossRef]
42. LoTurco, I.; Pereira, L.A.; Kobal, R.; Abad, C.C.C.; Komatsu, W.; Cunha, R.; Arliani, G.; Ejnisman, B.; Pochini, A.D.C.; Nakamura, F.Y.; et al. Functional Screening Tests: Interrelationships and Ability to Predict Vertical Jump Performance. *Int. J. Sports Med.* **2017**, *39*, 189–197. [CrossRef] [PubMed]
43. Bell, D.R.; Sanfilippo, J.L.; Binkley, N.; Heiderscheit, B.C. Lean Mass Asymmetry Influences Force and Power Asymmetry During Jumping in Collegiate Athletes. *J. Strength Cond. Res.* **2014**, *28*, 884–891. [CrossRef] [PubMed]
44. Hoffman, J.R.; Ratamess, N.A.; Klatt, M.; Faigenbaum, A.D.; Kang, J. Do Bilateral Power Deficits Influence Direction-Specific Movement Patterns? *Res. Sports Med.* **2007**, *15*, 125–132. [CrossRef]
45. Rohman, E.; Steubs, J.T.; Tompkins, M. Changes in Involved and Uninvolved Limb Function During Rehabilitation After Anterior Cruciate Ligament Reconstruction: Implications for Limb Symmetry Index measures. *Am. J. Sports Med.* **2015**, *43*, 1391–1398 [CrossRef] [PubMed]
46. Campa, F.; Semprini, G.; Júdice, P.B.; Messina, G.; Toselli, S. Anthropometry, Physical and Movement Features, and Repeated-sprint Ability in Soccer Players. *Int. J. Sports Med.* **2019**, *40*, 100–109. [CrossRef]

17. Whiteside, D.; Deneweth, J.M.; Pohorence, M.A.; Sandoval, B.; Russell, J.R.; McLean, S.G.; Zernicke, R.F.; Goulet, G.C. Grading the Functional Movement Screen: A Comparison of Manual (Real-Time) and Objective Methods. *J. Strength Cond. Res.* **2016**, *30*, 924–933. [CrossRef]
18. Bishop, C.; Read, P.; Chavda, S.; Jarvis, P.; Brazier, J.; Bromley, T.; Turner, A. Magnitude or Direction? Seasonal Variation of Interlimb Asymmetry in Elite Academy Soccer Players. *J. Strength Cond. Res.* **2020**. [CrossRef] [PubMed]
19. Maloney, S.J.; Fletcher, I.M.; Richards, J. A comparison of methods to determine bilateral asymmetries in vertical leg stiffness. *J. Sports Sci.* **2015**, *34*, 829–835. [CrossRef]
20. Menzel, H.-J.; Chagas, M.H.; Szmuchrowski, L.A.; Araujo, S.R.; de Andrade, A.G.; de Jesus-Moraleida, F.R. Analysis of Lower Limb Asymmetries by Isokinetic and Vertical Jump Tests in Soccer Players. *J. Strength Cond. Res.* **2013**, *27*, 1370–1377. [CrossRef] [PubMed]
21. Pardos-Mainer, E.; Lozano, D.; Torrontegui-Duarte, M.; Cartón-Llorente, A.; Roso-Moliner, A. Effects of Strength vs. Plyometric Training Programs on Vertical Jumping, Linear Sprint and Change of Direction Speed Performance in Female Soccer Players: A Systematic Review and Meta-Analysis. *Int. J. Environ. Res. Public Health* **2021**, *18*, 401. [CrossRef] [PubMed]
22. Atkins, S.J.; Bentley, I.; Hurst, H.T.; Sinclair, J.K.; Hesketh, C. The Presence of Bilateral Imbalance of the Lower Limbs in Elite Youth Soccer Players of Different Ages. *J. Strength Cond. Res.* **2016**, *30*, 1007–1013. [CrossRef] [PubMed]

Article

Muscle Oxygen Desaturation and Re-Saturation Capacity Limits in Repeated Sprint Ability Performance in Women Soccer Players: A New Physiological Interpretation

Aldo A. Vasquez-Bonilla [1,*], Alba Camacho-Cardeñosa [2], Rafael Timón [1], Ismael Martínez-Guardado [3], Marta Camacho-Cardeñosa [2] and Guillermo Olcina [1,*]

1 Faculty of Sports Sciences, University of Extremadura, 10003 Cáceres, Spain; rtimon@unex.es
2 Faculty of Languages and Education, University of Nebrija, 28015 Madrid, Spain; albacc@unex.es (A.C.-C.); mcamachocardenosa@unex.es (M.C.-C.)
3 Faculty of Life and Natural Sciences, University of Nebrija, 28015 Madrid, Spain; imartinezgu@nebrija.es
* Correspondence: alvasquezb@unex.es (A.A.V.-B.); golcina@unex.es (G.O.); Tel.: +34-927-257-461 (A.A.V.-B. & G.O.)

Abstract: Muscle oxygen consumption could provide information on oxidative metabolism in women soccer players. Therefore, the objective of this study was to analyze muscle oxygenation dynamics during repeated sprint ability (RSA): (8 sprint × 20 s recovery) by near-infrared spectroscopy (NIRS). The sample was made up of 38 professional women soccer players. To measure the external load, the best time, worst time, average time, individual speed, sprint decrement, and power were assessed. In connection with the internal load, the desaturation (sprint) and re-saturation (recovery) rates, as well as the oxygen extraction ($\nabla\%SmO_2$) in the gastrocnemius muscle and maximum heart rate (%HRmax) were measured. A repeated measures statistic was applied based on the inter-individual response of each subject from the baseline versus the other sprints, with linear regression and nonlinear regression analyses between variables. There was an increase in the SmO_2: desaturation rate after four sprints (Δ = 32%), in the re-saturation rate after six sprints (Δ = 89%), and in $\nabla\%SmO_2$ after four sprints (Δ = 72.1%). There was a linear association between the rates of desaturation and re-saturation relationships and the worst time (r = 0.85), and a non-linear association between $\nabla\%SmO_2$ and speed (r = 0.89) and between $\nabla\%SmO2$ and the sprint decrease (r = 0.93). The progressive increase in SmO_2 during RSA is a performance limitation to maintain a high speed; it depends on the capacity of fatigue resistance. Therefore, monitoring the muscle oxygenation dynamics could be a useful tool to evaluate the performance in women soccer players.

Keywords: NIRS; muscle oxygen saturation; workload; physiological adaptations; fatigue and sport performance

1. Introduction

Recent research has focused on speed as a performance parameter in sports teams, often using repeated sprint ability (RSA). RSA can dictate the ability to stay involved in the game due to the short maximum sprint distance and short recovery interval [1]. It may be considered an independent variable in the soccer training process, because it serves to develop acceleration, speed, explosive power of the legs, aerobic power, and high-intensity running performance. It is also directly involved in the performance of muscle metabolism to provide fatigue resistance, to maintain high speed, and to enhance recovery, all of which are crucial for the performance of sports teams [2–4]. However, RSA has been widely criticized in professional soccer, because the percentage of repeated sprint actions in a real soccer match is minimal [4].

The intensity during RSA can be measured through the speed performed in each of the sprints (external load). Generally, high-speed running is considered when the maximum aerobic speed (15–16 km/h for women) or the accumulation of blood lactate (> 90% speed at maximal oxygen uptake (VO2max)) is reached [5]. In addition, the heart rate (HR) is an indicator of internal load at a physiological level, which can discriminate the training zones reached during high-intensity running shown during sprints, where it is usually observed between 80% and 87% of the heart rate maximum (%HR max) [6]. Therefore, changes in workload can be reflected in the interplay between speed and HR.

Conversely, portable technology that uses non-invasive near-infrared spectroscopy (NIRS) takes measurements based on Lambert's laws, and allows the measurement of muscle oxygenation; it has been validated for use during dynamic exercise in adults [7]. Changes in muscle metabolism can be evaluated by the muscle oxygen saturation index, which is expressed as a percentage from 0% to 100% (SmO_2); this physiological variable determines muscle performance [8]. NIRS in soccer players has been used to examine oxygenation changes during recovery in small-sided games [9], where it has been observed that the longer the recovery time, the greater the amount of oxygen uptake. In repeated sprint activities, measuring the average rates of deoxygenation (during the sprint) and re-oxygenation (recovery between each sprint) as indicators of metabolic performance [10] has been proposed, due to the relationship between the best time (deoxygenation r = -0.76) and sprint times (re-oxygenation r = -0.84). Moreover, slower re-oxygenation is associated with poor performance [11]; this finding indicates that there is a slower recovery of high-energy intramuscular phosphates that are required for high-intensity exercise at levels prior to sprinting exercise. Therefore, improving muscle re-oxygenation capacity may increase sprint performance [12]. Most of these studies used portable wearable technology NIRS instruments, which are readily available to the sports population [7]. Nonetheless, there are scientific gaps regarding its application and interpretation as a method of controlling workload. Currently, the parameters used in a soccer game are usually HR and speed, and few studies report the muscle oxygenation dynamics with a practical approach that provides an easy-to-understand value of the physiological contribution to improve the performance of soccer players during high intensity performance.

Women's soccer has grown in popularity at all levels of play, and there has been increased interest from the Union of European Football Association (UEFA). Therefore, assessing a repeated sprint test is interesting, because it may discriminate performance level in women soccer players [13]. In addition, one of the latest investigations has proposed high-intensity tests to identify talents and performance differences among soccer players [14]. For this reason, we support this type of research in women's soccer, because this information will be applied by sports scientists and training specialists. The aim of this study was to interpret the role of muscle oxygen desaturation and re-saturation capacity on performance during a repeated sprint test in women soccer players. Therefore, our study is based on the following hypothesis: the muscle oxygen desaturation and re-saturation capacity is associated with the ability to maintain a high speed during repeated sprint in women soccer players.

2. Materials and Methods

2.1. Participants

Thirty-eight women soccer players (age 22.5 ± 3.8 years, body weight 60.7 ± 6.6 kg, height 165 ± 0.11 cm, medial calf skinfold 4.2 ± 1.8 mm, HR at rest 60.1 ± 11.2 ppm, experience 12 ± 5 years) were assessed. Participants competed in the same team in the second national division of Spain. The exclusion criteria included no presence of a disease or ailment or a recent skeletal muscle injury that could affect the evaluation of muscle oxygen. Both coaches and soccer players from the clubs signed the informed consent form to indicate that they understood the possible risks of this study. In addition, the protocol was approved by the Bioethical and Biosecurity Committee of the University of Extremadura with the registration code 131/2018, in accordance with the principles of the Declaration of Helsinki.

2.2. Experimental Design

This was a cross-sectional observational study aimed at characterizing the physiological response of HR, %HR, SmO2, and mechanical responses based on time and % individual speed during RSA. All tests were carried out on a heated sports court with an ambient temperature 16–19 °C and a relative humidity of 40–50%. Data were collected during a two-week preseason period. In the first week, the 20-m test was performed to estimate the % individual speed, and 72 h later, the subjects performed the RSA to become familiar with the performance. In the second week, the definitive RSA test was evaluated (see Figure 1). RSA stimuli were performed with the following criteria to avoid possible biases: (a) there was a minimum of 48 h of rest after the last training, which was a recovery load (i.e., evaluations were carried out on Tuesday or Wednesday, depending on the day a game was played (Saturday or Sunday)), and the test was carried out before training to guarantee maximum recovery; and (b) participants were instructed not to consume alcohol or caffeine 24 h before each test and maintain habitual sleep habits to avoid a decrease in performance [2]. The participants were divided into four work groups to guarantee considerable measurement time for each player.

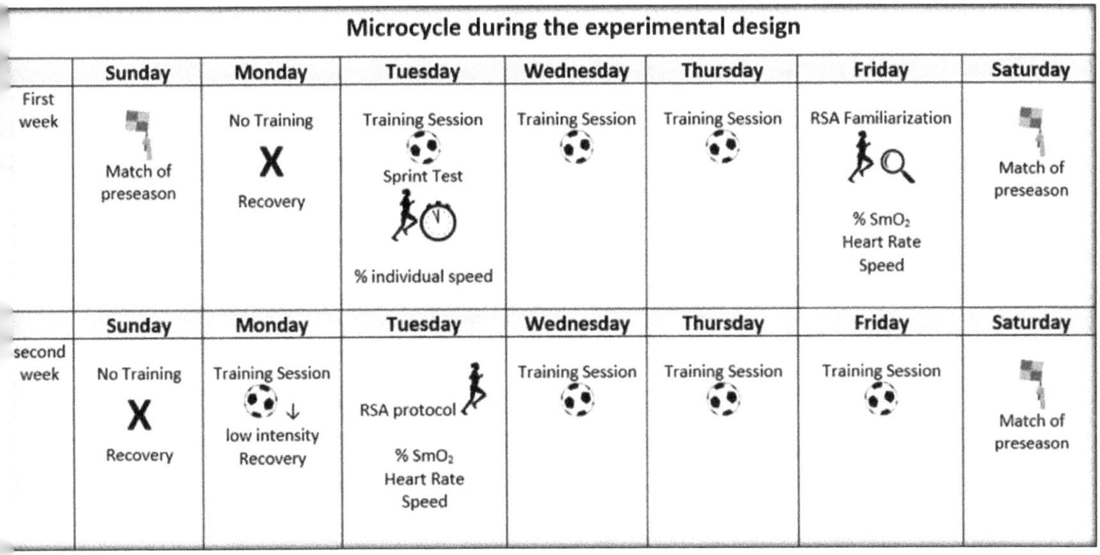

	Sunday	Monday	Tuesday	Wednesday	Thursday	Friday	Saturday
First week	Match of preseason	No Training ✗ Recovery	Training Session Sprint Test % individual speed	Training Session	Training Session	RSA Familiarization % SmO$_2$ Heart Rate Speed	Match of preseason
second week	No Training ✗ Recovery	Training Session ↓ low intensity Recovery	RSA protocol % SmO$_2$ Heart Rate Speed	Training Session	Training Session	Training Session	Match of preseason

Figure 1. Description of the preseason micro-cycle and RSA protocol measurements in women soccer players.

2.3. Assessment

2.3.1. Repeated Sprint Ability Test

The RSA test followed guidelines according to the University of Wolverhampton (United Kingdom), as previously reported [15]. First, the players performed a standardized warm-up as recommended by the fitness coach. Players were instructed to run at maximum speed for each sprint, and pacing was discouraged. RSA involved 8 × 20 m maximum straight-line sprints, followed by a 20 s recovery period. This protocol was proposed and validated by Aziz et al. [16]. Players were instructed to run through the time gates and to slow down only after being far away from the photocell gates (Witty, Microgate, Italy). The players then recovered by jogging around the 10 m recovery cone and returned to the finish line of the previous sprint, which was then the start line of the next sprint. During the recovery period, continuous verbal feedback of time was provided to ensure that the player adjusted their running recovery rate to allow themselves sufficient time (3–5 s) to be in position and ready for the next sprint.

The electronic photocell gates were adjusted according to the participant's hip height and placed 1.2 m above the ground. The doors were placed at the 0 and 20 m marks and connected to an electronic timer with an accuracy of ± 0.01 s. RSA times were evaluated using four scores: (a) best time, (b) worst time, (c) accumulated sprint time (sum of the eight sprints), and (d) sprint decrease score and/or fatigue %: Sdecr (%) = 100 − ((fastest sprint time × 8 (cumulative sprint times × times)) × 100) [3]. Absolute power in each race was determined through time, distance, and body mass (Power (W) = (body mass × distance^2/time^3). The mean power score was obtained from this equation. This protocol demonstrated that the total sprint time was highly reproducible (intra-class coefficient, $r = 0.98$, 95% confidence interval (CI): 0.96–0.99), with a typical error of 0.42 s (95% CI: 0.32–0.62 s) [15].

2.3.2. Individual Speed Zone

All players ran along a 20 m linear track on two occasions, starting from a standing position 0.3 m behind the starting line. A 5-min rest interval was allowed between each attempt, and the fastest time was considered for analysis. The individualized zone was then established based on the sprint speed threshold of > 90% average speed obtained in the 20 m sprint test [5]. Taking as a reference the best time within 40 m, this was calculated using the electronic photocell gates placed in parallel every 10 m. It is reasonable to consider the 20 m sprint as representative of a soccer player's sprint ability, and it further distinguishes the phases of acceleration (0–10 m) and top speed (10–20 m) [4,16]. In addition, the % individual speed was calculated based on 100% of each sprint during the RSA. For example, player 1 ran 20 m in 3.94 s, which was her 100%, making 4.33 s her 90%.

2.3.3. Heart Rate Zones

First, the resting heart rate was obtained after 10 min of resting in the supine position (Polar T31, Kempele, Finland). Then, indirect calculation of the training zones was performed based on the HR reserve percentage (%HRres) using the following formula: HRres = (coincidence of the mean HR − HR at rest)/(HRmax − HR at rest) × 100 [17]. In this formula, the HRmax of each player was previously reported as the peak HR reached in official matches monitored with a pulsometer. The calculated %HRes values were considered as the peak HR measured during each of the sprints, expressed as absolute values of %HRmax.

2.3.4. Relationship between External and Internal Load Measurements

Performance efficiency (Effindex) was used to quantify the match stimulus dose response, and was calculated as: (mean speed in m/min ÷ mean exercise intensity (%HRmax)) for the total test. This index integrates the average speed (the external load) with respect to the relative cardiovascular stress (the internal load) during exercise in a single parameter [6].

2.4. Muscle Oxygenation Dynamics

Measurements were carried out with the portable NIRS sensor (MOXY, Fortiori Design LLC, Hutchinson, MN USA). NIRS uses at modified form of the Beer−Lambert law to determine micro-molar changes in tissue oxyhemoglobin, deoxyhemoglobin, and total hemoglobin using differences in light absorption characteristics at 750 and 850 nm, calculated in terms of the index tissue saturation or SmO2 (TSI, expressed in % and calculated as oxyhemoglobin/(oxyhemoglobin + deoxyhemoglobin) × 100) [18]. These data were averaged based on 1 s, and a moving average (3 s) was applied to smooth the signal with the Golden Cheetah (version 3.4). The raw muscle O$_2$ saturation (SmO$_2$) signal was treated with a soft spline filter to reduce the noise created by movement [19] using Matlab (MathWorks Inc., Natick, MA, USA). In additional, real-time data were monitored (visible only to researchers) using the software with ANT + technology.

Muscle oxygenation dynamics analysis was performed in the gastrocnemius medialis (GM). The device was connected with adhesive tape and completely covered with a neoprene sleeve. Skinfold thickness was measured between the emitter and the detector using a skinfold caliper (Harpenden calipers, British Indicators, Hertfordshire, UK) to account for the thickness of the skin and adipose tissue covering the muscle. The thickness of the GM skinfold (4.25 ± 1.27 cm) was less than half of the distance between the emitter and the detector in all cases. In addition, the GM represents a good aerobic capacity index [20]. To calibrate and normalize values, the SmO_2 was on a functional scale of 0–100%, and the arterial occlusion method (AOM) was used with a pneumatic tourniquet (Rudolf Riester GmbH, DE) and a 96 × 13 cm cuff inflated to > 300 mmHg. The tourniquet was placed on the dominant leg of all participants. Arterial occlusion was performed with a passive test described by Feldmann et al. [21], where the tourniquet remained inflated for 6 min to find the minimum SmO_2 (SmO_2min), and was determined by means of the average of 10–20 visible points in the plateau. After 6 min, the pneumatic tourniquet was released, and an additional 3 min of measurement were taken to evaluate the hyperemia response and to find the maximum oxygen value (SmO_2max) in 10 or 5 data points at the end, after AOM.

Before the start of the RSA protocol, the subjects stopped for a period of 30 s, during which the reference SmO_2 was established. For the analysis of the RSA, well-differentiated phases were identified: (a) the execution phase (phase 1), where a desaturation process was observed, represented by a downward slope, and (b) a recovery phase (phase 2), where a re-saturation process was observed, represented by an upward slope.

For the analysis of muscle oxygenation dynamics (Figure 2), the following variables were calculated:

1. Raw SmO_2 values were calculated during desaturation and re-saturation of the last second of each of the eight sprints [10].
2. The muscle oxygen desaturation rate was evaluated as the difference between the maximum (work interval) and minimum SmO_2 values (rest interval) and divided by the duration of the work interval. Similarly, the muscle oxygen re-saturation rate was determined as the difference between the minimum (rest interval) and maximum SmO_2 (working interval), divided by the rest duration of the interval (20 s) [10].
3. The percentage of muscle oxygen extraction from the SmO_2 desaturation and re-saturation values was obtained during each sprint using the difference between SmO2 at the start and end of the sprint. The SmO_2 start value was considered 1 s before starting each series, while the SmO2 stop value was determined in the last second of the work interval of each sprint with the following formula: $\nabla\%SmO_2 = ((SmO2Stop \times 100/SmO2start) - 100) \times -1$ [22].

As a technical criterion for comparing SmO_2 during sprints, the second sprint was used as a baseline, because, at the beginning of the first sprint, a decrease in muscle oxygenation was observed. This is a standard physiological response, according to the study by Buchheit et al. [23].

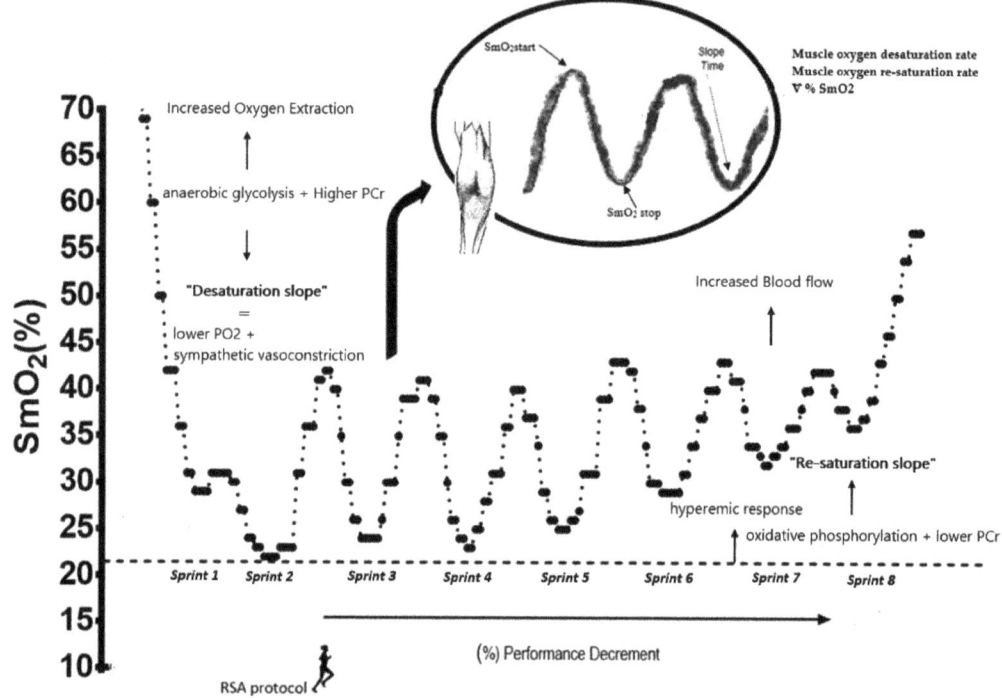

Figure 2. Example of the analysis and interpretation of desaturation and re-saturation muscle capacity during the sprinting exercise.

2.5. Statical Analysis

A descriptive analysis of the variables was performed, and the data are expressed as mean ± standard deviation (SD). The data were evaluated for clinical significance using a repeated measures approach based on the magnitude of differences [24]. This approach allowed us to make comparisons between the baseline (second sprint) and the other sprints, where the data shifted from classifying individuals based on their measured change scores to classifying the change scores themselves in order to identify the inter-individual response [24,25]. The possibility change was calculated based on the smallest practically significant difference (0.2 times the standard deviation between subjects), based on Cohen's effect size principle. The quantitative possibilities of higher or lower values were evaluated qualitatively as follows: < 1%, almost certainly not; 1–5%, very unlikely; 5–25%, unlikely; 25–75%, possible; 75–95%, very likely; and > 95%, almost certainly. If the possibility of having higher or lower values was > 5%, the difference was evaluated as unclear. In addition, the % change of each variable in each of the sprints is presented. The power of each variable was calculated using G * Power statistical software (Düsseldorf, Germany v3.1.3, 3). The interpretation of g power was calculated between 0.8 and 1, indicating sufficient statistical power. In addition, the partial eta square statistic (Np^2) was calculated to explain the proportion of variance determined by the effect within subjects. Furthermore, to analyze the influence of the muscle oxygen desaturation and re-saturation variables with variables of performance, multiple linear regression and non-linear regression analyses were performed. This was determined by the researcher based on the factor within subjects (behavior of the variable), Pearson's correlation coefficient > 0.50 and a p-value of < 0.05 (Supplementary Table S1), along with the percentage of prediction between variables with R2. Data were analyzed using SPSS Statistics Version 22.0 (IBM Corp, Armond, NY, USA).

3. Results

Below, we present the results of the mean values of the variable times during RSA: worst time = 4.35 ± 0.29 s; best time = 3.81 ± 0.17 s; mean time = 4.08 ± 0.21 s, and total time = 32.64 ± 1.75 s. Values of the intensity: % heart rate = 80 ± 4 and % individual speed = 92 ± 6; values of the workload: efficiency index = 3.60 ± 0.21 and sprint decrement (%) = 7 ± 3. More results with a correlation (r) analysis are presented in the Supplementary Table S1.

Table 1 describes the RSA test and the variables of internal load (HR) and external load (speed). Data were interpreted based on the true change (95%), and were expressed qualitatively in increases or decreases. First, in sprint time, a possible increase was observed from the sixth sprint (6S = 56%; 7S = 28%; 8S = 50%), and this variable presented a G power (0.973). The power showed a decrease from the fourth sprint (4S = 95%; 5S = 94%; 6S = 99%; 7S = 97%; 8S = 97%) with a G power of 0.837. As for the HR and %HRmax, they showed an increase from the beginning of the test to the end (2S = 100%), and the test continued in the same performance. Furthermore, the G power was 1000. As for speed, a decrease was shown from the third sprint (3S = 76%; 4S = 95%; 5S = 95%; 6S = 95%; 7S = 96%; 8S = 99%) with a G power of 0.972, and in individual speed (%), there was a decrease from the fourth sprint (4S = 92%; 5S = 85%; 6S = 98%; 7S = 99%; 8S = 98%) and a G power of 0.974. All variables had a better linear factor.

Table 2 describes the muscle oxygen desaturation and re-saturation variables during RSA. Data are interpreted based on the true change (95%), and were expressed qualitatively in increases or decreases. First, muscle oxygen desaturation and re-saturation showed a decrease after the first sprint, then, from the baseline second sprint, no changes occurred, with a G power of 0.893 and 0.858, respectively.

Regarding the muscle oxygen desaturation rate, it showed an increase from sprints one to two (S2: 96%), then, an increase was observed from the fourth sprint (S4 = 58%; S5 = 74%; S6 = 81%; S7 = 96%; S8 = 88%) with a G power of 0.643. The muscle oxygen desaturation rate showed a possible decrease from sprint one to two (S2 = 57%), then only showed a possible decrease from the sixth sprint (S6 = 36%; S7 = 67%; S8 = 38%), and a G power of 0.620. Regarding the $\nabla\%SmO_2$ values, an increase from sprint one to two was observed (S2 = 94%), then, it was observed that oxygen extraction increased from the fourth sprint (S4 = 72%; S5 = 82%; S6 = 79%; S7 = 87%; S8 = 86%), with a G power of 0.525. All variables had a better (quadratic) no-linear factor.

Figure 3 shows the multiple linear regression analysis between the SmO_2 ratios from four sprints to eight sprints for the muscle oxygen desaturation rate (graph a) and from six sprints to eight sprints for the muscle oxygen re-saturation rate (graph b). A linear increase of the oxygenation ratios was observed with a worse time during the RSA. The following values were obtained: independent variable: worst time = (k = 74,159 ± 0.101), dependent variables: desaturation rate = (S4 = 0.062 ± 0.076; B: 0.248), (S5 = −0.124 ± 0.136; B: −0.584), (S6= −0.109 ± 0.644; B = −0.631), (S7 = −0.554 ± 0.823; B: −4.470), and (S8 − 0.658 ± 0.753; B = 3.830), re-saturation rate = (S6 = −2.453 ± 3.385; B = −3.231), (S7 = −2.331 ± 4.17; B: −4.094), and (S8 = 3.609 ± 3.865; B = 5.089), a correlation value (r = 0.848), a prediction of (r^2 = 0.720), and an explanatory model with an F value (3.208) and a *p*-value (0.044).

Table 1. Analysis of repeated sprint ability, 20 m, power, heart rate, and speed in women soccer players.

Variables	Sprint 1	Sprint 2	Sprint 3	Sprint 4	Sprint 5	Sprint 6	Sprint 7	Sprint 8	N2 Partial/Factor
Time (s)	3.98 ± 0.28	3.94 ± 0.17	4.01 ± 0.26	4.11 ± 0.30	4.07 ± 0.20	4.19 ± 0.30	4.14 ± 0.33	4.18 ± 0.35	0.484
% Change	BL	−1.0	0.8	3.3	2.3	5.3 ↑↔ *	4 ↑↔ *	5 ↑↔ *	Linear
Power (w)	396 ± 97	399 ± 70	388 ± 96	359 ± 94	366 ± 72	343 ± 93	356 ± 107	348 ± 101	0.835
% Change	BL	0.8	−2	−9.3 ↓ **	−7.6 ↓ **	−13.4 ↓ ***	−10.1 ↓ ***	−12.1 ↓ ***	Linear
Heart Rate (pmm)	144 ± 13	159 ± 6	165 ± 6	170 ± 7	172 ± 4	174 ± 4	175 ± 5	173 ± 6	0.952
% Change	BL	10.4 ↑ ***	14.6 ↑ ***	18.1 ↑ ***	19.4 ↑ ***	21.2 ↑ ***	21.9 ↑ ***	20.6 ↑ ***	Linear
Heart Rate Zone (%)	61 ± 11	73 ± 5	78 ± 5	82 ± 6	84 ± 4	85 ± 3	87 ± 4	85 ± 5	0.952
% Change	BL	19.7 ↑ ***	27.9 ↑ ***	34.4 ↑ ***	37.7 ↑ ***	41 ↑ ***	42.6 ↑ ***	39.3 ↑ ***	Linear
Speed (km/h)	18.5 ± 1.2	18.7 ± 0.8	18.0 ± 1.2	17.6 ± 1.3 *	17.7 ± 0.9	17.3 ± 1.2 **	17.5 ± 1.3	17.3 ± 1.4	0.672
% Change	BL	1.1	−2.7	−4.9 ↓ ***	−4.3 ↓ **	−6.5 ↓ ***	−5.4 ↓ ***	−6.5 ↓ ***	Linear
Individual Speed (%)	95 ± 4	95 ± 3	94 ± 4	92 ± 5	93 ± 5	90 ± 5	91 ± 5	90 ± 6	0.672
% Change	BL	0	−1.1	−3.2 ↓ **	−2.1 ↓ **	−5.3 ↓ ***	−4.2 ↓ ***	−5.3 ↓ ***	Linear

Statistical analysis is based on the inter-individual responses of the subjects from the baseline (BL); SIE, smallest important effect. This is 0.2 for the between-subject SD and the percent change, a variable that has to be met to be considered a substantial change; ↑ indicates substantial increase; ↓ indicates substantial decrease; ↔ Indicates a substantial trivial. An asterisk indicates how clear the change is at the 99% confidence level, 25–75% * possible clear change, 75–95% ** likely clear change, >95% *** very likely clear change.

Table 2. Analysis of muscle desaturation and re-saturation during repeated sprint ability in women soccer players.

SmO₂ Dynamics	Sprint 1	Sprint 2	Sprint 3	Sprint 4	Sprint 5	Sprint 6	Sprint 7	Sprint 8	N2 Partial Square
Time Total (Sec)	3.98 ± 0.28	23.94 ± 0.17	47.95 ± 0.39	72.12 ± 0.65	96.14 ± 0.74	120.33 ± 0.98	144.47 ± 1.23	168.65 ± 1.52	0.742
SmO₂ desaturation	45 ± 22	34 ± 17	32 ± 16	32 ± 16	31 ± 16	32 ± 14	32 ± 14	33 ± 14	quadratic
% change		(BL) −24.4 ↓***	−5.9	−5.5	−8.8	−5.4	−5.9	−2.9	0.730
SmO₂ re-saturation	48 ± 20	38 ± 17	36 ± 16	37 ± 16	37 ± 16	38 ± 16	40 ± 17	41 ± 17	quadratic
% change		(BL) −20.8 ↓***	−5.3	2.8	0	−0.0	5.3	7.9	0.617
Desaturation rate	−0.22 ± 1.88	0.93 ± 1.21	1.13 ± 0.87	1.23 ± 1.19	1.47 ± 1.40	1.58 ± 1.73	2.07 ± 2.41	1.76 ± 1.74	quadratic
% change		(BL) −523 ↑***	21.5	32.3 ↑*	58.1 ↑**	69.9 ↑**	122.7 ↑***	89.2 ↑**	0.588
Re-saturation rate	0.04 ± 0.37	−0.18 ± 0.34	−0.23 ± 0.18	−0.25 ± 0.26	−0.30 ± 0.29	−0.34 ± 0.39	−0.43 ± 0.52	−0.38 ± 0.42	quadratic
% change		−550 ↓↔*	27.8	38.9	66.7	88.9 ↓↔*	138.9 ↓↔*	111.8 ↓↔*	0.305
∇%SmO₂	0.20 ± 17.1	14.3 ± 19.5	19.2 ± 20.5	24.7 ± 48.5	38.4 ± 85.7	26.1 ± 38.2	40.4 ± 84.4	28.1 ± 43.7	quadratic
% change		(BL) 6709 ↑**	36.4	72.7 ↑*	168.5 ↑**	82.5 ↑**	182.5 ↑***	96.5 ↑***	

Statistical analysis is based on the inter-individual responses of the subjects from the baseline (BL): SIE, smallest important effect. This is 0.2 for the between-subject SD and the percent change, a variable that has to be met to be considered a substantial change; ↑ indicates a substantial increase; ↓ indicates a substantial decrease; ↔ Indicates a substantial trivial. An asterisk indicates how clear the change is at the 99% confidence level: 25–75% * possible clear change, 75–95% ** likely clear change, >95% *** very likely clear change.

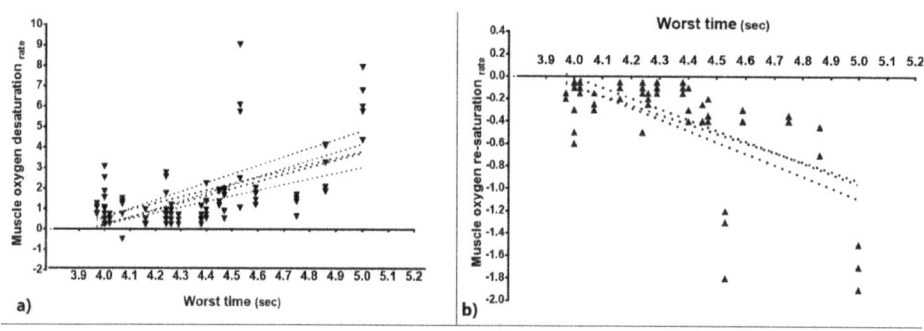

▼ Muscle oxygen desaturation from sprints: S4; S5; S6; S7 and S8   ▲ Muscle oxygen re-saturation from sprints: S6; S7 and S8

multiple regression analysis: r= 0.848; r2=0.720; F=3.208 and p=0.044

Figure 3. Association between the desaturation and re-saturation rates with the sprint time.

Figure 4 shows the analysis of association between the variables of individual speed and sprint decrement with muscle oxygen extraction and percentage of maximum heart rate. First, graphs a and b show the comparison between $\nabla\%SmO_2$ and $\%HRmax$ by means of non-linear regression analysis ($\nabla\%SmO_2$) and linear regression ($\%HRmax$) with the individual % of speed; the speed during the repeated sprints depended on the ability to oxygenate the muscles and not the $\%HRmax$. The following results were obtained: relationship between individual speed (%) (independent variable) and $\nabla\%SmO_2$ (dependent variable): (k = −194.979; b1 = 5.276; b2: −0.025), a correlation (r = 0.889), a prediction of (r2 = 0.809), and an explanatory model with an F value of (33.952) and p-value of (0.000).

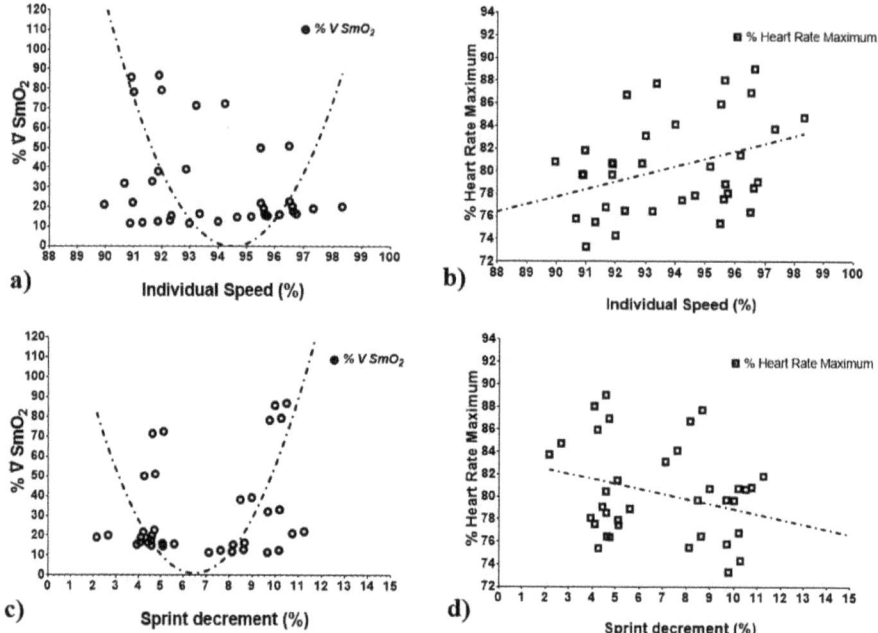

Figure 4. Association of individual speed and sprint decrement (%) with muscle oxygen extraction and maximum heart rate (%). Graphs a) Non-linear regression analysis between $\nabla\% SmO2$ and individual speed (%). Graphs b) Linear regression analysis between $\%HRmax$ and individual speed (%). Graphs c) Non-linear regression analysis between $\nabla\%SmO2$ and sprint decrement (%). Graphs d) linear regression analysis between $\%HRmax$ and sprint decrement (%).

Graphs c and d show the comparison between ∇%SmO$_2$ and %HRmax, using nonlinear regression analysis (∇%SmO$_2$) and linear regression (%HRmax) with the sprint decrease (%). The bearing fatigue (% Sdecr) due to high speed during repeated sprints depended on the ability to oxygenate and not on %HRmax. The following results were obtained: relationship between sprint decrease (%) (independent variable) and ∇%SmO$_2$ (dependent variable) = (k = 172.912; b1 = −55.108; b2 = 4.396), a correlation of (r = 0.934), a prediction of (r2 = 0.872), and an explanatory model with an F value of (53.977) and a *p*-value of (0.000) for this model.

4. Discussion

This study demonstrated that: (a) there is a gradual increase in SmO$_2$ observed in all RSA tests, which is a performance-limiting factor in maintaining high speed during RSA in women soccer players, and (b) the desaturation and re-saturation slopes are dependent on fatigue caused by high speed during the repeated sprint exercises.

First, the decrease in speed was different from the baseline in the third sprint and the % individual speed in the fourth sprint. This coincides with the HR values, which from the fourth sprint enter a zone of real competition > 80% [26]. Although the trend of the HR was to increase from the first sprint, it was only after the fourth sprint that it was considered high intensity. After this, the HR stabilized, and only small changes occurred. At the same time, there was a decrease in % individual speed. This phenomenon can be supported by the latest study by Beato and Drust [27], where the intensity measured with HR was affected by speed during the repeated sprint.

The exercise time reached in the first four sprints (72 s) is considered as a factor causing fatigue accumulation > 1 min, which is where increases in the variables ∇%SmO2 and desaturation rate were observed. This fact could be explained by the predominance of the energy system, where first sprints depend to a greater extent on the phosphocreatine (PCr) system and anaerobic glycolysis. During the RSA protocol, a progressive depletion of ATP and PCr reserves began in the course of a repeated multiple sprint effort [19,28]. Subsequently, there is a greater interaction between the anaerobic and aerobic systems, which is due to an inability to restore high-energy phosphates within 20 s of recovery [29], followed by the progressive increase in PCr decomposition and accumulation of inorganic phosphate (Pi) during the high-intensity sprints with limited rest periods. As a result, an increase in muscle oxygen from the first sprint to the end is observed [30]. This is supported by the fact that the availability of PCr is critical for RSA and that aerobic oxidations and PCr become the main sources of energy as sprints are repeated, while the contribution of anaerobic glycolysis gradually fades (for a review, see Billaut and Bishop, [31]).

The lower ∇%SmO$_2$, which indicates a greater extraction of muscle oxygen by the anaerobic pathway during sprints and greater ∇%SmO$_2$, may suggest a metabolic shift towards aerobic/anaerobic activity to maintain ATP and mechanical power [32]. Consequently, there was a non-linear relationship between ∇%SmO$_2$ and the ability to withstand fatigue and maintain better performance (r = 0.943, r^2 = 0.871), which in this study is expressed by (% Sdecr). Likewise, Figure 3 shows the multiple linear relationship of the rates of desaturation and re-saturation, where there were important changes, with the worst time in the fourth and sixth sprints, respectively; it is at these points where the change in the metabolic pathway occurred, although most studies have focused on correlations with the best sprint [11].

We also found an association between muscle oxygen desaturation and re-saturation with the worst time (r = 0.848). In this sense, the protocol used by Brocherie et al. [11] is more focused on the measurement of anaerobic capacity with a shorter RSA test, because it is less specific in observing changes in metabolic pathways. A limitation of high speed on sprinting is evidenced at desaturation and re-saturation, when the energy system becomes dependent on oxidative metabolism (oxidative phosphorylation) within the muscle [33].

During this metabolic process, the difference in the inter-individual response of the subjects will depend on the capacity of the cardiovascular system and the hemodynamics of capillary beds to maintain the supply of oxygen in the muscle [34]. For example, the accumulation of metabolites within the interstitial fluid (K+, lactate) contributes towards vasomotor relaxation and greater hyperemia during exercise [35]. This mechanism attenuates sympathetic vasoconstriction in active muscles by metabolic events in contracting skeletal muscle, in part by the activation of ATP-sensitive potassium (KATP) channels. The sympathetic vasoconstriction is mediated by the endogenous vasodilator nitric oxide (NO), which is necessary to optimize muscle O2 perfusion [36]. Therefore, in this study, a progressive increase in the hyperemic response and greater blood flow were observed.

Likewise, a greater activation capacity of the type II fibers to extract oxygen through the glycolytic pathway is necessary to achieve better performance in high-intensity zones and to maintain greater force and power production, because type II fibers need less oxygen to function [37]. Therefore, RSA improvement through training can be favorable for success in soccer matches, because it is related to covering longer running distances at very high intensity [38], and it is a complement to technical and tactical game demands.

Finally, some studies provided %HR data in soccer players as an indicator of internal load, but no significant changes in %HRmax occur during high-speed protocols [39]. In our study, $\nabla\%SmO_2$ showed changes during high-intensity repeated sprints, so it could be a promising indicator of internal load. Nevertheless, more research is needed to develop software or spreadsheets that use individual $\nabla\%SmO2$ values. Likewise, future studies could encapsulate the muscle oxygenation dynamics with GPS and accelerometry systems to obtain a better efficiency index in high-intensity zones.

There are a few limitations in this study. First, there was no direct measurement of local oxygen absorption in active musculature, so it cannot be determined whether the rate of muscle blood flow or the delivery/utilization ratio of O_2 is greater. Second, GPS was not incorporated to detect changes in acceleration and deceleration during the test, especially at 5–10 m. Lastly, acute fatigue and lactic acid were not measured, and these factors may influence muscle oxygenation capacity.

5. Conclusions

The tendency to increase SmO_2 during repeated sprints is a performance limitation because muscle oxygen desaturation and re-saturation capacity is dependent on the fatigue and maintenance of high speed in the women soccer players. In addition, more studies are needed with portable NIRS instruments that correlate workload with vascular hemodynamic and metabolic energy pathways. With this study, we propose to interpret the new parameter $\nabla\%SmO_2$, which integrates the SmO_2 desaturation and re-saturation slopes in short, high-intensity periods to observe physiological adaptations within the muscles in women soccer players.

Supplementary Materials: The following are available online at https://www.mdpi.com/article/10.3390/ijerph18073484/s1, Table S1: Correlation between muscle oxygen desaturation and resaturation variables with workload variables during repeated sprint ability in women soccer players.

Author Contributions: Conceptualization, A.A.V.-B. and G.O.; Methodology, A.C.-C., M.C.-C., and I.M.-G.; Software, A.A.V.-B.; Formal Analysis, A.A.V.-B. and R.T.; Investigation, A.A.V.-B., A.C.-C., R.T., M.C.-C., I.M.-G., and G.O.; Resources, R.T. and G.O.; Writing—Original Draft Preparation A.A.V.-B.; Writing—Review & Editing, R.T. and G.O.; Supervision; R.T. and G.O.; Project Administration, A.A.V.-B.; Funding Acquisition, R.T. and G.O. All authors have read and agreed to the published version of the manuscript.

Funding: This study has been supported by the Government of Extremadura with funding from the European Regional Development Fund under grant (Ref: GR18003).

Institutional Review Board Statement: In this section, please add the Institutional Review Board Statement and approval number for studies involving humans or animals. Please note that the Editorial Office might ask you for further information. Please add "The study was conducted according to the guidelines of the Declaration of Helsinki, and approved by the Institutional Review Board (or Ethics Committee) of NAME OF INSTITUTE (protocol code XXX and date of approval)." OR "Ethical review and approval were waived for this study, due to REASON (please provide a detailed justification)." OR "Not applicable." for studies not involving humans or animals. You might also choose to exclude this statement if the study did not involve humans or animals. The study was conducted according to the guidelines of the Declaration of Helsinki. The protocol was approved by the Bioethical and Biosecurity Committee of the University of Extremadura with the registration code 131/2018

Informed Consent Statement: Any research article describing a study involving humans should contain this statement. Please add "Informed consent was obtained from all subjects involved in the study." OR "Patient consent was waived due to REASON (please provide a detailed justification)." OR "Not applicable." for studies not involving humans. You might also choose to exclude this statement if the study did not involve humans. Written informed consent for publication must be obtained from participating patients who can be identified (including by the patients themselves). Please state "Written informed consent has been obtained from the patient(s) to publish this paper" if applicable. Informed consent was obtained from all subjects involved in the study.

Data Availability Statement: In this section, please provide details regarding where data supporting reported results can be found, including links to publicly archived datasets analyzed or generated during the study. Please refer to suggested Data Availability Statements in section "MDPI Research Data Policies" at https://www.mdpi.com/ethics. You might choose to exclude this statement if the study did not report any data. The data presented in this study are available on request from the corresponding author. The data are not publicly available due to privacy.

Acknowledgments: The authors gratefully acknowledge the collaboration of the Caceres women's soccer club.

Conflicts of Interest: The authors declare no conflict of interest.

References

1. Lockie, R.G.; Moreno, M.R.; Orjalo, A.J.; Stage, A.A.; Liu, T.M.; Birmingham-Babauta, S.A.; Hurley, J.M.; Torne, I.A.; Beiley, M.D.; Risso, F.G.; et al. Repeated-Sprint Ability in Division i Collegiate Male Soccer Players: Positional Differences and Relationships with Performance Tests. *J. Strength Cond. Res.* **2019**. [CrossRef] [PubMed]
2. Taylor, J.M.; Macpherson, T.W.; Spears, I.R.; Weston, M. Repeated sprints: An independent not dependent variable. *Int. J. Sports Physiol. Perform.* **2016**, *11*, 693–696. [CrossRef] [PubMed]
3. Girard, O.; Mendez-Villanueva, A.; Bishop, D. Repeated-Sprint Ability—Part I. *Sport. Med.* **2011**. [CrossRef]
4. Nakamura, F.Y.; Pereira, L.A.; Loturco, I.; Rosseti, M.; Moura, F.A.; Bradley, P.S. Repeated-Sprint Sequences during Female Soccer Matches Using Fixed and Individual Speed Thresholds. *J. Strength Cond. Res.* **2017**. [CrossRef] [PubMed]
5. Bradley, P.S.; Vescovi, J.D. Velocity thresholds for women's soccer matches: Sex specificity dictates high-speed-running and sprinting thresholds-female athletes in motion (FAiM). *Int. J. Sports Physiol. Perform.* **2015**, *10*, 112–116. [CrossRef] [PubMed]
6. Suarez-Arrones, L.; Torreño, N.; Requena, B.; Sáez De Villarreal, E.; Casamichana, D.; Barbero-Alvarez, J.C.; Munguía-Izquierdo, D. Match-play activity proile in professional soccer players during oficial games and the relationship between external and internal load. *J. Sports Med. Phys. Fitness* **2015**, *55*, 1417–1422. [PubMed]
7. McManus, C.J.; Collison, J.; Cooper, C.E. Performance comparison of the MOXY and PortaMon near-infrared spectroscopy muscle oximeters at rest and during exercise. *J. Biomed. Opt.* **2018**, *23*, 1. [CrossRef]
8. Azevedo, R.D.A.; Béjar Saona, J.E.; Inglis, E.C.; Iannetta, D.; Murias, J.M. The effect of the fraction of inspired oxygen on the NIRS-derived deoxygenated hemoglobin "breakpoint" during ramp-incremental test. *Am. J. Physiol. Integr. Comp. Physiol.* **2020**, *318*, R399–R409. [CrossRef]
9. McLean, S.; Kerhervé, H.; Lovell, G.P.; Gorman, A.D.; Solomon, C. The effect of recovery duration on vastus lateralis oxygenation, heart rate, perceived exertion and time motion descriptors during small sided football games. *PLoS ONE* **2016**. [CrossRef]
10. Buchheit, M.; Cormie, P.; Abbiss, C.R.; Ahmaidi, S.; Nosaka, K.K.; Laursen, P.B. Muscle deoxygenation during repeated sprint running: Effect of active vs. Passive recovery. *Int. J. Sports Med.* **2009**. [CrossRef]
11. Brocherie, F.; Millet, G.P.; Girard, O. Neuro-mechanical and metabolic adjustments to the repeated anaerobic sprint test in professional football players. *Eur. J. Appl. Physiol.* **2015**. [CrossRef]
12. Haseler, L.J.; Hogan, M.C.; Richardson, R.S. Skeletal muscle phosphocreatine recovery in exercise-trained humans is dependent on O_2 availability. *J. Appl. Physiol.* **1999**. [CrossRef] [PubMed]

13. Gabbett, T.J. The development of a test of repeated-sprint ability for elite women's soccer players. *J. Strength Cond. Res.* **2010**. [CrossRef] [PubMed]
14. Datson, N.; Weston, M.; Drust, B.; Gregson, W.; Lolli, L. High-intensity endurance capacity assessment as a tool for talent identification in elite youth female soccer. *J. Sports Sci.* **2019**. [CrossRef] [PubMed]
15. Zagatto, A.M.; Beck, W.R.; Gobatto, C.A. Validity of the running anaerobic sprint test for assessing anaerobic power and predicting short-distance performances. *J. Strength Cond. Res.* **2009**. [CrossRef] [PubMed]
16. Aziz, A.R.; Mukherjee, S.; Chia, M.Y.H.; Teh, K.C. Validity of the running repeated sprint ability test among playing positions and level of competitiveness in trained soccer players. *Int. J. Sports Med.* **2008**. [CrossRef]
17. Karvonen, M.J.; Kentala, E.; Mustala, O. The effects of training on heart rate; a longitudinal study. *Ann. Med. Exp. Biol. Fenn.* **1957**, *35*, 307–315.
18. Ihsan, M.; Watson, G.; Lipski, M.; Abbiss, C.R. Influence of postexercise cooling on muscle oxygenation and blood volume changes. *Med. Sci. Sports Exerc.* **2013**. [CrossRef]
19. Rodriguez, R.F.; Townsend, N.E.; Aughey, R.J.; Billaut, F. Influence of averaging method on muscle deoxygenation interpretation during repeated-sprint exercise. *Scand. J. Med. Sci. Sport.* **2018**. [CrossRef]
20. Bangde, W.; Guodong, X.; Qingping, T.; Jinyan, S.; Bailei, S.; Lei, Z.; Qingming, L.; Hui, G.; Wang, B.; Xu, G.; et al. Differences between the vastus lateralis and gastrocnemius lateralis in the assessment ability of breakpoints of muscle oxygenation for aerobic capacity indices during an incremental cycling exercise. *J. Sport. Sci. Med.* **2012**, *11*, 606–613.
21. Feldmann, A.; Schmitz, R.W.; Erlacher, D. Near-infrared spectroscopy-derived muscle oxygen saturation on a 0% to 100% scale: Reliability and validity of the Moxy Monitor. *J. Biomed. Opt.* **2019**, *24*, 115001. [CrossRef] [PubMed]
22. Gómez-Carmona, C.D.; Bastida-Castillo, A.; Rojas-Valverde, D.; de la Cruz Sánchez, E.; García-Rubio, J.; Ibáñez, S.J.; Pino-Ortega, J. Lower-limb Dynamics of Muscle Oxygen Saturation During the Back-squat Exercise: Effects of Training Load and Effort Level. *J. strength Cond. Res.* **2019**. [CrossRef] [PubMed]
23. Buchheit, M.; Abbiss, C.R.; Peiffer, J.J.; Laursen, P.B. Performance and physiological responses during a sprint interval training session: Relationships with muscle oxygenation and pulmonary oxygen uptake kinetics. *Eur. J. Appl. Physiol.* **2012**. [CrossRef]
24. Hecksteden, A.; Pitsch, W.; Rosenberger, F.; Meyer, T. Repeated testing for the assessment of individual response to exercise training. *J. Appl. Physiol.* **2018**. [CrossRef]
25. Ross, R.; Goodpaster, B.H.; Koch, L.G.; Sarzynski, M.A.; Kohrt, W.M.; Johannsen, N.M.; Skinner, J.S.; Castro, A.; Irving, B.A.; Noland, R.C.; et al. Precision exercise medicine: Understanding exercise response variability. *Br. J. Sports Med.* **2019**. [CrossRef]
26. Alexiou, H.; Coutts, A.J. A comparison of methods used for quantifying internal training load in women soccer players. *Int. J. Sports Physiol. Perform.* **2008**. [CrossRef] [PubMed]
27. Beato, M.; Drust, B. Acceleration intensity is an important contributor to the external and internal training load demands of repeated sprint exercises in soccer players. *Res. Sport. Med.* **2020**. [CrossRef]
28. McGawley, K.; Bishop, D.J. Oxygen uptake during repeated-sprint exercise. *J. Sci. Med. Sport* **2015**. [CrossRef]
29. Dawson, B.; Goodman, C.; Lawrence, S.; Preen, D.; Polglaze, T.; Fitzsimons, M.; Fournier, P. Muscle phosphocreatine repletion following single and repeated short sprint efforts. *Scand. J. Med. Sci. Sports* **2007**. [CrossRef]
30. Whipp, B.J.; Ward, S.A.; Rossiter, H.B. Pulmonary O2 uptake during exercise: Conflating muscular and cardiovascular responses. *Med. Sci. Sports Exerc.* **2005**, *37*, 1574–1585. [CrossRef]
31. Billaut, F.; Bishop, D. Muscle fatigue in males and females during multiple-sprint exercise. *Sport. Med.* **2009**, *39*, 257–278. [CrossRef]
32. Woorons, X.; Mucci, P.; Aucouturier, J.; Anthierens, A.; Millet, G.P. Acute effects of repeated cycling sprints in hypoxia induced by voluntary hypoventilation. *Eur. J. Appl. Physiol.* **2017**. [CrossRef]
33. Lapointe, J.; Paradis-Deschênes, P.; Woorons, X.; Lemaître, F.; Billaut, F. Impact of Hypoventilation Training on Muscle Oxygenation, Myoelectrical Changes, Systemic [K+], and Repeated-Sprint Ability in Basketball Players. *Front. Sport. Act. Living* **2020**, *2*, 29 [CrossRef] [PubMed]
34. Rodriguez, R.F.; Townsend, N.E.; Aughey, R.J.; Billaut, F. Muscle oxygenation maintained during repeated-sprints despite inspiratory muscle loading. *PLoS ONE* **2019**. [CrossRef] [PubMed]
35. Murias, J.M.; Spencer, M.D.; Keir, D.A.; Paterson, D.H. Systemic and vastus lateralis muscle blood flow and O2 extraction during ramp incremental cycle exercise. *Am. J. Physiol. Regul. Integr. Comp. Physiol.* **2013**. [CrossRef]
36. Thomas, G.D.; Victor, R.G. Nitric oxide mediates contraction-induced attenuation of sympathetic vasoconstriction in rat skeletal muscle. *J. Physiol.* **1998**. [CrossRef]
37. Calaine Inglis, E.; Iannetta, D.; Murias, J.M. The plateau in the NIRS-derived [HHb] signal near the end of a ramp incremental test does not indicate the upper limit of O2 extraction in the vastus lateralis. *Am. J. Physiol. Regul. Integr. Comp. Physiol.* **2017**. [CrossRef]
38. Rampinini, E.; Bishop, D.; Marcora, S.M.; Ferrari Bravo, D.; Sassi, R.; Impellizzeri, F.M. Validity of simple field tests as indicators of match-related physical performance in top-level professional soccer players. *Int. J. Sports Med.* **2007**. [CrossRef] [PubMed]
39. Bendiksen, M.; Pettersen, S.A.; Ingebrigtsen, J.; Randers, M.B.; Brito, J.; Mohr, M.; Bangsbo, J.; Krustrup, P. Application of the Copenhagen Soccer Test in high-level women players—Locomotor activities, physiological response and sprint performance. *Hum. Mov. Sci.* **2013**. [CrossRef]

The Influence of Stretching the Hip Flexor Muscles on Performance Parameters. A Systematic Review with Meta-Analysis

Andreas Konrad [1,*], Richard Močnik [1], Sylvia Titze [1], Masatoshi Nakamura [2] and Markus Tilp [1]

1. Institute of Human Movement Science, Sport and Health, University of Graz, A-8010 Graz, Austria; richard.mocnik@uni-graz.at (R.M.); sylvia.titze@uni-graz.at (S.T.); markus.tilp@uni-graz.at (M.T.)
2. Institute for Human Movement and Medical Sciences, Niigata University of Health and Welfare, 1398 Shimami-cho, Kita-ku, Niigata 950-3198, Japan; masatoshi-nakamura@nuhw.ac.jp
* Correspondence: andreas.konrad@uni-graz.at; Tel.: +43-316-380-8336; Fax: +43-316-380-9790

Abstract: The hip flexor muscles are major contributors to lumbar spine stability. Tight hip flexors can lead to pain in the lumbar spine, and hence to an impairment in performance. Moreover, sedentary behavior is a common problem and a major contributor to restricted hip extension flexibility. Stretching can be a tool to reduce muscle tightness and to overcome the aforementioned problems. Therefore, the purpose of this systematic review with meta-analysis was to determine the effects of a single hip flexor stretching exercise on performance parameters. The online search was performed in the following three databases: PubMed, Scopus, and Web of Science. Eight studies were included in this review with a total of 165 subjects (male: 111; female 54). In contrast to other muscle groups (e.g., plantar flexors), where 120 s of stretching likely decreases force production, it seems that isolated hip flexor stretching of up to 120 s has no effect or even a positive impact on performance-related parameters. A comparison of the effects on performance between the three defined stretch durations (30–90 s; 120 s; 270–480 s) revealed a significantly different change in performance ($p = 0.02$) between the studies with the lowest hip flexor stretch duration (30–90 s; weighted mean performance change: −0.12%; CI (95%): −0.49 to 0.41) and the studies with the highest hip flexor stretch duration (270–480 s; performance change: −3.59%; CI (95%): −5.92 to −2.04). Meta-analysis revealed a significant (but trivial) impairment in the highest hip flexor stretch duration of 270–480 s (SMD effect size = −0.19; CI (95%) −0.379 to 0.000; Z = −1.959; $p = 0.05$; $I^2 = 0.62\%$), but not in the lowest stretch duration (30–90 s). This indicates a dose-response relationship in the hip flexor muscles. Although the evidence is based on a small number of studies, this information will be of great importance for both athletes and coaches.

Keywords: iliopsoas; rectus femoris; mobility; flexibility

1. Introduction

Stretching is commonly used as a warm-up routine prior to physical activities, with the goal being to increase the range of motion (ROM) of a joint [1]. With regard to the impact on performance parameters (i.e., strength, speed) there is a debate as to whether stretching can be helpful as a warm-up. In their review, Behm et al. [2] reported mean performance impairments of 3.7% and 4.4% immediately after static stretching and proprioceptive neuromuscular facilitation (PNF) stretching, respectively, but an increase in performance of 1.3% after dynamic stretching. Both muscle tightness and muscle stiffness can be reduced by single stretching exercises [3,4]. However, whilst muscle tightness is defined as a limited range of motion, muscle stiffness is defined as the resistance to stretch [5].

The hip flexor muscles (e.g., musculus iliopsoas, rectus femoris) are major contributors to lumbar spine stability [6]. While a minimum amount of tightness is required for lumbar spine stability and health, hip flexors that are too tight pose a risk for lower back pain [7].

Hence, an optimum amount of ROM in the hip flexors is required. Hip flexors are defined as being tight if full hip extension in the end position of the modified Thomas test cannot be reached [8]. In addition to lower back pain, tight hip flexors can also compromise isometric trunk strength [9], which likely has detrimental effects on sports performance. Endo and Sakamoto [10] also reported relationships between tight hip flexors and reduced dynamic balance, as assessed by star excursion balance tests in the lateral direction. Hip flexor tightness can also lead to muscle fatigue and can negatively affect movement patterns [11,12]. Furthermore, reduced gluteus maximus activation and lower gluteus maximus to biceps femoris co-activation were reported in female soccer players with lower hip extension ROM, indicating adapted neuromuscular strategies that negatively influence movement patterns, and hence can lead to decreased performance and injury [13]. In summary, there is a body of evidence that hip flexors that are too tight likely have a negative effect on several performance parameters.

Sedentary behavior reduces hip extension flexibility and hence increases flexor tightness. An average of ≥ 8 h mean sedentary time has been reported in a youth population [14] and also in an elderly population [15]. It is therefore likely that most of the sedentary population have tight hip flexors. This is underlined by the findings of Mettler et al. [16], who reported that two-thirds of the investigated population had limited hip extension flexibility, and hence tight hip flexors.

Similar to the other muscles of the lower leg (i.e., plantar flexors [17]), hip flexor stretching decreases tightness (and hence increases hip extension ROM) following an acute bout of stretching [12]. This will likely counteract the aforementioned problems when applied repeatedly [16]. Thus, frequent hip flexor stretching could be a beneficial strategy to sustain or even increase hip extension ROM. This might also imply a reduction in lower back pain and the prevalence of injuries and likely lead to an increase in performance [18]. However, to date, no review has summarized the literature about the effects of a single hip flexor stretching exercise on sports performance.

Therefore, this systematic review with meta-analysis was aimed at identifying if a single bout of stretching of the hip flexors has an impact on performance parameters. Since isokinetic, balance, and sport-specific parameters describe the different skills and dimensions of performance, we divided the analyzed parameters into the following three groups. Group 1: isokinetic parameters (*peak torque, mean power output, work, joint angle at peak torque, acceleration*); Group 2: balance and proprioception parameters (*Y-balance test, joint position sense*); Group 3: sport-specific parameters (*sprint time, countermovement jump height, foot speed*).

2. Materials and Methods

2.1. Search Strategy and Risk of Bias Assessment

This review is based on the suggestions from Munn et al. [19] for systematic reviews with meta-analysis. This review considered studies where the participants stretched the hip flexor muscles exclusively. However, as the biarticular rectus femoris is responsible for hip flexion and knee extension, specific leg extensor stretches were also considered.

An electronic literature search was performed in the following three databases: PubMed, Scopus, and Web of Science. The search period ranged from 1990 until the end of May 2020. The keywords for the online search remained unchanged for all databases and were applied within the title and abstract. The detailed search strategy for each database is presented in Appendix A.

A systematic search was done by two independent researchers (A.K., R.M.). In the first step, all hits were screened by their title. If the content of a study remained unclear, the abstract (and if necessary the full text) was screened to identify relevant papers. Following this independent screening process, the researchers compared their findings. Disagreements were resolved by jointly reassessing the studies against the eligibility criteria. Overall, 2344 papers were screened, from which finally eight papers were found to be eligible for this review. The full search process is illustrated as a flowchart in Figure 1. Additionally, a risk of bias assessment was conducted with the Cochrane risk of bias assessment tool [20]. Table 1 shows a high risk of bias in three out of the eight included studies. Two studies [21,22] had a high risk of selection bias because they followed an intervention protocol without a control group. Moreover, in one study, 10 out of 35 participants could not complete the whole study setup (4 visits) due to sore muscles from the previous visits [23]. Thus, a high risk of attrition bias has to be reported.

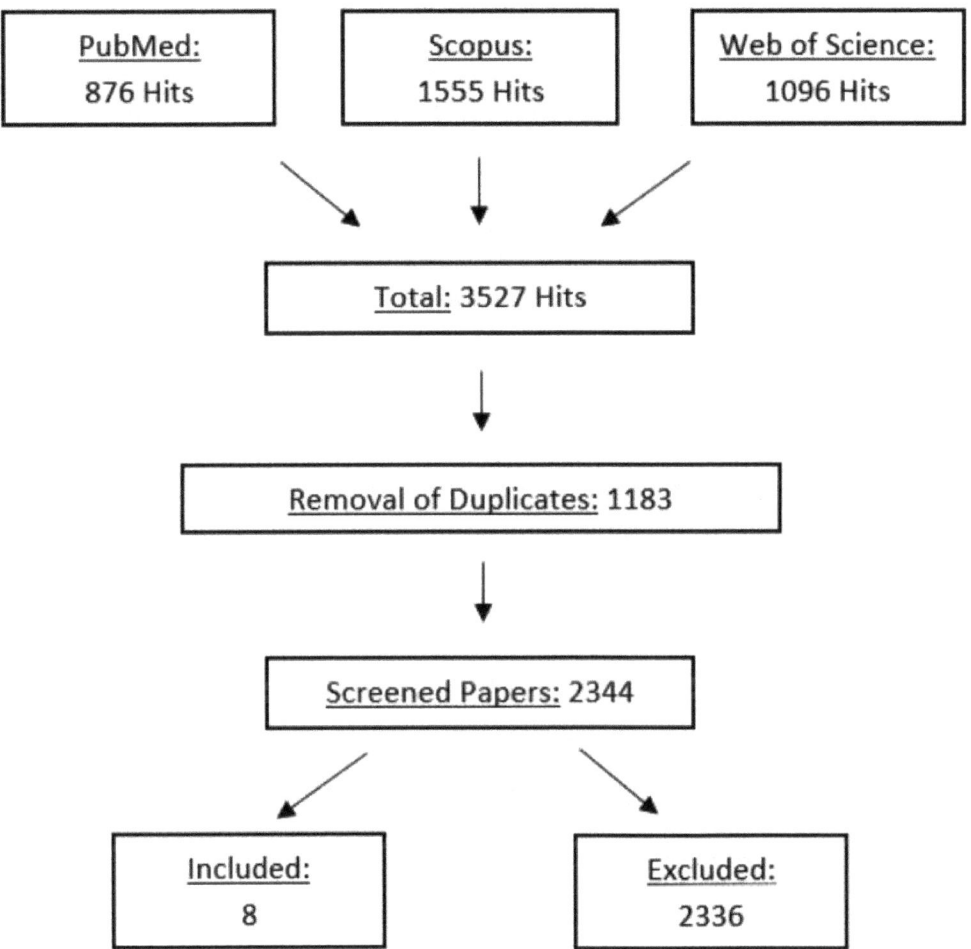

Figure 1. Flowchart of the systematic screening process (PRISMA).

Table 1. Risk of Bias Assessment with the Cochrane Tool.

	Random Sequence Generation (Selection Bias)	Allocation Concealment (Selection Bias)	Blinding of Participants and Personnel (Performance Bias)	Blinding of Outcome Assessment (Detection Bias)	Incomplete Outcome Data (Attrition Bias)	Selective Reporting (Reporting Bias)	Other Bias
Aslan et al. [12]	🟢	🔴	🟡	🟡	🟢	🟡	🟢
Cramer et al. [21]	🔴	🟢	🟡	🟡	🟢	🟡	🟢
Cramer et al. [22]	🟢	🟢	🟡	🟡	🟢	🟡	🟢
Marek et al. [24]	🟢	🟢	🟡	🟡	🔴	🟡	🟢
Wakefield et al. [25]	🟢	🟢	🟢	🟢	🟢	🟡	🟢
Wallmann et al. [23]	🟢	🟢	🟡	🟡	🟢	🟡	🟢
Young et al. [26]	🟢	🟢	🟡	🟡	🟢	🟡	🟢
Zakas et al. [27]	🟢	🟢	🟡	🟡	🟢	🟡	🟢

🟢 Low risk of bias
🟡 Unclear risk of bias
🔴 High risk of bias

2.2. Inclusion/Exclusion Criteria

To be considered useful and therefore selected for this review, a study had to meet the following inclusion criteria: (1) the study was written in English and published after 1990 as an article in a peer-reviewed journal; (2) the study examined the effects of stretching (static, dynamic, PNF, or ballistic) on the hip flexor muscles exclusively; (3) the study was executed with healthy and pain-free individuals; (4) the results must include sport-specific performance parameters (e.g., peak torque, running speed, force production, balance, jump height, and others); and (5) the study had a pre/post stretching intervention design.

Studies were excluded if: (1) the intervention was performed on children or an elderly population; (2) muscles other than the hip flexors were stretched (except for leg extensors in combination with the rectus femoris); and (3) the study only focused on the effects of stretching on flexibility or ROM.

We then categorized the analyzed parameters into the following three groups. Group 1: isokinetic parameters (*peak torque, mean power output, work, joint angle at peak torque, acceleration* tested with an isokinetic dynamometer); Group 2: balance and proprioception parameters (*Y-balance test* [Y-Balance test kit], *joint position sense* [iPod touch device]); Group 3: sport-specific parameters (*sprint time* [electronic timing system], *countermovement jump height* [Vertec system], *foot speed* [high-frequency video camera]). We believed that this classification scheme would help to make the results more applicable, and would therefore allow a better understanding of which kind of sports/performance may be benefited by stretching the hip flexors. The applied tests are standard measures in sport science and showed (where assessable) a high reliability (e.g., isokinetic measures the ICC was >0.93 [21] or Vertex system for counter-movement jump assessment the ICC was 0.88 [25]).

2.3. Data Analysis

Percentage and/or absolute changes of the relevant parameters were extracted from the included studies. Mean values represent the means of the percentage changes weighted by the sample sizes of the respective studies. The 95% confidence interval (CI) and the median (since some data was not normally distributed) were calculated. Individual effect sizes were calculated when absolute mean values and standard deviations were reported based on the suggestions of Cohen [28]. The effect sizes 0.2, 0.5, and 0.8 were defined for a small, medium, and large effect, respectively [28].

Since the Shapiro-Wilk test was significant, a Kruskal-Wallis-test was used to determine the effect between the three stretching durations (defined in clusters. 30–90 s; 120 s; 270–480 s). If the Kruskal-Wallis-test was significant, a Mann-Whitney-U-test was used for pairwise comparisons between these groups. The meta-analysis was performed with the software Comprehensive Meta-Analysis according to the recommendations of Borenstein et al. [29]. Using a random-effects meta-analysis, we assessed the effect in terms of standardized mean difference (SMD). According to the recommendations of Hopkins et al. [30], we defined the effect for the SMD <0.2, 0.2–0.6, 0.6–1.2, 1.2–2.0, 2.0–4.0, >4.0 as trivial, small, moderate, large, very large, extremely large, respectively. I^2 statistics were calculated to assess the heterogeneity among the included studies and thresholds of 25%, 50%, and 75% were defined to be a low, moderate, and high level of heterogeneity, respectively [31,32]. A meta-analysis was only conducted if a sufficient amount of studies ($n \geq 3$) was involved in the analysis. An alpha level of 0.05 was defined for the statistical significance of all the tests.

3. Results

Eight studies of the acute effects of hip flexor stretching were included in this review. These studies included a total of 165 subjects (male: 111; female 54) and applied an average stretching duration of 242 ± 205 s (30 s to 480 s).

Table 2 reports detailed information about the population and the stretching exercises used in the included studies. Table 3 shows the outcomes for all the measured parameters.

Table 2. Summary of the Participants and Intervention Characteristics of the Studies which Investigated the Acute Effects of Hip Flexor Stretching on Performance.

Study	Population			Stretching Intervention			
	Subjects (m/f)	n	Age (Years)	Stretching Type	Stretching Method	Stretching Duration (Total Time)	Stretching Intensity
Aslan et al. [12]	m/f	36 (25/11)	22.37 ± 1.63	PNF (hold-relax)	6 × 20 s [10 s rest]	2 min/leg	<POD
				Dynamic	6 × 10 reps [10 s rest]	2 min/leg	<POD
Cramer et al. [21]	m/f	21 (7/14)	21.5 ± 1.3	Static	Unassisted: 4 × 30 s [20 s rest] + 3 × assisted: 4 × 30 s [20 s rest]	8 min/leg	POMD
Cramer et al. [22]	m/f	18 (8/10)	21.4 ± 3.0/ 23.0 ± 2.9	Static	Unassisted: 4 × 30 s [20 s rest] + 3 × assisted: 4 × 30 s [20 s rest]	8 min/leg	POMD
Marek et al. [24]	m/f	19 (9/10)	21 ±3/23 ± 3	Static	Unassisted: 4 × 30 s [20 s rest] + 3 × assisted: 4 × 30 s [20 s rest]	8 min/leg	POD
				PNF (contract-relax)	Unassisted: 4 × 30 s [20 s rest] + 3 × assisted: 4 × 30 s [20 s rest]	8 min/leg	POD
Wakefield et al. [25]	m	15	24.1 ± 2.4	Static	Assisted: 3 × 30 s [30 s rest]	90 s/leg	POMD
Wallmann et al. [23]	m/f	25 (16/9)	26.76 ± 2.42	Static	2 × 30 s	30 s/leg	<POD
				Dynamic	4 × 15 s	30 s/leg	<POD
				Ballistic	4 × 15 s	30 s/leg	<POD
Young et al. [26]	m	16	18–33	Static	2 × assisted: 6 × 30 s [30 s rest] + unassisted: 6 × 30 s [30 s rest]	4.5 min/leg	<POD
Zakas et al. [27]	m	15	25 ± 1.5	Static	Unassisted: 4 × 15 s [15 s rest]	1 min/leg	<POD
					Unassisted: 4 × 15 s [15 s rest] + assisted: 28 × 15 s [15 s rest]	8 min/leg	<POD

POD = point of discomfort, POMD = point of mild discomfort.

Table 3. Summary of the Results of the Studies which Investigated the Acute Effects of Stretching of the Hip Flexor Muscles.

Study	Stretching Type	Results (Performance)		Results (Range of Motion [°])	
		Outcome (Change in %)	Outcome (Δ-Values)	Hip	Knee
Aslan et al. [12]	PNF (hold-relax)	JPS 30°: ↑15.57% JPS 60°: ↓25.94% Y-Test-A: ↑1.38% Y-Test-PM: ↑2.78% * Y-Test-PL: ↑1.02% *	JPS 30°: ↑0.97 PS 60°: ↓0.55 Y-Test-A: ↑0.94 Y-Test-PM: ↑2.92 * Y-Test-PL: ↑1.15 *	pROM: ↑13.1 *	-
	Dynamic	JPS 30°: ↑7.01% JPS 60°: ↓72.82% Y-Test-A: ↑1.66% Y-Test-PM: ↑5.23% * Y-Test-PL: ↑3.65% *	JPS 30°: ↑0.42 JPS 60°: ↓0.75 Y-Test-A: ↑1.07 Y-Test-PM: ↑5.36 * Y-Test-PL: ↑3.97 *	pROM: ↑5.2 *	-

Table 3. Cont.

Study	Stretching Type	Results (Performance)		Results (Range of Motion [°])	
		Outcome (Change in %)	Outcome (Δ-Values)	Hip	Knee
Cramer et al. [21]	Static	PT 60° s^{-1}: ↓2.72% * PT 240° s^{-1}: ↓4.18% * JAPT 60° s^{-1}: ↓1.56% JAPT 240° s^{-1}: ↑5.97% MP 60° s^{-1}: ↓7.93% MP 240° s^{-1}: ↑2.51%	PT 60° s^{-1}: ↓5.5 * PT 240° s^{-1}: ↓5.7 * JAPT 60° s^{-1}: ↓1.0 JAPT 240° s^{-1}: ↑3.1 MP 60° s^{-1}: ↓10.5 MP 240° s^{-1}: ↑5.9	-	-
Cramer et al. [22]	Static	PT: ↓3% * JAPT: no sign. change MP: no sign. change Acc.: ↓ 17.5% * Results presented as marginal means	nr	-	pROM 60° s^{-1}: no sign. change; pROM 300° s^{-1}: no sign. change
Marek et al. [24]	Static	PT 60° s^{-1}: ↓0.16% PT 300° s^{-1}: ↓1.68% MP 60° s^{-1}: ↓0.37% MP 300° s^{-1}: ↓2.62%	PT 60° s^{-1}: ↓0.3 PT 300° s^{-1}: ↓2.9 MP 60° s^{-1}: ↓0.6 MP 300° s^{-1}: ↓13.4	-	aROM: ↑1.8 * pROM: ↑1.8 *
	PNF (contract-relax)	PT 60° s^{-1}: ↓5.96% * PT 300° s^{-1}: ↓3.17% MP 60° s^{-1}: ↓4.06% MP 300° s^{-1}: ↓4.48%	PT 60° s^{-1}: ↓10.9 PT 300° s^{-1}: ↓3.7 MP 60° s^{-1}: ↓6.6 MP 300° s^{-1}: ↓22.9	-	aROM: ↑1.6 * pROM: ↑0.5 *
Wakefield et al. [25]	Static	CMJ: ↑1.74% *	CMJ: ↑1.02 *	pROM: ↑6.54% *	-
Wallmann et al. [23]	Static	40-yard sprint time: ↓0.17%	40-yard sprint time: ↓0.01	-	-
	Dynamic	40-yard sprint time: ↓0.87%	40-yard sprint time: ↓0.05	-	-
	Ballistic	40-yard sprint time: ↑0.34%	40-yard sprint time: ↑0.02	-	-
Young et al. [26]	Static	Foot speed: ↑0.49%	Foot speed: ↑0.1	pROM: ↑1.4	pROM: ↓1.7
Zakas et al. [27]	Static/1 min	PT 60° s^{-1}: ↓0.28% PT 90° s^{-1}: ↑0.05% PT 150° s^{-1}: ↓0.46% PT 210° s^{-1}: ↓0.61% PT 270° s^{-1}: ↓0.56%	PT 60° s^{-1}: ↓0.6 PT 90° s^{-1}: ↑0.1 PT 150° s^{-1}: ↓0.8 PT 210° s^{-1}: ↓0.9 PT 270° s^{-1}: ↓0.7	-	pROM: ↑4.1
	Static/8 min	PT 60° s^{-1}: ↓5.54% * PT 90° s^{-1}: ↓5.92% * PT 150° s^{-1}: ↓7.22% * PT 210° s^{-1}: ↓6.57% * PT 270° s^{-1}: ↓8.19% *	PT 60° s^{-1}: ↓11.7 * PT 90° s^{-1}: ↓11.8 * PT 150° s^{-1}: ↓12.7 * PT 210° s^{-1}: ↓9.8 * PT 270° s^{-1}: ↓10.4 *	-	pROM: ↑4.3

* = significant change; ↓ = performance decrease; ↑ = performance increase; Acc. = acceleration (ms); aROM = active range of motion (°); CMJ = countermovement jump height (cm); JAPT = joint angle at peak torque (°); JPS = joint position sense; MP = mean power output (W); OL-CMJ = one-leg countermovement jump height (cm); pROM = passive range of motion (°); PT = peak torque (Nm); VI = vascularity index (%); W = work (J); Y-Test-A = Y-balance test anterior (%); Y-Test-PL = Y-balance test posterolateral (%); Y-Test-PM = Y-balance test posteromedial (%); nr = not reported; Note that e.g., °/s = ° s^{-1}.

3.1. Effect of Stretching Duration

The mean, median, and confidence intervals of the weighted percentage changes in performance in the defined clusters of 30–90 s, 120 s, and 270–480 s were −0.12%; −0.28%; CI (95%): −0.49 to 0.41, −5.90%; 2.22%; CI (95%): −22.95 to 5.89, and −3.59%; −3.62% CI (95%): −5.92 to −2.04, respectively. The Kruskal-Wallis-test showed a significant effect between the three stretch durations ($p = 0.006$; H = 10.3). The post-hoc Mann-Whitney-U-test revealed a significant difference between the cluster 30–90 s and 270–480 s ($p = 0.02$), but no significant effect between the other groups. Within the cluster of 30–90 s, one parameter was significantly improved (sport-specific parameters), while the remaining eight were unchanged (5 isokinetic and 3 sport-specific parameters) (see also Table 4 for more information). Within the cluster of 120 s (only balance and proprioception parameters within one study; [12]), four parameters were significantly improved while the remaining six were unchanged. Within the cluster of 270–480 s, seven parameters were unchanged (1 sport-specific parameter and 6 isokinetic parameters), while the remaining 17 showed an impairment (isokinetic parameters only). Figure 2 shows boxplots of the percentage change in the performance parameters (including non-significant results), comparing pre and post values in relation to the stretching durations (30–90 s; 120 s; 270–480 s). In accordance, the meta-analysis showed no significant changes in performance in the cluster 30–90 s stretching, however, a significant decrease in performance in the cluster with a stretching duration between 270 and 480 s (trivial effect size) with all included parameters as well as for peak torque only (small effect size) (see Table 5). Note that 120 s stretching was applied in only one study and hence, no meta-analysis was performed. Moreover, due to technical reasons, the study of Young et al. [26] could not be implemented in the meta-analysis because the authors compared only between the intervention and control group but not within the intervention group.

Table 4. Summary of the Results of the Studies which Investigated the Acute Effects of Stretching of the Hip Flexor Muscles.

Study	Stretching Duration (s)	Stretching Type	Related Group of the Parameter	Change in %	Effect Size
Wallmann et al. [23]	30	Dynamic	sport-specific parameters	−0.87%	0.1
	30	Static	sport-specific parameters	−0.17%	0.02
	30	Ballistic	sport-specific parameters	0.34%	0.04
Zakas et al. [27] *	60	Static	isokinetic parameters	−0.28%	0.02
	60	Static	isokinetic parameters	0.05%	0.003
	60	Static	isokinetic parameters	−0.46%	0.03
	60	Static	isokinetic parameters	−0.61%	0.04
	60	Static	isokinetic parameters	−0.56%	0.04
Wakefield et al. [25]	90	Static	sport-specific parameters	1.74%	na
Aslan et al. [12]	120	Dynamic	balance and proprioception parameters	7.01%	0.14
	120	Dynamic	balance and proprioception parameters	−72.82%	0.28
	120	Dynamic	balance and proprioception parameters	1.66%	0.17
	120	Dynamic	balance and proprioception parameters	5.23%	0.61
	120	Dynamic	balance and proprioception parameters	3.65%	0.44
	120	PNF (hold-relax)	balance and proprioception parameters	15.57%	0.23
	120	PNF (hold-relax)	balance and proprioception parameters	−25.94%	0.15
	120	PNF (hold-relax)	balance and proprioception parameters	1.38%	0.17
	120	PNF (hold-relax)	balance and proprioception parameters	2.78%	0.25
	120	PNF (hold-relax)	balance and proprioception parameters	1.02%	0.11

Table 4. Cont.

Study	Stretching Duration (s)	Stretching Type	Related Group of the Parameter	Change in %	Effect Size
Young et al. [26]	270	Static	sport-specific parameters	0.49%	0.12
Marek et al. [24]	480	PNF (contract-relax)	isokinetic parameters	−5.96%	0.18
	480	PNF (contract-relax)	isokinetic parameters	−3.17%	0.07
	480	PNF (contract-relax)	isokinetic parameters	−4.06%	0.12
	480	PNF (contract-relax)	isokinetic parameters	−4.48%	0.11
	480	Static	isokinetic parameters	−0.16%	0.005
	480	Static	isokinetic parameters	−1.68%	0.04
	480	Static	isokinetic parameters	−0.37%	0.01
	480	Static	isokinetic parameters	−2.62%	0.06
Zakas et al. [27] *	480	Static	isokinetic parameters	−5.54%	0.4
	480	Static	isokinetic parameters	−5.92%	0.41
	480	Static	isokinetic parameters	−7.22%	0.52
	480	Static	isokinetic parameters	−6.57%	0.46
	480	Static	isokinetic parameters	−8.19%	0.65
Cramer et al. [21]	480	Static	isokinetic parameters	−2.72%	0.11
	480	Static	isokinetic parameters	−4.18%	0.14
	480	Static	isokinetic parameters	−1.56%	0.2
	480	Static	isokinetic parameters	5.97%	0.29
	480	Static	isokinetic parameters	−7.93%	0.32
	480	Static	isokinetic parameters	2.51%	0.08
Cramer et al. [22]	480	Static	isokinetic parameters	Not reported	na
	480	Static	isokinetic parameters	Not reported	na
	480	Static	isokinetic parameters	−3.00%	na
	480	Static	isokinetic parameters	−17.50%	na

The results are sorted according to the stretch duration. Green color = significant improvement; Red color = significant impairment; Grey color = no significant Change; na = not available. * = Zakas et al. [27] had two stretch durations (60 s and 480 s).

Table 5. Meta-Analysis of the Effects of the Different Stretching Durations (Clusters 30–90 s and 270–480 s) on Performance Parameters. SDM = Standardized Difference in Means; * = Significant Effect for SDM.

Stretching Duration	N Studies	N Measures	Effect Size				Heterogeneity
			SDM	95% CI	Z	p	I^2
30–90 s	3	9	0.135	[−0.168 to 0.438]	0.874	0.382	11.95%
270–480 s	4	24	−0.19	[−0.379 to 0.000]	−1.959	0.05 *	0.62%
270–480 s (only peak torque)	4	12	−0.206	[−0.385 to −0.027]	−2.257	0.02 *	0.97%

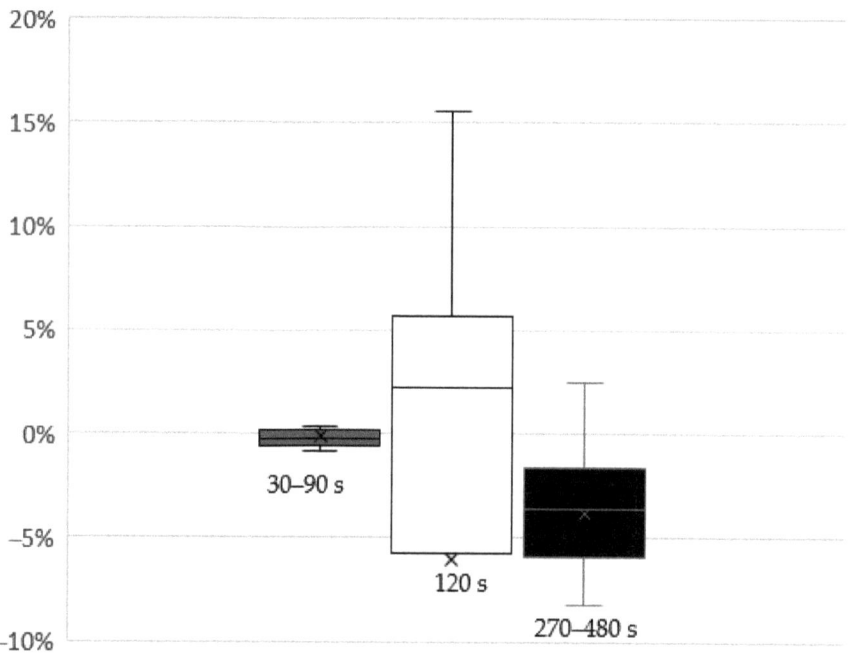

Figure 2. Boxplot diagram of the percentage change in performance parameters in relation to the stretching duration. The grey boxplot represents the parameter changes following a stretching duration of between 30 and 90 s. The white boxplot represents the parameter changes following a stretching duration of 120 s. The black boxplot represents the parameter changes following a stretching duration of between 270 and 480 s. Weighted means are represented by the "×" in or next to the box.

3.2. Effect of Stretching Method

While 27 out of the 43 parameters were tested following a static stretching exercise (in seven studies), nine parameters were tested following PNF stretching (in two studies), and seven were tested following dynamic stretching (in two studies) (see Table 6 for details). With regard to static stretching, only a single measure of vertical jump performance (sport specific parameter) was significantly improved [25], while 13 parameters did not change (11 isokinetic parameters and 2 sport-specific parameters), and 13 parameters (isokinetic parameters only) showed an impairment following the single static stretching exercise. Thus, in summary, the included studies (n = 7) which investigated the effects of static stretching on performance (isokinetic parameters and sport-specific parameters) revealed an average impairment of −2.54% (median: −1.56% CI (95%): −4.48 to −1.05) (see Table 6 for details). A meta-analysis with the static stretching studies showed no significant effect of a single static stretching exercise of the hip flexors on performance (effect size = −0.070 CI (95%) −0.202 to 0.061; Z = −1.048; p = 0.29; I^2 = 27.75%). With regard to PNF stretching two balance and proprioception parameters (*Y-balance test posteromedial* and *Y-balance test posterolateral*) showed a significant improvement, while three showed no change (*joint position sense at 30°, joint position sense at 60°*, and *Y-balance test anterior*) (all balance parameters out of one study), and four isokinetic parameters (*peak torque 60°/s* and *peak torque 300°/s*, *mean power 60°/s*, and *mean power 300°/s*) showed an impairment (all isokinetic measures out of one study). The included studies (n = 2) which investigated the effects of PNF stretching on performance (balance and proprioception parameters and isokinetic parameters revealed an average impairment of −2.59% (median: −3.17% CI (95%): −9.54 to 3.63) (see Table 6 for details). Dynamic stretching led to a significant improvement in two parameters (*Y-balance test posteromedial* and *Y-balance test posterolateral*) and no significant change in the other five tested parameters (*40-yard sprint time, joint position sense at 30°, joint position sense at 60°*, and *Y-balance test anterior*). The included studies (n = 2) which investigated the effects of dynamic stretching on performance (balance and proprioception parameters and sport-specific parameters) revealed an average impairment of −7.06% (median: 1.66% CI (95%): −30.45 to 4.36) (see Table 6 for details). Since only two studies investigated the effects of PNF stretching, dynamic stretching, respectively, no meta-analysis was performed in these groups.

Table 6. Summary of the Results of the Studies which Investigated the Acute Effects of Stretching of the Hip Flexor Muscles.

Study	Stretching Duration (s)	Stretching Type	Related Group of the Parameter	Change in %	Effect Size
Wallmann et al. [23]	30	Ballistic	sport-specific parameters	0.34%	0.04
	30	Dynamic	sport-specific parameters	−0.87%	0.1
Aslan et al. [12]	120	Dynamic	balance and proprioception parameters	7.01%	0.14
	120	Dynamic	balance and proprioception parameters	−72.82%	0.28
	120	Dynamic	balance and proprioception parameters	1.66%	0.17
	120	Dynamic	balance and proprioception parameters	5.23%	0.61
	120	Dynamic	balance and proprioception parameters	3.65%	0.44
	120	PNF (hold-relax)	balance and proprioception parameters	15.57%	0.23
	120	PNF (hold-relax)	balance and proprioception parameters	−25.94%	0.15
	120	PNF (hold-relax)	balance and proprioception parameters	1.38%	0.17
	120	PNF (hold-relax)	balance and proprioception parameters	2.78%	0.25
	120	PNF (hold-relax)	balance and proprioception parameters	1.02%	0.11
Marek et al. [24]	480	PNF (contract-relax)	isokinetic parameters	−5.96%	0.18
	480	PNF (contract-relax)	isokinetic parameters	−3.17%	0.07
	480	PNF (contract-relax)	isokinetic parameters	−4.06%	0.12
	480	PNF (contract-relax)	isokinetic parameters	−4.48%	0.11
Wallmann et al. [23]	30	Static	sport-specific parameters	−0.17%	0.02
Zakas et al. [27]	60	Static	isokinetic parameters	−0.28%	0.02
	60	Static	isokinetic parameters	0.05%	0.003
	60	Static	isokinetic parameters	−0.46%	0.03
	60	Static	isokinetic parameters	−0.61%	0.04
	60	Static	isokinetic parameters	−0.56%	0.04
Wakefield et al. [25]	90	Static	sport-specific parameters	1.74%	na
Young et al. [26]	270	Static	sport-specific parameters	0.49%	0.12

Table 6. Cont.

Study	Stretching Duration (s)	Stretching Type	Related Group of the Parameter	Change in %	Effect Size
Marek et al. [24]	480	Static	isokinetic parameters	−0.16%	0.005
	480	Static	isokinetic parameters	−1.68%	0.04
	480	Static	isokinetic parameters	−0.37%	0.01
	480	Static	isokinetic parameters	−2.62%	0.06
Zakas et al. [27]	480	Static	isokinetic parameters	−5.54%	0.4
	480	Static	isokinetic parameters	−5.92%	0.41
	480	Static	isokinetic parameters	−7.22%	0.52
	480	Static	isokinetic parameters	−6.57%	0.46
	480	Static	isokinetic parameters	−8.19%	0.65
Cramer et al. [21]	480	Static	isokinetic parameters	−2.72%	0.11
	480	Static	isokinetic parameters	−4.18%	0.14
	480	Static	isokinetic parameters	−1.56%	0.2
	480	Static	isokinetic parameters	5.97%	0.29
	480	Static	isokinetic parameters	−7.93%	0.32
	480	Static	isokinetic parameters	2.51%	0.08
Cramer et al. [22]	480	Static	isokinetic parameters	Not reported	na
	480	Static	isokinetic parameters	Not reported	na
	480	Static	isokinetic parameters	−3.00%	na
	480	Static	isokinetic parameters	−17.50%	na

The results are sorted according to the stretching technique. Green color = significant improvement; Red color = significant impairment; Grey color = no significant change; na = not available.

3.3. Effects of Hip Flexor Stretching on Different Aspects/Dimensions of Performance

The eight included studies investigated 43 different performance-related parameters Performance parameters were defined in this review as isokinetic parameters (e.g., *peak torque* and *mean power*), balance and proprioception parameters (e.g., *Y-balance test*), and sport-specific parameters (e.g., *sprint time, countermovement jump height*), but not flexibility (*ROM*). While five parameters showed a significant improvement following a hip flexor stretching exercise (4 balance and proprioception parameters and 1 sport-specific parameter), 21 showed no change (11 isokinetic parameters, 6 balance and proprioception parameters, and 4 sport-specific parameters), and 17 showed impairment in performance (isokinetic parameters only).

3.3.1. Isokinetic Parameters

Four studies investigated the effects of a hip flexor stretching exercise on isokinetic strength parameters. The investigated parameters were *peak torque, mean power output, work, joint angle at peak torque*, and *acceleration*. All four studies reported either a significant decrease (17×) in the measured parameter or no change (11×). On average, the included studies revealed an impairment of −3.22% (median: −2.86%; CI (95%): −5.11 to −1.79). A meta-analysis revealed a significant trivial effect of a single stretching exercise on isokinetic performance parameters (effect size = −0.123; CI (95%) −0.209 to −0.037; Z = −2.812; $p = 0.005$; $I^2 = 0\%$).

3.3.2. Sport-Specific Parameters

Three studies considered sport-specific parameters. These were *sprint time, countermovement jump height*, and *foot speed*. The studies showed either a significant improvement (1×) or no change (4×) in the measured parameters following a single stretching exercise of the hip flexors. The sport-specific parameters revealed an average improvement of 0.16% (median: 0.34%; CI (95%): −0.45 to 1.11). Since only two studies investigated the effects of stretching on sport-specific parameters (the study of Young et al. [26] could have not been included due to technical reasons) no meta-analysis was performed.

3.3.3. Balance and Proprioception Parameters

Only one study tested the effects of a single stretching exercise of the hip flexors on balance and proprioception parameters. The investigated parameters were the *Y-balance test* and *joint position sense*. The study reported either a significant improvement (4×) or no change (6×) following a single stretching exercise of the hip flexors. These parameters revealed an average impairment of −5.90% (median: 2.22%; CI (95%): −22.95 to 5.89) Since only one study investigated the effects of stretching on balance and proprioception parameters, no meta-analysis was performed.

4. Discussion

4.1. Effect of Stretching Duration

With regard to static stretching, Behm and Chaouachi [33] showed in their review that static stretching (independent of which muscle) for more than 90 s has a high probability of decreasing force production and jump height. To rule out the likelihood of strength deficits, the authors suggested limiting static stretching exercises to 30 s or less for each muscle group prior to a task that requires "springiness". A more recent review by Behm et al. [2] reported a greater loss in performance with static stretching of ≥60 s (−4.6%) compared to static stretching of <60 s (−1.1%). In addition, Kay and Blazevich [34] pointed out in their review that, in three-quarters of the involved studies, a static stretching exercise of less than 45 s did not affect muscle strength in terms of measured peak torque. In the studies considered in this review that included stretching for ≤90 s (n = 3), one parameter was significantly improved (sport-specific parameter), while the remaining eight parameters did not change (5 isokinetic parameters and 3 sport-specific parameters) (see also Table 4 for more detail). The average percentage change of all nine parameters with stretching durations for ≤90 s was −0.12% (median: −0.28%; CI (95%): −0.49 to 0.41). Additionally, the meta-analysis showed no significant effect in these nine parameters (see Table 5), which indicates that stretching the hip flexor for ≤90 s will result in neither an improvement nor an impairment in performance parameters. Only one study [12] investigated an intermediate stretching duration of 120 s and included the effects of both dynamic and PNF stretching exercises on balance and proprioception (see also Table 4 for more detail). In this review, out of the 10 considered measures, four showed a significant improvement (*Y-balance test posteromedial and Y-balance test posterolateral* in the dynamic stretching group, PNF stretching group, respectively), while the remaining six were unchanged (*joint position sense at 30°, joint position sense at 60°, and Y-balance test anterior* in the dynamic stretching group, PNF stretching group, respectively). However, on average, there was an average impairment of all 10 parameters (mean: −5.90%; median: 2.22%; CI (95%): −22.95 to 5.89). This can be explained by the high percentage changes (however not significant) since the baseline values of the *joint position sense* parameter were close to zero. Thus, minor absolute changes of this parameter led to high percentage changes. Hence, the averaged results of this review, with regard to balance and proprioception, and also PNF and dynamic stretching, should be viewed with caution. By excluding the *joint position sense* parameter, the average change due to hip flexor stretching on balance and proprioception would be an improvement of 3.44% (median: 2.22%; CI (95%): 1.54 to 3.95), instead of an impairment of −5.90% (median: 2.22%; CI (95%): −22.95 to 5.89). When longer stretching durations (270–480 s) were applied, seven out of the 24 parameters showed no significant change and 17 parameters showed a significant impairment, which is reflected in the average percentage change of −3.59 (median −3.62% CI (95%): −5.92 to −2.04) (see also Table 4 for details) and a significant effect in the meta-analysis (see also Table 5). However, the results of the meta-analysis revealed a trivial effect (SMD = −0.19) only, and hence, caution must be taken to not overemphasize this result. Zakas et al. [27] was the only study that compared the effect of a single short-duration static stretching exercise (60 s) to that of a longer-duration exercise (480 s). They reported no significant changes in quadriceps isokinetic peak torque following the short hip flexor stretching exercise, whereas they did find significant decreases in isokinetic peak torque following the longer-duration exercise. This result was confirmed by the comparison of the effects on performance between the three defined stretch durations (30–90s; 120 s; 270–480 s) in this review. The shortest stretch duration (30–90 s) was significantly different from the longest stretch duration (270–480 s) (see Figure 2). This finding, the findings from the meta-analysis (see Table 5), and the findings from Zakas et al. [27] suggest a similar dose-response relationship between stretching duration and performance for the hip flexor muscle and other lower leg muscles (e.g., plantar flexor muscles), as reported by several reviews [2,33,34]. A possible mechanism for such a dose-response relationship might be found in the decrease in muscle stiffness following stretching durations ≥120 s (e.g., [35,36]), whilst shorter durations (e.g. 60 s) did not lead to changes in muscle stiffness [37].

In summary, the existing data provide evidence that a single bout of hip flexor stretching of up to 120 s can have a positive effect on balance [12] and jump performance [25]. Moreover, up to a stretching duration of 120 s, no detrimental effect has been reported in the studies dealing with a sport-specific performance [23], balance [12], or isokinetic parameters [27], regardless of the stretching techniques used. In contrast to other muscle groups where 120 s of stretching likely decreases force production (e.g., plantar flexors [38]), it seems likely that isolated hip flexor stretching with a moderate duration of up to 120 s has no detrimental effect or even a positive impact on performance-related parameters. This difference might at one hand be explained in the special characteristic of the hip flexor muscles. Compared to other lower limb muscles the hip flexor muscles, especially the iliopsoas, have a major function in lumbar spine stability [6] and hence, too-tight hip flexors can lead to a disadvantageous position of the pelvis. Consequently, this can cause muscle fatigue and can negatively affect movement patterns [11,12] and hence lead to major impairment in performance [9]. On the other hand, the tested movements that showed improvements (running, jumping) are rather characterized by hip extensions than hip flexing. Therefore, the hip flexors are not the main contributors but rather improve the movement conditions for the agonist muscles. It should be, however, noted that hip flexor stretching led to decreases, when tests directly measured hip flexion performance, e.g. peak torque. It can be therefore assumed that even longer stretching durations (≥60 s [2]) of the hip flexors, which are generally suggested to decrease performance do not necessarily lead to detrimental effects in movements where hip flexors are not the main movers.

Although the evidence is based on a small number of studies, this information will be of great importance for both athletes and coaches.

4.2. Effect of Stretching Method

All three investigated stretching techniques can lead to an impairment in performance following a single hip flexor stretching exercise. While dynamic stretching showed the greatest average impairment of all the parameters (−7.06% (median: 1.66% CI (95%): −30.45 to 4.36); average stretch duration: 94.2 s), PNF stretching and static stretching showed similar average impairments (PNF: −2.59% (median: −3.17% CI (95%): −9.54 to 3.63); average stretch duration: 280 s; static: −2.54% (median: −1.56% CI (95%): −4.48 to −1.05); average stretch duration: 363.3 s). At first glance, this goes against the findings of Behm et al. [2], who reported mean performance impairments of 3.7% and 4.4% immediately after static stretching and PNF stretching, respectively, but an increase in performance of 1.3% after dynamic stretching. However, removing the results of the *joint position sense* parameter, because of its high and misleading percentage change (since the values are close to zero), leads to more credible average changes of −2.54%, +1.64%, and −1.878% for static, dynamic, and PNF stretching, respectively. Thus, this small increase in performance following dynamic stretching and impairments following static and PNF stretching would underline the findings of Behm et al. [2].

Two studies included in this review compared the effects of different stretching methods. Wallmann et al. [23] compared the effects of single bouts of static, dynamic, or ballistic stretching of the hip flexors on the *40-yard sprint time* (sport-specific parameter). They found no significant difference between pre and post values within the two techniques, but a significant reduction in *sprint time* following a conventional warm-up without stretching. Aslan et al. [12] compared the effects of 120 s of dynamic and PNF stretching of the hip flexors on the *Y-balance test* (balance and proprioception parameter). Although both techniques were shown to be an effective way to improve balance parameters, the PNF technique provided greater positive effects than dynamic stretching [12]. This is in contrast to the findings of Behm et al. [2] on strength tasks, who reported an impairment of 4.4% following PNF stretching, but an increase in performance following a dynamic stretching protocol. Although strength and balance are related [39], an acute bout of stretching has different impacts on balance and strength parameters [40]. Thus, it can be assumed that the findings of Behm et al. [2] about strength tasks and the findings of Aslan et al. [12] about balance tasks are not totally comparable. Moreover, in the review of Behm et al. [2], the results were based on the stretching of several lower leg muscles, and this might not be valid for isolated stretching exercises for the hip flexor muscles, as presented in this review.

Most of the included studies (six out of eight) investigated the effects of a static stretching exercise of the hip flexors on performance and reported an average decrease of −2.54% (median: −1.56% CI (95%): −4.48 to −1.05 (see also Table 6 for more detail). However, no significant effect was shown in the meta-analysis (effect size = −0.070; CI (95%) −0.202 to 0.061; $Z = -1.048$; $p = 0.29$; $I^2 = 27.75\%$), indicating that this impairment was not significant. With regard to dynamic stretching the exclusion of the *joint position sense* parameter from the analysis in the study of Aslan et al. [12] changes the result substantially into an average improvement of 1.64%. However, since only five parameters (3 balance and proprioception parameters and 2 sport-specific parameters) out of two studies [12,23] were included in this analysis, these results should not be generalized and have to be interpreted with caution.

4.3. Effects of Hip Flexor Stretching on Different Aspects/Dimensions of Performance

4.3.1. Isokinetic Parameters

The included studies which investigated the effects of a hip flexor stretching exercise on isokinetic strength parameters [21,22,24,27] reported either a decrease in the measured parameters or no change. This resulted in an average impairment of −3.22% (median: −2.86%; CI (95%): −5.11 to −1.79). Although the meta-analysis revealed that this change was significant, the magnitude showed a trivial effect only (effect size = −0.123; CI (95%) −0.209 to −0.037; $Z = -2.812$; $p = 0.005$; $I^2 = 0\%$). However, it should be mentioned that the studies which included isokinetic parameters mainly used stretching durations of 480 s [21,22,24], which was likely the underlying reason for the decrease in performance (see the review of Behm et al. [2]). This is supported by the study of Zakas et al. [27], who reported no change in quadriceps isokinetic performance following 60 s of static stretching, while 480 s of static stretching caused a decrease in performance. This has also been observed in similar studies of the plantar flexors, where static stretching of the calf muscles for 1 min [37] and 3 min [36] did not induce changes in maximum voluntary isometric contraction (MVC), while 5 min of static stretching caused a decrease [41].

4.3.2. Sport-Specific Parameters

The sport-specific parameters such as *sprint time, countermovement jump height*, and *foot speed* investigated in three studies showed either an improvement or no change in performance, which resulted in an average improvement of 0.16% (median: 0.34%; CI (95%): −0.45 to 1.11). Since only five parameters were considered in the different stretching techniques (static (n = 3); dynamic (n = 2)), and durations ranging from 30 to 270 s were tested, no general conclusion should be made from this data. Wallmann et al. [23] compared the effects of single bouts of static, dynamic, or ballistic stretching of the hip flexors on the *40-yard sprint time*. They found no significant difference between pre and post values within the techniques, but a significant reduction in *sprint time* following a conventional warm-up without stretching. This result suggests that a warm-up including stretching of the hip flexors increases the chance of performance improvement. In addition,

Behm et al. [2] concluded that post-stretching dynamic activities are able to counteract possible detrimental effects on performance following stretching, leading to a positive effect on performance. Thus, several authors have suggested including post-stretching dynamic activities in the warm-up regimes of athletes (see Behm et al. [2] for a review).

4.3.3. Balance and Proprioception Parameters

The data of one study [12] showed that 120 s of hip flexor stretching can either improve or does not change balance and proprioception parameters. The average change of −5.90% (median: 2.22%; CI (95%): −22.95 to 5.89) indicates an overall impairment due to stretching. However, the results were substantially affected by the *joint position sense* parameter, due to its high percentage change (since the values were close to zero). Excluding this parameter changes the average impairment of −5.90% (median: 2.22%; CI (95%): −22.95 to 5.89) to an improvement of 3.44% (median: 2.22%; CI (95%): 1.54 to 3.95). Behm et al. [41] reported a decrease in balance and proprioception (compared to the control condition) following a 3 × 45 s static stretching exercise of the quadriceps, but also the hamstrings and plantar flexors. Since Aslan et al. [12] reported an improvement in some balance parameters following 120 s of stretching of the hip flexors, it can be speculated that stretching of the hip flexors has no adverse effect on balance. This is supported by Costa et al. [42], who found an improvement in the balance score following short-duration stretches (3 × 15 s), while the more prolonged stretching duration (3 × 45 s) did not cause balance performance changes.

A possible limitation of this review was that three out of the eight studies showed a high risk of bias (see Table 1 for details). Two studies [21,22] followed an intervention protocol without a control group which represents a high risk of selection bias. Moreover, in one study 10 out of 35 participants could not complete the whole study setup (4 visits) due to sore muscles from the previous visits [23]. Thus, a high risk of attrition bias has to be reported. However, these studies reported high reliability of their data, and hence, at least the measurement itself can be considered of high quality. Although significant effects were reported in some meta-analyses, the magnitudes of the effects were only trivial or small. Thus, caution must be taken not to overemphasize these results. However, we are confident that this systematic review with meta-analysis will be of great importance to get an overview on this topic and helps to develop further research hypotheses and projects.

5. Conclusions

The existing data provides evidence that a single bout of hip flexor stretching of up to 120 s can have a positive effect on balance (following dynamic stretching or PNF stretching) [12] and jump performance (following static stretching) [25]. Moreover, up to a stretching duration of 120 s, no detrimental effect has been reported in the studies dealing with sports-related performances [23], balance [12], or isokinetic parameters [27], regardless of the stretching techniques used. In contrast to other muscle groups such as the plantar flexors [38], where 120 s of stretching likely decreases force production, it seems likely that isolated hip flexor stretching of up to 120 s has no effect or even a positive impact on performance-related parameters. This difference might be explained by the specific function of the hip flexor muscles for lumbar spine stability. While too-tight hip flexors can lead to a disadvantageous position of the pelvis, stretching will lead to a more advantageous position of the lumbar spine and the pelvis. A comparison of the effects on performance between the three defined stretch durations (30–90 s; 120 s; 270–480 s) revealed a significantly different change in performance ($p = 0.02$) between the lowest hip flexor stretch duration (30–90 s; performance change: mean: −0.12%; median: −0.28%; CI (95%): −0.49 to 0.41) and the highest hip flexor stretch duration (270–480 s; performance change: mean −3.59%; median: −3.62% CI (95%): −5.92 to −2.04). Moreover, meta-analysis reported a significant impairment (but with a trivial effect size only) in the highest hip flexor stretch duration (270–480 s), whilst no significant effect was reported in the lowest hip flexor stretch duration (30–90 s) (see Table 5). This additionally indicates a dose-response relationship in the hip flexor muscles. Although the evidence is based on a small amount of studies, this information will be of great importance for both athletes and coaches. Based on our findings it can be recommended to stretch the hip flexor up to 120 s to improve performance, especially in sports where a high range of motion in the hip extension is required (e.g., dancing, gymnastics). Additionally, hip flexor stretching can be a preventive approach against injuries. Especially soccer players with tight hip flexors might benefit since tight hip flexors lead to greater activation of the synergistic rectus femoris which likely leads to overloads and/or fatigue of the muscle [43].

However, the limited amount of studies about the acute effects of PNF stretching (n = 2) and dynamic stretching (n = 2) on performance does not allow a clear conclusion to be made as to which stretching technique should be preferably applied to avoid performance impairment.

6. Perspective

While this review has shed some light on the effects of hip flexor stretching on performance, including some positive but also negative effects, more studies are needed to obtain a clearer picture of the effects of the various techniques and the dose-response relationship.

In addition to the immediate effect of a bout of stretching, it is also of great importance to understand the long-term effect of prolonged stretching training. Especially with regard to flexibility, it has been shown that repeated single stretches of a muscle-tendon unit can lead to enhanced flexibility in the long term. However, to date, only one study has investigated the effects of a hip flexion stretching intervention over 3 weeks on passive and sport-related flexibility and related kinematic changes of the lumbo-pelvic-hip complex during running [16]. The authors reported that an increase in passive hip extension flexibility cannot be transferred to an active movement during running. No studies are available that have investigated long-term hip flexor stretching training and its effects on lower back pain, the prevalence of injuries, and performance. Therefore, we strongly recommend long-term studies of hip flexor stretching in the future.

Author Contributions: A.K., R.M., and M.N. collaborated in the literature review and producing figures and tables. A.K., M.N., and M.T. collaborated in writing the manuscript. S.T., A.K. contributed in the meta-analysis. All authors contributed to the article and approved the submitted version. All authors have read and agreed to the published version of the manuscript.

Funding: This study was supported by a grant (Project P 32078-B) from the Austrian Science Fund FWF.

Institutional Review Board Statement: Not applicable.

Informed Consent Statement: Not applicable.

Data Availability Statement: All data generated or analyzed during this study are included in this published article.

Acknowledgments: Open Access Funding by the Austrian Science Fund (FWF) from by a grant (Project P 32078-B).

Conflicts of Interest: The authors declare no conflict of interest.

Appendix A

PubMed:

(((stretch * [Title/Abstract] OR mobility [Title/Abstract] OR flexibility [Title/Abstract] OR "range of motion" [Title/Abstract] OR rom [Title/Abstract]) AND ("hip joint" [Title/Abstract] OR pelvis [Title/Abstract] OR iliacus [Title/Abstract] OR "psoas major" [Title/Abstract] OR "rectus femoris" [Title/Abstract] OR iliopsoas [Title/Abstract] OR "hip flexor *" [Title/Abstract] OR "hip extension" [Title/Abstract])) AND (sport * [Title/Abstract] OR performance [Title/Abstract] OR jump * [Title/Abstract] OR run * [Title/Abstract] OR swim * [Title/Abstract] OR cycl * [Title/Abstract] OR bike * [Title/Abstract] OR strength [Title/Abstract] OR activation [Title/Abstract] OR sprint * [Title/Abstract] OR economy [Title/Abstract] OR mvc [Title/Abstract] OR "maximum voluntary contraction" [Title/Abstract] OR power [Title/Abstract] OR "stride length" [Title/Abstract] OR force [Title/Abstract] OR speed [Title/Abstract])) NOT (disease [Title/Abstract] OR palsy [Title/Abstract] OR syndrome [Title/Abstract] OR elderly [Title/Abstract] OR "back pain" [Title/Abstract]).

Scopus:

TITLE-ABS-KEY (*stretch* *) OR TITLE-ABS-KEY (*mobility*) OR TITLE-ABS-KEY (*flexibility*) OR TITLE-ABS-KEY (*"range of motion"*) OR TITLE-ABS-KEY (*rom*) AND TITLE-ABS-KEY (*"hip joint"*) OR TITLE-ABS-KEY (*pelvis*) OR TITLE-ABS-KEY (*iliacus*) OR TITLE-ABS-KEY (*"psoas major"*) OR TITLE-ABS-KEY (*"rectus femoris"*) OR TITLE-ABS-KEY (*iliopsoas*) OR TITLE-ABS-KEY (*"hip flexor *"*) OR TITLE-ABS-KEY (*"hip extension"*) AND TITLE-ABS-KEY (*sport* *) OR TITLE-ABS-KEY (*performance*) OR TITLE-ABS-KEY (*jump* *) OR TITLE-ABS-KEY (*run* *) OR TITLE-ABS-KEY (*swim* *) OR TITLE-ABS-KEY (*cycl* *) OR TITLE-ABS-KEY (*bike* *) OR TITLE-ABS-KEY (*strength*) OR TITLE-ABS-KEY (*activation*) OR TITLE-ABS-KEY (*sprint* *) OR TITLE-ABS-KEY (*economy*) OR TITLE-ABS-KEY (*mvc*) OR TITLE-ABS-KEY (*"maximum voluntary contraction"*) OR TITLE-ABS-KEY (*power*) OR TITLE-ABS-KEY (*"stride length"*) OR TITLE-ABS-KEY (*force*) OR TITLE-ABS-KEY (*speed*), AND NOT TITLE-ABS-KEY (*disease*) OR TITLE-ABS-KEY (*palsy*) OR TITLE-ABS-KEY (*syndrome*) OR TITLE-ABS-KEY (*elderly*) OR TITLE-ABS-KEY (*"back pain"*) AND (EXCLUDE (SUBJAREA, "ENGI") OR EXCLUDE (SUBJAREA, "COMP") OR EXCLUDE (SUBJAREA, "AGRI") OR EXCLUDE (SUBJAREA, "MATE") OR EXCLUDE (SUBJAREA, "CENG") OR EXCLUDE (SUBJAREA, "SOCI") OR EXCLUDE (SUBJAREA, "MATH") OR EXCLUDE (SUBJAREA, "VETE") OR EXCLUDE (SUBJAREA, "PHYS") OR EXCLUDE (SUBJAREA, "ENVI") OR EXCLUDE (SUBJAREA, "IMMU") OR EXCLUDE (SUBJAREA, "ARTS") OR EXCLUDE (SUBJAREA, "PHAR") OR EXCLUDE (SUBJAREA, "CHEM") OR EXCLUDE (SUBJAREA, "EART") OR EXCLUDE (SUBJAREA, "ENER") OR EXCLUDE (SUBJAREA, "DENT") OR EXCLUDE (SUBJAREA, "BUSI") OR EXCLUDE (SUBJAREA, "DECI") OR EXCLUDE (SUBJAREA, "BIOC")) AND (LIMIT-TO (PUBYEAR, 2020) OR LIMIT-TO (PUBYEAR, 2019) OR LIMIT-TO (PUBYEAR, 2018) OR LIMIT-TO (PUBYEAR, 2017) OR LIMIT-TO (PUBYEAR, 2016) OR LIMIT-TO (PUBYEAR, 2015) OR LIMIT-TO (PUBYEAR, 2014) OR LIMIT-TO (PUBYEAR, 2013) OR LIMIT-TO (PUBYEAR, 2012) OR LIMIT-TO (PUBYEAR, 2011) OR LIMIT-TO (PUBYEAR, 2010) OR LIMIT-TO (PUBYEAR, 2009) OR LIMIT-TO (PUBYEAR, 2008) OR LIMIT-TO (PUBYEAR, 2007) OR LIMIT-TO (PUBYEAR, 2006) OR LIMIT-TO (PUBYEAR, 2005) OR LIMIT-TO (PUBYEAR, 2004) OR LIMIT-TO (PUBYEAR, 2003) OR LIMIT-TO (PUBYEAR, 2002) OR LIMIT-TO (PUBYEAR, 2001) OR LIMIT-TO (PUBYEAR, 2000) OR LIMIT-TO (PUBYEAR, 1999) OR LIMIT-TO (PUBYEAR, 1998) OR LIMIT-TO (PUBYEAR, 1997) OR LIMIT-TO (PUBYEAR, 1996) OR LIMIT-TO (PUBYEAR, 1995) OR LIMIT-TO (PUBYEAR, 1994) OR LIMIT-TO (PUBYEAR, 1993) OR LIMIT-TO (PUBYEAR, 1992) OR LIMIT-TO (PUBYEAR, 1991) OR LIMIT-TO (PUBYEAR, 1990)) AND (LIMIT-TO (LANGUAGE, "English")).

Web of Science:

TS = (stretch * OR mobility OR flexibility OR "range of motion" OR rom) AND TS = ("hip joint" OR pelvis OR iliacus OR "psoas major" OR "rectus femoris" OR iliopsoas OR "hip flexor*" OR "hip extension") AND TS = (sport * OR performance OR jump * OR run * OR swim * OR cycl * OR bike * OR strength OR activation OR sprint * OR economy OR mvc OR "maximum voluntary contraction" OR power OR "stride length" or force OR speed) NOT TS = (disease OR palsy OR syndrome OR elderly OR "back pain").

References

1. McHugh, M.P.; Cosgrave, C.H. To Stretch or Not to Stretch: The Role of Stretching in Injury Prevention and Performance. *Scand. J. Med. Sci. Sports* **2010**, *20*, 169–181. [CrossRef]
2. Behm, D.G.; Blazevich, A.J.; Kay, A.D.; McHugh, M. Acute Effects of Muscle Stretching on Physical Performance, Range of Motion, and Injury Incidence in Healthy Active Individuals: A Systematic Review. *Appl. Physiol. Nutr. Metab.* **2016**, *41*, 1–11. [CrossRef]

3. Konrad, A.; Budini, F.; Tilp, M. Acute Effects of Constant Torque and Constant Angle Stretching on the Muscle and Tendon Tissue Properties. *Eur. J. Appl. Physiol.* **2017**, *117*, 1649–1656. [CrossRef]
4. Salamh, P.A.; Kolber, M.J.; Hegedus, E.J.; Cook, C.E. The Efficacy of Stretching Exercises to Reduce Posterior Shoulder Tightness Acutely in the Postoperative Population: A Single Blinded Randomized Controlled Trial. *Physiother. Theory Pract.* **2018**, *34*, 111–120. [CrossRef] [PubMed]
5. Bhimani, R.; Gaugler, J.E.; Felts, J. Consensus Definition of Muscle Tightness from Multidisciplinary Perspectives. *Nurs. Res.* **2020**, *69*, 109–115. [CrossRef] [PubMed]
6. Juker, D.; McGill, S.; Kropf, P.; Steffen, T. Quantitative Intramuscular Myoelectric Activity of Lumbar Portions of Psoas and the Abdominal Wall During a Wide Variety of Tasks. *Med. Sci. Sports Exerc.* **1998**, *30*, 301–310. [CrossRef]
7. Ingber, R.S. Iliopsoas Myofascial Dysfunction: A Treatable Cause of "Failed" Low Back Syndrome. *Arch. Phys. Med. Rehabil.* **1989**, *70*, 382–386.
8. Avrahami, D.; Potvin, J.R. The Clinical and Biomechanical Effects of Fascialmuscular Lengthening Therapy on Tight Hip Flexor Patients with and without Low Back Pain. *J. Can. Chiropr. Assoc.* **2014**, *58*, 444–455.
9. Masset, D.F.; Piette, A.G.; Malchaire, J.B. Undefined Relation between Functional Characteristics of the Trunk and the Occurrence of Low Back Pain: Associated Risk Factors. *Spine* **1998**, *23*, 359–365. [CrossRef] [PubMed]
10. Endo, Y.; Sakamoto, M. Relationship between Lower Extremity Tightness and Star Excursion Balance Test Performance in Junior High School Baseball Players. *J. Phys. Ther. Sci.* **2014**, *26*, 661–663. [CrossRef]
11. Krivickas, L.S.; Feinberg, J.H. Lower Extremity Injuries in College Athletes: Relation between Ligamentous Laxity and Lower Extremity Muscle Tightness. *Arch. Phys. Med. Rehabil.* **1996**, *77*, 1139–1143. [CrossRef]
12. Younis Aslan, H.I.; Buddhadev, H.H.; Suprak, D.N.; San Juan, J.G. Acute Effects of Two Hip Flexor Stretching Techniques on Knee Joint Position Sense and Balance. *Int. J. Sports Phys. Ther.* **2018**, *13*, 846–859. [CrossRef]
13. Mills, M.; Frank, B.; Goto, S.; Blackburn, T.; Cates, S.; Clark, M.; Aguilar, A.; Fava, N.; Padua, D. Effect of Restricted Hip Flexor Muscle Length on Hip Extensor Muscle Activity and Lower Extremity Biomechanics in College-Aged Female Soccer Players. *Int. J. Sports Phys. Ther.* **2015**, *10*, 946–954.
14. Pate, R.R.; Mitchell, J.A.; Byun, W.; Dowda, M. Sedentary Behaviour in Youth. *Br. J. Sports Med.* **2011**, *45*, 906–913. [CrossRef]
15. Harvey, J.A.; Chastin, S.F.M.; Skelton, D.A. Prevalence of Sedentary Behavior in Older Adults: A Systematic Review. *Int. J. Environ. Res. Public Health* **2013**, *10*, 6645–6661. [CrossRef]
16. Mettler, J.H.; Shapiro, R.; Pohl, M.B. Effects of a Hip Flexor Stretching Program on Running Kinematics in Individuals With Limited Passive Hip Extension. *J. Strength Cond. Res.* **2019**, *33*, 3338–3344. [CrossRef] [PubMed]
17. Konrad, A.; Tilp, M. Increased Range of Motion after Static Stretching Is Not due to Changes in Muscle and Tendon Structures. *Clin. Biomech.* **2014**, *29*, 636–642. [CrossRef] [PubMed]
18. Starrett, K.; Cordoza, G. *Becoming a Supple Leopard 2nd Edition: The Ultimate Guide to Resolving Pain, Preventing Injury, Andoptimizing Athletic Performance*; Victory Belt Publishing: Las Vegas, NV, USA, 2015.
19. Munn, Z.; Peters, M.D.J.; Stern, C.; Tufanaru, C.; McArthur, A.; Aromataris, E. Systematic Review or Scoping Review? Guidance for Authors When Choosing between a Systematic or Scoping Review Approach. *BMC Med. Res. Methodol.* **2018**, *18*. [CrossRef] [PubMed]
20. Higgins, J.P.T.; Altman, D.G.; Gøtzsche, P.C.; Jüni, P.; Moher, D.; Oxman, A.D.; Savović, J.; Schulz, K.F.; Weeks, L.; Sterne, J.A.C. The Cochrane Collaboration's Tool for Assessing Risk of Bias in Randomised Trials. *Bmj* **2011**, *18*, 143. [CrossRef]
21. Cramer, J.T.; Housh, T.J.; Weir, J.P.; Johnson, G.O.; Coburn, J.W.; Beck, T.W. The Acute Effects of Static Stretching on Peak Torque, Mean Power Output, Electromyography, and Mechanomyography. *Eur. J. Appl. Physiol.* **2005**, *93*, 530–539. [CrossRef]
22. Cramer, J.; Beck, T.; Housh, T.; Massey, L.; Marek, S.; Danglemeier, S.; Purkayastha, S.; Culbertson, J.; Fitz, K.; Egan, A. Acute Effects of Static Stretching on Characteristics of the Isokinetic Angle-Torque Relationship, Surface Electromyography, and Mechanomyography. *J. Sports Sci.* **2007**, *25*, 687–698. [CrossRef]
23. Wallmann, H.W.; Christensen, S.D.; Perry, C. The Acute Effects of Various Types of Stretching Static, Dynamic, Ballistic, and No Stretch of the Iliopsoas on 40-Yard Sprint Times in Recreational Runners. *Int. J. Sports Phys. Ther.* **2012**, *7*, 540–547.
24. Marek, S.M.; Cramer, J.T.; Fincher, A.L.; Massey, L.L.; Dangelmaier, S.M.; Purkayastha, S.; Fitz, K.A.; Culbertson, J.Y. Acute Effects of Static and Proprioceptive Neuromuscular Facilitation Stretching on Muscle Strength and Power Output. *J. Athl. Train.* **2005**, *40*, 94–103. [PubMed]
25. Wakefield, C.B.; Cottrell, G.T. Changes in Hip Flexor Passive Compliance Do Not Account for Improvement in Vertical Jump Performance after Hip Flexor Static Stretching. *J. Strength Cond. Res.* **2015**, *29*, 1601–1608. [CrossRef]
26. Young, W.; Clothier, P.; Otago, L.; Bruce, L.; Liddell, D. Acute Effects of Static Stretching on Hip Flexor and Quadriceps Flexibility, Range of Motion and Foot Speed in Kicking a Football. *J. Sci. Med. Sport* **2004**, *7*, 23–31. [CrossRef]
27. Zakas, A.; Galazoulas, C.; Doganis, G.; Zakas, N. Effect of Two Acute Static Stretching Durations of the Rectus Femoris Muscle on Quadriceps Isokinetic Peak Torque in Professional Soccer Players. *Isokinet. Exerc. Sci.* **2006**, *14*, 357–362. [CrossRef]
28. Cohen, J. *Statistical Power Analysis for the Behavioral Sciences*, 2nd ed.; Department of Psychology, New York University: New York, NY, USA, 1988.
29. Borenstein, M.; Hedges, L.V.; Higgins, J.P.T.; Rothstein, H.R. *Introduction to Meta-Analysis*; Borenstein, M., Ed.; Wiley: Hoboken, NJ, USA, 2009; ISBN 9780470057247.

30. Hopkins, W.G.; Marshall, S.W.; Batterham, A.M.; Hanin, J. Progressive Statistics for Studies in Sports Medicine and Exercise Science. *Med. Sci. Sport. Exerc.* **2009**, *41*, 3–13. [CrossRef] [PubMed]
31. Higgins, J.P.T.; Thompson, S.G.; Deeks, J.J.; Altman, D.G. Measuring Inconsistency in Meta-Analyses. *Br. Med. J.* **2003**, *327*, 557–560. [CrossRef] [PubMed]
32. Behm, D.G.; Alizadeh, S.; Anvar, S.H.; Drury, B.; Granacher, U.; Moran, J. Non-Local Acute Passive Stretching Effects on Range of Motion in Healthy Adults: A Systematic Review with Meta-Analysis. *Sports Med.* **2021**. [CrossRef]
33. Behm, D.G.; Chaouachi, A. A Review of the Acute Effects of Static and Dynamic Stretching on Performance. *Eur. J. Appl. Physiol.* **2011**, *111*, 2633–2651. [CrossRef]
34. Kay, A.D.; Blazevich, A.J. Effect of Acute Static Stretch on Maximal Muscle Performance: A Systematic Review. *Med. Sci. Sport. Exerc.* **2012**, *44*, 154–164. [CrossRef] [PubMed]
35. Konrad, A.; Reiner, M.M.; Thaller, S.; Tilp, M. The Time Course of Muscle-Tendon Properties and Function Responses of a Five-Minute Static Stretching Exercise. *Eur. J. Sport Sci.* **2019**, *19*. [CrossRef]
36. Konrad, A.; Tilp, M. The Time Course of Muscle-Tendon Unit Function and Structure Following Three Minutes of Static Stretching. *J. Sports Sci. Med.* **2020**, *19*, 52–58.
37. Konrad, A.; Tilp, M. The Acute Time Course of Muscle and Tendon Tissue Changes Following One Minute of Static Stretching. *Curr. Issues Sport Sci.* **2020**, *5*, 63–78. [CrossRef]
38. Konrad, A.; Stafilidis, S.; Tilp, M. Effects of Acute Static, Ballistic, and PNF Stretching Exercise on the Muscle and Tendon Tissue Properties. *Scand. J. Med. Sci. Sports* **2017**, *27*, 1070–1080. [CrossRef] [PubMed]
39. Wilson, B.R.; Robertson, K.E.; Burnham, J.M.; Yonz, M.C.; Ireland, M.L.; Noehren, B. The Relationship Between Hip Strength and the Y Balance Test. *J. Sport Rehabil.* **2018**, *27*, 445–450. [CrossRef]
40. Lee, C.L.; Chu, I.H.; Lyu, B.J.; Chang, W.D.; Chang, N.J. Comparison of Vibration Rolling, Nonvibration Rolling, and Static Stretching as a Warm-Up Exercise on Flexibility, Joint Proprioception, Muscle Strength, and Balance in Young Adults. *J. Sports Sci.* **2018**, *36*, 2575–2582. [CrossRef] [PubMed]
41. Behm, D.G.; Bambury, A.; Cahill, F.; Power, K. Effect of Acute Static Stretching on Force, Balance, Reaction Time, and Movement Time. *Med. Sci. Sports Exerc.* **2004**, *36*, 1397–1402. [CrossRef]
42. Costa, P.B.; Graves, B.S.; Whitehurst, M.; Jacobs, P.L. The Acute Effects of Different Durations of Static Stretching on Dynamic Balance Performance. *J. Strength Cond. Res.* **2009**, *23*, 141–147. [CrossRef]
43. Mendiguchia, J.; Alentorn-Geli, E.; Idoate, F.; Myer, G.D. Rectus Femoris Muscle Injuries in Football: A Clinically Relevant Review of Mechanisms of Injury, Risk Factors and Preventive Strategies. *Br. J. Sports Med.* **2013**, *47*, 359–366. [CrossRef]

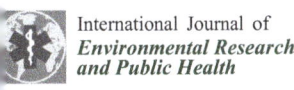

Article

Key Physical Factors in the Serve Velocity of Male Professional Wheelchair Tennis Players

Alejandro Sánchez-Pay [1,*], Rafael Martínez-Gallego [2], Miguel Crespo [3] and David Sanz-Rivas [4]

1. Department of Physical Activity and Sport, Faculty of Sport Sciences, University of Murcia, C/Argentina, s/n, 30720 San Javier, Spain
2. Department of Physical Education and Sport, Faculty of Sport Sciences, University of Valencia, Av. Blasco Ibáñez, 13, 46010 Valencia, Spain; rafael.martinez-gallego@uv.es
3. International Tennis Federation, London SW15 5XZ, UK; Miguel.crespo@itftennis.com
4. Tennis Research Group, 28080 Madrid, Spain; dsanzrivas@gmail.com
* Correspondence: aspay@um.es; Tel.: +34-868-88-92-97

Abstract: The aim of this study was to identify the physical factors related to serve speed in male professional wheelchair tennis players (WT). Nine best nationally-ranked Spanish male wheelchair tennis players (38.35 ± 11.28 years, 63.77 ± 7.01 kg) completed a neuromuscular test battery consisting of: isometric handgrip strength; serve velocity; 5, 10 and 20 m sprint (with and without racket); agility (with and without racket); medicine ball throw (serve, forehand and backhand movements); and an incremental endurance test specific to WT. Significantly higher correlations were observed in serve (r = 0.921), forehand (r = 0.810) and backhand (r = 0.791) medicine ball throws showing a positive correlation with serve velocity. A regression analysis identified a single model with the medicine ball throw serve as the main predictor of serve velocity ($r^2 = 0.847$, $p < 0.001$). In conclusion, it is recommended that coaches and physical trainers include medicine ball throw workouts in the training programs of WT tennis players due to the transfer benefits to the serve speed.

Keywords: tennis; movement; biomechanics; physical tests

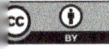

1. Introduction

Wheelchair tennis (WT) is the adapted modality of conventional tennis (CT) [1]. WT is one of the most popular Paralympic sports [2]. This progress has increased the competitive level of the players and has driven the professionalization of the best-ranked ones [3]. In order to assist WT players in their quest for performance improvement and professionalization, creating specific training situations that simulate the reality of the competition has been indicated as a key factor in the design of the sessions [4]. For this, it is vitally important for coaches and physical trainers to better understand the factors that specifically affect WT performance in order to achieve the best results.

WT competition is divided into two categories: Open and Quad. In the Open category, there are two draws: women and men [1]. In this category players have a wide range of disabilities, including spinal cord injury, single amputees, double amputees or spina bifida. In the Quad category, men and women play together and they also have a disability in their upper limbs as well [5].

Most of the studies conducted on WT match analysis have focused on the Open category. These research have concluded that WT rally length has been shown to last between six to ten seconds, with three to four shots per rally [6,7]. Serve and return of serve seem to be the most important strokes in a WT match. In conventional tennis (CT) the serve has been described as the most potentially dominant stroke in the modern game [8,9], although in WT it does not seem to have the same positive influence than in TC [10,11]. Serve velocity (SV) is undoubtedly one of the determining factors for standing players [12] and its relationships with other factors related to the physical condition of the players has been widely studied [13]. Some research has used different isometric tests such as wrist, elbow or shoulder flexion-extension [14], whereas other studies have used dynamic strength tests such as the isokinetic shoulder test [15] to find the relationships between physical condition and service speed. On the other hand, studies have also used functional field tests related to medicine ball throwing as possible predictors of service speed [13,16,17]. In general, it seems that knee flexion before extension is a prerequisite for an efficient execution of the serve as well as to achieve a higher jump [18,19] aspects that cannot be considered in adapted tennis because it is played sitting on the wheelchair (Figure 1).

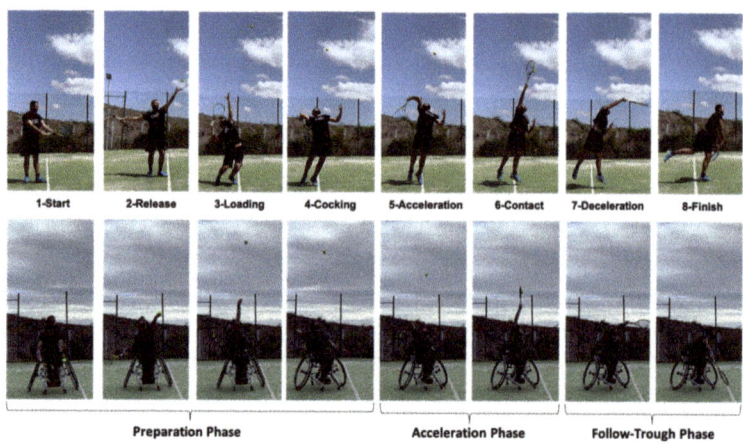

Figure 1. Service sequence in conventional and wheelchair tennis.

Some studies conducted by national tennis associations have used a battery of physical tests to know the evolution of their athletes [20,21], as well as to establish relationships between the measurements [13,22,23]. In general, anthropometric measurements, strength, speed, agility, endurance and flexibility are usually included in these tests.

From a biomechanics perspective, the serve movement is commonly divided into three phases (preparation, acceleration and follow-through) including eight stages (start, release, loading, cocking, acceleration, contact, deceleration and finish) [24]. The loading stage or the lower body has been described as the 'loaded position' the dominant elbow adopts at its lowest vertical position, it coincides with the maximal knee flexion [24] and it occurs at the end of the eccentric phase of the movement. In the case of WT, the players have a lower hitting plane as compared to the standing players, as well as a lower force generation due to the deficit in the production of force of the lower body [25]. In addition, the functional limitation of the WT players implies that the Quad category players, who have a high functional limitation, impact the ball closer to the body and generate a lower hitting power than those of the Open category [26]. An increasing serve speed reduces the time for the opponent to successfully return the ball and increases the probability of the server's dominance in the rally or of winning a direct point [27]. Due to the fact that, in CT, there are studies that show a relationship between physical parameters and service speed [13–16] and that the service technique is similar between both disciplines, our hypothesis is that there will be a relationship between some physical parameters and the service speed in WT players. Despite this, to the authors' knowledge there is no research on how the serve speed is related to the WT athlete's physical parameters, where field tests have become a reliable option to establish the performance level of players [28]. Therefore, the objective of this research was to identify the physical factors related to the velocity of the serve in WT players using different reliable and valid field tests previously utilized in research.

2. Materials and Methods

2.1. Participats and Procedures

Nine of the top ten male wheelchair tennis players in the Spanish national ranking participated in this research (mean ± SD age: 38.35 ± 11.28 years, weight: 63.77 ± 7.01 kg). All of them played national and international competitions and were among the top 150 international WT ranking ITF (Open category). Eight of the nine players were right-handed, and one was left-handed. Players had 10.2 ± 6.2 years of playing experience and practised an average of 9.3 ± 4.8 hours of tennis per week. The characteristics of the participants are shown in Table 1. The players were informed of the characteristics of the study and signed an informed consent to participate in it. All the procedures followed in this study were in accordance with the ethical standards of the Declaration of Helsinki of 1975, revised in 2008, and were approved by the ethics committee of the Royal Spanish Tennis Federation (RFET_CE17.3).

Table 1. Characteristics of the sample of wheelchair tennis players participating in the study.

n	National Ranking	International WT Ranking (ITF)	Age	Weight (kg)	Playing Training hours per week	WT Playing Experience (years)
1	1	Top 15	24	61	20	12
2	2	Top 15	18	65	15	8
3	3	Top 40	34	67	8	5
4	4	Top 50	45	57	3	24
5	5	Top 60	39	52	6	9
6	6	Top 100	35	72	10	2
7	8	Top 100	50	73	8	17
8	9	Top 150	50	70	6	8
9	10	Top 150	41	57	8	7

The players were summoned at the same time of day to perform the tests [29]. First, a standardized 10-min directed warm-up was performed consisting of joint mobility, linear movements with the chair, circular movements and turns simulating hitting, and low-intensity accelerations and decelerations [30]. The tests were carried out on two consecutive days in the following order: Day 1: Sprint test (5, 10 and 20 m), agility test (T-test), service speed test, and medicine ball throw test (forehand, backhand and serve); Day 2: Incremental resistance test (Hit and Turn Tennis Test) and manual dynamometry test. The scores of the different tests were collected during their development by the researchers themselves. All tests were conducted on an indoor hard tennis court.

2.2. Measurements Collected

Different reliable and valid field tests used previously in research were selected. The characteristics of each of the tests were the following [28,30–32]:

- Sprint test: Four gates at 0, 5, 10 and 20 m were used to measure the speed of the WT players. Subjects started from a line 0.5 m behind the first gate. Each participant performed the test three times without a racket, and three times with a racket, with a 2 min rest time between each repetition. The best value of the three attempts was recorded. The time was counted in seconds (s) and thousandths of a second (ms) with an error of ± 0.001 s through Chronojump photocell® (Chronojump, Barcelona, Spain) and Chronojump software version 1.7.1.8 (Chronojump, Barcelona, Spain) for MAC.
- Agility test (T-Test): This agility test is adapted for wheelchair sports [31] and has previously been used in WT players [33]. The test includes accelerations and decelerations, as well as turns for both sides. The participant started in the centre of the court behind the baseline, they had to move to the intersections of the singles line with the service line, always passing through the central area of the court (T) until returning to the starting area (Figure 2). Each participant performed the test three times without a racket, and three times with a racket, with a 2 min rest time

between each repetition. The best value of the three attempts was recorded. Time was measured using the Chronojump Photocell® (Chronojump, Barcelona, Spain) and the Chronojump software version 1.7.1.8 for MAC with a gate located on the baseline to record the start and the end of the test.
- Serve velocity test: A radar gun (Stalker Pro Inc., Plano, Texas, USA) was used to measure serve velocity. The player performed 10 services at maximum velocity directed to the wide area of the service box from the advantage side for the right-handed players, and from the deuce side for the left-handed player [34]. The radar was positioned behind the player at the same hitting height and oriented in the same direction as the ball. The average value of 10 serves in km·h^{-1} was recorded.
- Upper body strength: Explosive strength was evaluated through three medicine ball through tests, simulating the forehand, the backhand and the serve shots [35,36]. The participants stood behind the throwing line in a 45° position. A 15 m long measuring tape was placed on the court perpendicular to the throwing line and two evaluators marked the bounce zone of the recorded ball in 0.10 m sections. A 2-kilogram medicine ball was used for the test. Participants performed each type of throw three times, with a 2 min rest time between each repetition. The players had to throw the ball simulating the technical gesture of the backhand (Figure 3a), the forehand (Figure 3b) and the serve (Figure 3c).
- Isometric handgrip strength: The hand dynamometry test was carried out to assess the maximum isometric force in the flexors of the fingers with a Smedley III T-18A dynamometer (Takei, Tokyo, Japan) and a range between 0 and 100 kg in 0.5 kg increments and an accuracy of ±2 kg. The test was carried out in the wheelchair sitting position with the arm extended and glued to the wheel without actually contacting it [30]. Each subject made three maximum attempts with each hand after a familiarization phase with the instrument with sub-maximum repetitions. The rest time between each attempt was 2 min. The best value of three attempts was recorded in N·kg^{-1}.
- Anaerobic endurance test (Hit and Turn Tennis Test): This test is an adaptation of the one developed for conventional tennis to evaluate the specific anaerobic endurance of the player through the level reached [32]. The test consists of simulating a hit on top of a cone located at the intersection of the doubles line with the baseline line, coinciding with the sound signals emitted by the sound of the test. After that hit, the player must simulate another hit on the opposite side and so on until the end of the series. In this adaptation, the hitting had to be made close to a cone located between the intersection of the singles line with the doubles line, thus reducing the distance of displacement for the WT players. As an incremental test, it ended when the player was unable to reach the cone at the rate set by the sound signals. The period reached by each player was recorded when he was no longer able to simulate hitting in the designated area at the same time as the acoustic signal sounded.

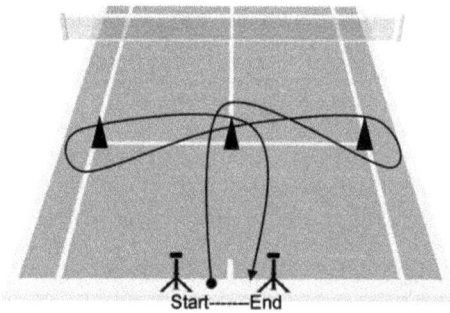

Figure 2. Agility test (T-Test).

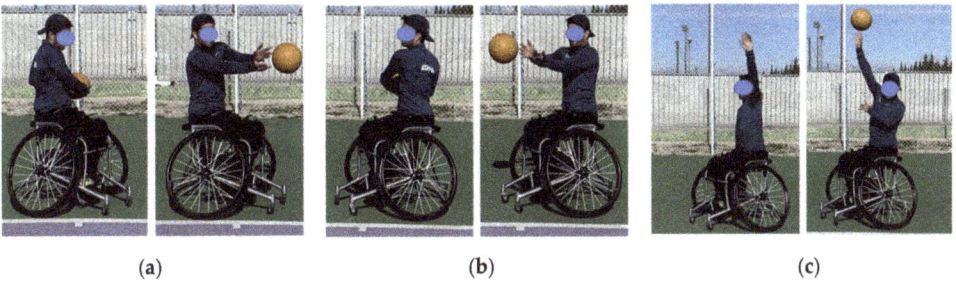

Figure 3. Medicine ball through backhand (**a**), forehand (**b**), and serve (**c**).

Table 2 shows the physical variables measured as well as the different tests used.

Table 2. Physical variable and test event.

Physical Variable	Test	Characteristic
Strength	Grip strength (2)	1-Dominant 2-Non-Dominant
	Medicine ball through (3)	1-Forehand 2-Backhand 3-Serve
	Serve velocity	Average value of 10 serves
Sprint	5 m 10 m 20 m	With and without racket
Agility	T-Test	With and without racket
Endurance	Hit and Turn Tennis Test	With racket

2.3. Data Analysis

Due to the small size of the sample, the Shapiro–Wilk and Levene tests were used to contrast the normality and homogeneity of variances for each variable (sprint, agility, strength and anaerobic endurance). All the variables obtained p-values > 0.05 except in the dynamometry with the dominant arm. A Pearson correlation analysis (Kendall's Tau-b for dominant dynamometry) was performed to identify those variables related to serve speed. Values were classified as trivial (0–0.1), small (0.1–0.3), moderate (0.3–0.5), large (0.5–0.7), very large (0.7–0.9), almost perfect (0.9) and perfect (1.0) [37]. Subsequently, a multiple linear regression analysis (stepwise) was performed to identify the parameters with the greatest influence on SV. The SV was used as a dependent variable, while the rest of the variables that had previously shown significance operated as independent. Significance was established at $p < 0.05$. All data were analyzed with the IBM SPSS 25.0 statistical package for Macintosh (IBM Corp, Armonk, NY, USA).

3. Results

Table 3 shows the descriptive analysis of test measurement in wheelchair tennis players.

Table 4 shows the correlation coefficients of the different physical tests performed with the serve speed. Figure 4 shows the relationship between statistically significant variables and serve velocity. Significantly higher correlations were observed in medicine ball throws for service ($r = 0.921$), forehand ($r = 0.810$) and backhand ($r = 0.791$) showing a positive correlation. The 20-meter racket test showed significance ($p = 0.012$) and negatively correlated with serve velocity ($r = -0.788$).

Table 3. Mean (M), standard deviation (SD) and confidence interval (CI) of physical test measurements.

Test	M	SD	CI 95%
Grip strength. Dom. (N·kg^{-1})	46.33	4.13	43.11;49.54
Grip strength. No Dom. (N·kg^{-1})	38.61	6.26	33.79;43.43
Service velocity (km·h^{-1})	114.90	10.06	107.16;122.63
Sprint 5m NR (s)	1.555	0.16	1.42;1.68
Sprint 10m NR (s)	2.977	0.27	2.76;3.18
Sprint 20m NR (s)	5.403	0.50	5.01;5.78
Sprint 5m R (s)	1.657	0.21	1.49;1.82
Sprint 10m R (s)	3.021	0.37	2.73;3.31
Sprint 20m R (s)	5.456	0.51	5.05;5.85
T-Test NR (s)	12.426	0.99	11.66;13.19
T-Test R (s)	12.681	1.20	11.75;13.6
MBT F (m)	5.91	1.93	4.42;7.4
MBT B (m)	5.81	1.81	4.42;7.21
MBT S (m)	7.16	1.42	6.06;8.26
Hit and Turn (n)	15.22	2.99	12.92;17.52

Dom: Dominant. No Dom.: Non-dominant. NR: no racquet. R: racquet. MBT: medicine ball throw. F: Forehand. B: Backhand.

Table 4. Correlation coefficient of physical tests with serve velocity.

Test	r	p
Grip strength. Dom. (N·kg^{-1})	0.582	0.100
Grip strength. No Dom. (N·kg^{-1})	0.297	0.438
Sprint 5m NR (s)	−0.613	0.079
Sprint 10m NR (s)	−0.518	0.154
Sprint 20m NR (s)	−0.523	0.148
Sprint 5m R (s)	−0.502	0.168
Sprint 10m R (s)	−0.599	0.089
Sprint 20m R (s)	−0.788	0.012
T-Test NR (s)	−0.623	0.073
T-Test R (s)	−0.585	0.098
MBT F (m)	0.810	0.008
MBT B (m)	0.791	0.011
MBT S (m)	0.921	<0.001
Hit and Turn (n)	0.608	0.082

Dom: Dominant. No Dom.: Non-dominant. NR: no racquet. R: racquet. MBT: medicine ball throw. F: Forehand. B: Backhand. S: Serve.

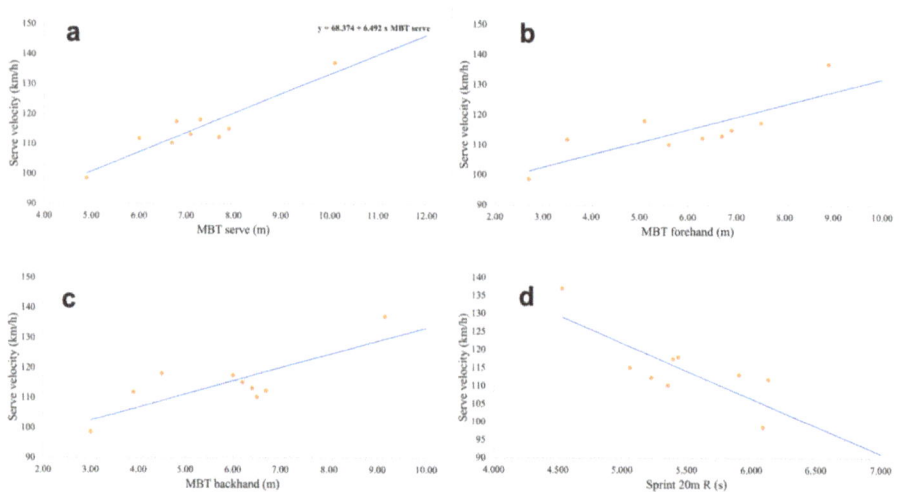

Figure 4. Relationship between the medicine ball throw test simulating a serve (**a**), forehand (**b**), backhand (**c**) and sprint of 20 meters with racket (**d**) with the serve velocity (km/h).

Table 5 shows the results of the multiple regression analysis. The medicine ball throw simulating a serve was shown as the main and only predictor measure of the speed of the serve ($r^2 = 0.847$, $p < 0.001$) with a positive relationship.

Table 5. Statistics of multiple regression analysis.

	R	R^2	R^2 Adjust	F	Sig F.	Regression Equation
Model	0.921	0.847	0.826	38.953	<0.001	
			Beta	T	Sig. T.	y = 68.374 + 6.492 × MBT S
MBT S			0.921	6.241	<0.001	

MBT: medicine ball throw. S: Serve.

4. Discussion

Knowing how the physical demands of WT are related, as well as identifying which are the variables that determine any of them, can help coaches and physical trainers in the design of exercises adapted to the specific needs of the game. The aim of this research was to determine the relationship of different physical demands evaluated through a field test battery with the serve velocity in professional WT players. In general, it was observed that medicine ball throws simulating the forehand, the backhand and the serve strokes showed the highest correlation with SV, while the serve medicine ball throw was the test that best predicted the model.

Coaches and physical trainers often use batteries of tests (related to speed, agility, maximum strength or functional movements) to understand the evolution of their athletes and to prescribe training, among other goals [38]. Medicine ball throws both in the forehand and the backhand showed a positive and statistically significant correlation with service speed (Table 4). These throws have been useful to examine the rotational power of the trunk of athletes in general [39] and in tennis players in particular [38].

The tennis serve includes the activation of the abdominal muscles (rectum and obliques) to perform a trunk flexion with a rotation [25]. Furthermore, the forehand MBT had a higher correlation with serve velocity than the backhand MBT ($r = 0.810$ vs. $r = 0.791$). It is worth noting that the forehand MBT includes a rotation of the trunk towards the player's dominant side, as does the serve, which could explain the greater correlation between both. In addition, the 20-m sprint showed a negative correlation with service speed ($r = -0.788$). In this sense, a greater throw distance is related to a higher displacement speed (less time) over long distances (20 m) (Figure 4d). The abdominal muscles have a great implication in the generation of force in the service [25], and also in the stabilization of the trunk for the propulsion tasks [40], which could explain the observed correlation.

The biomechanical requirements of the serve have been specifically analysed using an 8-stage model (star, release, loading, cocking, acceleration, contact, deceleration and finish) [24]. Due to the considerably low contribution of the lower body to generate force in the kinetic chain of the service movement in WT players, it could be indicated that from the loading phase (semi-side position, elbow of the racket arm at its lowest position, free arm stretched up, etc.) the movement of the upper body in the serve is similar to the service MBT in both standing and chair players. This could explain that the medicine ball throw simulating a serve is the main variable predicting the speed of serve (Table 5) showing a high correlation (Figure 4a). In addition, this loading position in both shots has specific biomechanical implications that do not occur in the forehand and the backhand MBT (shoulder over shoulder work, action-reaction of free arm, line of force in the direction of throw/impact, asynchronous movements between both arms, etc.) [41,42].

In fact, it is known that one of the movements that generates greater power in the hitting action is the torque or rotation component of the trunk to increase the acceleration distance with respect to the point of impact, as well as to add a greater number of elements of the kinetic chain in the corresponding stroke action [43]. Therefore, this action is very clear in the forehand and backhand strokes, but it also has a very relevant role in the serve movement. In this study, it has been observed that from a kinematic point of view, actions that resemble the forehand, the backhand and the serve strokes have a high correlation with serve speed (Figure 4a–c). Specifically, and from a kinematic point of view, the action of MBT serve reproduces the serve movement in its setup and advance-impact phases (Figure 1). Even wheelchair tennis players who have a spinal cord injury and functional deficit in the trunk musculature, can use their non-dominant hand as a support in the hitting action, in a similar way to that which occurs in the serve movement of standing players. In fact, the serve requires multiarticular recruitment and a high rotation speed during the shot [41,42].

Due to the fact that the serve and, specifically, the SV have been reported as the most powerful and dominant stroke feature in tennis, involving various factors such as the strength and power of the upper body and the range of motion of the shoulder [24]; and without considering other elements of the kinetic chain such as the lower body (which also has its influence), it can be considered that this stroke is also decisive in WT. Therefore, and as per the results obtained, it seems reasonable to think that specific strength training prescription, simulating the kinematics of the serve gesture with medicine balls, can help to achieve speed increases especially in the serve, and also in the forehand and backhand strokes. Therefore, it is recommended that coaches and physical trainers incorporate this type of specific work in their training plans to assist players in improving these strokes. These workouts should be done in neuromuscular working conditions, in the absence of fatigue and at the beginning of the training sessions, to avoid the practice of serve stroke workouts in the final parts of the training sessions as usual.

The results obtained in this study present a series of limitations that should be considered. On the one hand, although the sample includes the top nine national players in the Open category, the small size of the sample does not allow for divisions according to their functional limitation, since the strength of the relationship between the variables would have been very light. Therefore, future research should include a larger sample of WT players, players from different WT categories (Quad and Open), as well as female and male players to compare this relationship (SV with physical tests), both due to functional limitation and between genders. In addition, other anthropometric variables, such as height or body segments, were not measured, which have shown a correlation with service speed in CT players. On the other hand, the SV test was carried out in a training environment and taking measurements in a competition setting using a radar gun could provide different data.

5. Conclusions

Medicine ball throws simulating the forehand, the backhand and the serve strokes showed a high correlation with SV in WT. The MBT serve is the test that best predicts SV in WT. Therefore, and given the similarity of the movements between the two gestures, coaches and physical trainers are encouraged to include medicine ball throws workouts as a service transfer exercises within the training programs of WT players. Likewise, it is advisable to work with medicine ball throws for the forehand and backhand, given the importance of trunk rotation for the serve.

Author Contributions: Conceptualization: A.S.-P., D.S.-R.; methodology: A.S.-P., and D.S.-R.; software: A.S.-P., R.M.-G., M.C. and D.S.-R.; validation: A.S.-P., R.M.-G., M.C. and D.S.-R.; formal analysis: A.S.-P. and D.S.-R.; investigation: A.S.-P., R.M.-G., M.C. and D.S.-R.; resources: A.S.-P. and D.S.-R.; data curation: A.S.-P. and D.S.-R.; writing—original draft preparation: A.S.-P., R.M.-G., M.C and D.S.-R.; writing—review and editing: A.S.-P., R.M.-G., M.C. and D.S.-R.; visualization: A.S.-P., R.M.-G., M.C. and D.S.-R.; supervision: A.S.-P. and D.S.-R. All authors have read and agreed to the published version of the manuscript.

Funding: This research received no external funding.

Institutional Review Board Statement: The study was conducted according to the guidelines of the Declaration of Helsinki, and approved by the Ethics Committee of Royal Spanish Tennis Federation (RFET_CE17.3).

Informed Consent Statement: Informed consent was obtained from all subjects involved in the study.

Data Availability Statement: The data presented in this study are available on request from the corresponding author. The data are not publicly available due to privacy.

Acknowledgments: We are grateful for the cooperation of the wheelchair tennis players.

Conflicts of Interest: The authors declare no conflict of interest.

References

1. International Tennis Federation. *Rules of Tennis*; International Tennis Federation: London, UK, 2020.
2. Diaper, N.J.; Goosey-Tolfrey, V.L. A physiological case study of a paralympic wheelchair tennis player: Reflective practise. *J. Sport. Sci. Med.* **2009**, *8*, 300–307.
3. Sánchez-Pay, A. Analysis of scientific production in wheelchair tennis [Análisis de la producción científica sobre el tenis en silla de ruedas]. *Rev. Iberoam. Cienc. Act. Física Deport.* **2019**, *8*, 13–25. [CrossRef]
4. Reid, M.; Morgan, S.; Whiteside, D. Matchplay characteristics of Grand Slam tennis: Implications for training and conditioning. *J. Sport. Sci.* **2016**, *34*, 1791–1798. [CrossRef]
5. Sánchez-Pay, A.; Sanz-Rivas, D. Wheelchair tennis, from health to competitive analysis: A narrative review. *J. Hum. Sport Exerc.* **2020**, in press. [CrossRef]
6. Mason, B.S.; van der Slikke, R.M.A.; Hutchinson, M.J.; Goosey-Tolfrey, V.L. Division, result and score margin alter the physical and technical performance of elite wheelchair tennis players. *J. Sports Sci.* **2020**, *38*, 937–944. [CrossRef]
7. Sánchez-Pay, A.; Sanz-Rivas, D.; Torres-Luque, G. Match analysis in a wheelchair tennis tournament. *Int. J. Perform. Anal. Sport* **2015**, *15*, 540–550. [CrossRef]
8. O'Donoghue, P.; Brown, E. The importance of service in Grand Slam singles tennis. *Int. J. Perform. Anal. Sport* **2008**, *8*, 70–78. [CrossRef]
9. Fitzpatrick, A.; Stone, J.A.; Choppin, S.; Kelley, J. Important performance characteristics in elite clay and grass court tennis match-play. *Int. J. Perform. Anal. Sport* **2019**, *19*, 942–952. [CrossRef]
10. Sánchez-Pay, A.; Torres-Luque, G.; Fernandéz-Garcia, Á.I.; Sanz-Rivas, D.; Palao, J.M. Differences in game statistics between winning and losing for male wheelchair tennis players in Paralympics Games. *Mot. Rev. Educ. Física* **2017**, *23*. [CrossRef]
11. Sánchez-Pay, A.; Palao, J.M.; Torres-Luque, G.; Sanz-Rivas, D. Differences in set statistics between wheelchair and conventional tennis on different types of surfaces and by gender. *Int. J. Perform. Anal. Sport* **2015**, *15*, 1177–1188. [CrossRef]
12. Brown, E.; O'Donoghue, P. Efecto del género y la superficie en la estrategia del tenis de élite. *Coach. Sport Sci. Rev.* **2008**, *15*, 11–13.
13. Fett, J.; Ulbricht, A.; Ferrauti, A. Impact of physical performance and anthropometric characteristics on serve velocity in elite junior tennis players. *J. Strength Cond. Res.* **2020**, *34*, 192–202. [CrossRef]
14. Baiget, E.; Corbi, F.; Fuentes, J.P.; Fernández-Fernández, J. The relationship between maximum isometric strength and ball velocity in the tennis serve. *J. Hum. Kinet.* **2016**, *53*, 63–71. [CrossRef]
15. Cohen, D.B.; Mont, M.A.; Campbell, K.R.; Vogelstein, B.N.; Loewy, J.W. Upper extremity physical factors affecting tennis serve velocity. *Am. J. Sports Med.* **1994**, *22*, 746–750. [CrossRef]
16. Colomar, J.; Baiget, E.; Corbi, F. Influence of strength, power, and muscular stiffness on stroke velocity in junior tennis players. *Front. Physiol.* **2020**, *11*, 1–9. [CrossRef]
17. Kramer, T.; Huijgen, B.C.H.; Elferink-Gemser, M.T.; Visscher, C. Prediction of tennis performance in junior elite tennis players. *J. Sport. Sci. Med.* **2017**, *16*, 14–21.
18. Girard, O.; Micallef, J.P.; Millet, G.P. Lower-limb activity during the power serve in tennis: Effects of performance level. *Med. Sci. Sports Exerc.* **2005**, *37*, 1021–1029. [CrossRef] [PubMed]
19. Dossena, F.; Rossi, C.; LA Torre, A.; Bonato, M. The role of lower limbs during tennis serve. *J. Sports Med. Phys. Fitness* **2018**, *58*, 210–215. [CrossRef] [PubMed]
20. Kramer, T.; Huijgen, B.C.H.; Elferink-Gemser, M.T.; Visscher, C. A longitudinal study of physical fitness in elite junior tennis players. *Pediatr. Exerc. Sci.* **2016**, *28*, 553–564. [CrossRef]
21. Van Den Berg, L.; Coetzee, B.; Pienaar, A.E. The influence of biological maturation on physical and motor performance talent identification determinants of U-14 provincial girl tennis players. *J. Hum. Mov. Stud.* **2006**, *50*, 273–290.
22. Fernandez-Fernandez, J.; Nakamura, F.Y.; Moreno-Perez, V.; Lopez-Valenciano, A.; Del Coso, J.; Gallo-Salazar, C.; Barbado, D.; Ruiz-Perez, I.; Sanz-Rivas, D. Age and sex-related upper body performance differences in competitive young tennis players. *PLoS ONE* **2019**, *14*. [CrossRef] [PubMed]
23. Ulbricht, A.; Fernandez-Fernandez, J.; Mendez-Villanueva, A.; Ferrauti, A. Impact of fitness characteristics on tennis performance in elite junior tennis players. *J. Strength Cond. Res.* **2016**, *30*, 989–998. [CrossRef]
24. Kovacs, M.S.; Ellenbecker, T.S. A performance evaluation of the tennis serve: Implications for strength, speed, power, and flexibility training. *Strength Cond. J.* **2011**, *33*, 22–30. [CrossRef]
25. Reid, M.; Elliott, B.C.; Alderson, J. Shoulder joint kinetics of the elite wheelchair tennis serve. *Br. J. Sports Med.* **2007**, *41*, 739–744. [CrossRef] [PubMed]
26. Cavedon, V.; Zancanaro, C.; Milanese, C. Kinematic analysis of the wheelchair tennis serve: Implications for classification. *Scand. J. Med. Sci. Sport.* **2014**, *24*, 381–388. [CrossRef]

27. Whiteside, D.; Reid, M. Spatial characteristics of professional tennis serves with implications for serving aces: A machine learning approach. *J. Sports Sci.* **2017**, *35*, 648–654. [CrossRef]
28. De Groot, S.; Balvers, I.J.M.; Kouwenhoven, S.M.; Janssen, T.W.J. Validity and reliability of tests determining performance-related components of wheelchair basketball. *J. Sports Sci.* **2012**, *30*, 879–887. [CrossRef]
29. López-Samanes, Á.; Moreno-Pérez, D.; Maté-Muñoz, J.L.; Domínguez, R.; Pallarés, J.G.; Mora-Rodriguez, R.; Ortega, J.F. Circadian rhythm effect on physical tennis performance in trained male players. *J. Sports Sci.* **2017**, *35*, 2121–2128. [CrossRef] [PubMed]
30. Granados, C.; Yanci, J.; Badiola, A.; Iturricastillo, A.; Otero, M.; Olasagasti, J.; Bidaurrazaga-Letona, I.; Gil, S.M. Anthropometry and performance in wheelchair basketball. *J. Strength Cond. Res.* **2015**, *29*, 1812–1820. [CrossRef] [PubMed]
31. Yanci, J.; Granados, C.; Otero, M.; Badiola, A.; Olasagasti, J.; Bidaurrazaga-Letona, I.; Iturricastillo, A.; Gil, S.M. Sprint, agility strength and endurance capacity in wheelchair basketball players. *Biol. Sport* **2015**, *32*, 71–78. [CrossRef]
32. Ferrauti, A.; Kinner, V.; Fernandez-Fernandez, J. The Hit & Turn Tennis Test: An acoustically controlled endurance test for tennis players. *J. Sports Sci.* **2011**, *29*, 485–494.
33. Sánchez-Pay, A.; Sanz-Rivas, D. Assessment of the physical condition of the high-level wheelchair tennis player according to competitive level and kind of injury. *RICYDE Rev. Int. Ciencias del Deport.* **2019**, *57*, 235–248. [CrossRef]
34. Hernández-Davó, J.L.; Moreno, F.J.; Sanz-Rivas, D.; Hernández-Davó, H.; Coves, Á.; Caballero, C. Variations in kinematic variables and performance in the tennis serve according to age and skill level. *Int. J. Perform. Anal. Sport* **2019**, *19*, 749–762 [CrossRef]
35. Negrete, R.J.; Hanney, W.J.; Kolber, M.J.; Davies, G.J.; Ansley, M.K.; Mcbride, A.B.; Overstreet, A.L. Reliability, minimal detectable change, and normative values for tests of upper extremity function and power. *J. Strength Cond. Res.* **2010**, *24*, 3318–3325 [CrossRef]
36. Roetert, E.P.; McCormick, T.J.; Brown, S.W.; Ellenbecker, T.S. Relationship between isokinetic and functional trunk strength in elite junior tennis players. *Isokinet. Exerc. Sci.* **1996**, *6*, 15–20. [CrossRef]
37. Hopkins, W.G. Measures of reliability in sports medicine and science. *Sport. Med.* **2000**, *30*, 1–15. [CrossRef]
38. Roetert, P.; Ellenbecker, T.S. *Complete Conditioning for Tennis*; Human Kinetics: Champaign, IL, USA, 2007.
39. Ikeda, Y.; Kijima, K.; Kawabata, K.; Fuchimoto, T.; Ito, A. Relationship between side medicine-ball throw performance and physical ability for male and female athletes. *Eur. J. Appl. Physiol.* **2007**, *99*, 47–55. [CrossRef]
40. Yang, Y.-S.; Koontz, A.M.; Triolo, R.J.; Mercer, J.L.; Boninger, M.L. Surface electromyography activity of trunk muscles during wheelchair propulsion. *Clin. Biomech.* **2006**, *21*, 1032–1041. [CrossRef]
41. Reid, M.; Elliot, B.; Alderson, J. Lower-limb coordination and shoulder joint mechanics in the tennis serve. *Med. Sci. Sports Exerc* **2008**, *40*, 308–315. [CrossRef]
42. Reid, M.; Schneiker, K. Strength and conditioning in tennis: Current research and practice. *J. Sci. Med. Sport* **2008**, *11*, 248–256 [CrossRef]
43. Herring, R.M.; Chapman, A.E. Effects of changes in segmental values and timing of both torque and torque reversal in simulated throws. *J. Biomech.* **1992**, *25*, 1173–1184. [CrossRef]

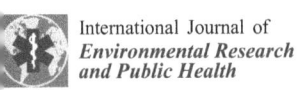

Article
The Development Strategy of Home-Based Exercise in China Based on the SWOT-AHP Model

Hanming Li [1], Xingquan Chen [1,*] and Yiwei Fang [2]

1 College of Physical Education, Sichuan University, Chengdu 610065, China; lhm@stu.scu.edu.cn
2 Department of Materials Science and Chemical Engineering, Stony Brook University, Stony Brook, NY 11794, USA; yiwei.fang@stonybrook.edu
* Correspondence: cxq@scu.edu.cn

Abstract: In view of the increasing importance of sports to people and the impact of COVID-19 on people's lives, home-based exercise has become a popular choice for people to keep fit due to its unique advantages and its popularity is expected to keep growing in the future. Therefore, it is necessary to determine the development direction of home-based exercise and put in the corresponding efforts. However, there is currently a lack of research on all aspects of home-based exercise. The purpose of this research was to investigate the effective sustainable development strategy of home-based exercise in China through a SWOT (Strengths, Weaknesses, Opportunities and Threats) and AHP (Analytic Hierarchy Process) hybrid model. Thirteen factors corresponding to the SWOT analysis were identified through a literature review and expert opinions. The results show that in China the advantages and potential outweigh the weaknesses and threats of home-based exercise. Home-based exercise should grasp the external development opportunities and choose the SO development strategic type that combines internal strengths and external opportunities. As the core for the development of home-based exercise, this strategy should be given priority. To sum up, home-based exercise is believed to have a bright future.

Keywords: home-based exercise; sustainable development; SWOT-AHP; physical activities; public health; COVID-19; intelligent sports

1. Introduction

At the end of 2019, the COVID-19 epidemic broke out and spread all over the world. During the prevention and control period of the pandemic, various sports venues were not open. This scenario where all sports venues are shut down is challenging to everyone who needs exercise. In January 2020, the General Administration of Sports of China issued the "Notice on Vigorously Promoting Scientific Home-based Exercise Methods", requesting local sports departments to introduce simple, scientific, and effective home-based exercise methods based on local conditions. Since then, "home-based exercise" has gradually become a hot topic in China.

The idea of home-based exercise is to fully utilize the space in your home and make it act as a sports venue, with your own or family members, with your hands or using some portable equipment, to perform a series of applicable sports to strengthen your physical fitness and mentality. Home-based exercise is popular among people of all ages due to its convenience and is one of the important ways to stay healthy. People carry out various forms of sports at home, which not only strengthen their physical fitness and improve their own immunity, but also help relieve a series of psychological problems caused by COVID-19 [1–4].

Before the outbreak of the epidemic, home-based exercise was mainly used as aids for patient treatment or as means to restore physical function after surgery. Existing researches show that home-based exercise has good auxiliary effects on the treatment of fractures, osteoarthritis, and other musculoskeletal system diseases [5–10], cardio-cerebral vascular system diseases [11–16], respiratory system diseases [17–19], and even cancers [20–23]. Home-based exercise also has effects on supporting the treatment of nervous system diseases such as depression and Parkinson's disease [24–28].

After the outbreak of the epidemic, in order to reduce people going out and avoid too much contact with each other to cause infection, home-based exercise replaced sports outdoors or in specific venues and became an inevitable choice to meet people's needs. According to the study of Bo Pu et al. [29], during the epidemic, people mainly carried out the five aspects of home-based exercise, that is, gymnastics, walking or jogging, stretching exercises, housework, etc. It shows that male, married, and more than 25-year-old participants are more likely to do home-based exercise [29–32].

As COVID-19 still poses a huge threat to the public health, more and more people around the world have adopted home-based exercise. Home-based exercise has the prospect of becoming a common way for people to participate in physical activities. This study will employ a SWOT (Strengths, Weaknesses, Opportunities and Threats) and AHP (Analytic Hierarchy Process) hybrid model to provide a certain reference for the sustainable development of home-based exercise in China, and also it can provide some references for the development of home-based exercise in other countries.

1.1. SWOT Analysis

The SWOT analysis is a widely used tool for analyzing internal and external environments in order to attain a systematic approach and support for decision situations [33]. By applying the SWOT analysis in scientific research, people are able to draw a series of conclusions from the research objects including the main strengths, weaknesses, opportunities, and threats. Most articles on the SWOT analysis only presented a literal description of the analysis and a few conducted quantified analysis and as planning processes are often complicated by numerous criteria and interdependencies, it may lead to the insufficient use of this analytical method [33–35].

1.2. Analytic Hierarchy Process (AHP)

The analytical hierarchy process (AHP) is a multiple criteria decision analysis (MCDA) method which helps in addressing the complicated decision problems [36,37]. The advantages of AHP include its ability to qualitatively and quantitatively analyze decision attributes, and its flexibility with regard to the setting of objectives [38]. It does so by structuring the problem, identifying decision making factors, measuring the importance of the factors, and synthesizing all the decision-making factors [39–41]. At present, AHP has been widely used in various areas, such as operations management [42], health care [43], project risk assessment [44], etc. [45,46]. However, AHP also has some defects, for example, it is criticized for its possible rank reversal phenomenon [47].

1.3. SWOT-AHP Model

Since the SWOT analysis includes no quantitative analysis, AHP can be integrated with the SWOT analysis [48–50]. Research by Mika Marttunen et al. shows that SWOT is most often used in combination with MCDA methods, and the mixed use of SWOT and AHP is the most common one [51]. Using AHP, each group of SWOT can be created as a pairwise comparison matrix, the weights and intensities of the SWOT groups and factors can be measured [50]. In this way, the reliability of the SWOT analysis can be improved. Many studies in different disciplines have already achieved good results by utilizing the SWOT-AHP hybrid model [38,48,52,53], and this method has also been applied in sports science and physical education [39,54–56].

2. Methods

2.1. Factors Generation

In order to determine the factors, the expert panel of sports science and medical science conducts a SWOT analysis. First, 10 expert panel members leading by Prof. Xingquan Chen from the Physical Education College of Sichuan University and West China Hospital of Sichuan University conducted the SWOT analysis. Every member of the panel was asked to identify various strengths and weaknesses, opportunities and threats related to the development of home-based exercise. Based on the SWOT analysis, the authors selected 13 factors. Then, these factors were grouped into each SWOT category and were given a brief description (Table 1).

Table 1. Strengths, weaknesses, opportunities and threats-analytical hierarchy process (SWOT-AHP) factors and description.

SWOT Group	SWOT Factor	Description of Factor
Strengths (S)	S1 Construction of a leading sports nation	The issuance of various policies has promoted China's sports industry [57,58].
	S2 Increased awareness of exercise	People have gradually realized the importance of physical health.
	S3 Time Freedom	Home-based exercise can meet the demand of most office workers to do sports.
	S4 Low cost and convenient	People can complete the sports with light equipment or just with hands, and home-based exercise is not affected by the weather and is more convenient.
Weaknesses (W)	W1 Limited space leads to fewer sports methods	The equipment that can be used is basically simple and lightweight and there are fewer options to do sports at home, which are more restrictive.
	W2 Monotonous and boring form of exercise	Home-based exercise is less interesting and easy to cause boredom.
	W3 Less theoretical research and insufficient professional talents	There are relatively few theoretical studies and there is still a lack of innovative talents who can cross-study sports with other disciplines.
Opportunities (O)	O1 Support provided by the government	"Notice on Vigorously Promoting Scientific Home-based Exercise Methods" issued by the General Administration of Sports of China provides strong support for the future development of home-based exercise [59].
	O2 The stable development of sports industry	The output value of China's sports industry and the scale of the online sports market have grown steadily every year, laying a solid foundation for the development of home-based exercise [60,61].
	O3 The rapid development of intelligent sports	Wearable devices, intelligent sports equipment, intelligent sports entertainment products, virtual reality technology, artificial intelligence motion algorithms and various new environmentally friendly materials used in sports equipment are also key projects for the development of the intelligent sports industry [62–66].
Threats (T)	T1 Noise	It is very likely that excessive noise will be produced, affecting neighbors.
	T2 Easy to be slack at home	Exercise at home can easily make people slack and become lazy.
	T3 Fading enthusiasm for home-based exercise	After the epidemic, the enthusiasm for home exercise easily fades.

2.2. AHP Instrument

Based on the factors obtained by the SWOT analysis method, the AHP hierarchy was constructed (Figure 1). In order to carry out the analytic hierarchy process, a questionnaire was compiled that required a series of paired comparisons of factors. The respondents were asked to give answers by comparing two given factors according to his or her own preferences. They were asked to evaluate the factors based on the AHP scale (Table 2) [40].

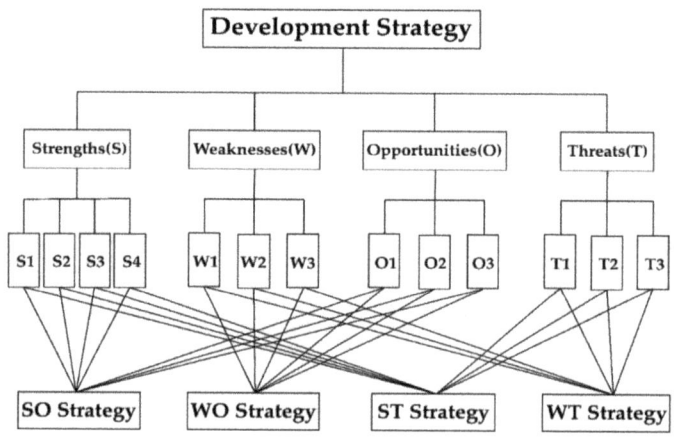

Figure 1. Hierarchical analysis structure graph.

Table 2. The fundamental scale of absolute numbers.

Intensity of Importance	Definition	Explanation
1	Equal Importance	Two activities contribute equally to the objective
3	Moderate importance	Experience and judgement slightly favor one activity over another
5	Strong importance	Experience and judgement strongly favor one activity over another
7	Very strong or demonstrated importance	An activity is favored very strongly over another; its dominance is demonstrated in practice
9	Extreme importance	The evidence favoring one activity over another is of the highest possible order of affirmation
2,4,6,8	Importance between the above levels	
Reciprocals of the above	If activity i has one of the above non-zero numbers assigned to it when compared with activity j, then j has the reciprocal value when compared with i	A reasonable assumption

2.3. Weight and Consistency Check

Since people tend to make inconsistent decisions, decision making science should judge the consistency of decision making, a consistency ratio (CR) test is a measurement of the validity of the survey respondents' responses [39–41]. IBM SPSS Statistics 23 and MATLAB R2018b were used for statistics and calculations. The calculation methods and steps are as follows [40,53,54]:

1. Construct comparison matrix A.

$$A = (a_{ij}) = \begin{bmatrix} a_{11} & a_{12} & \cdots & a_{1n} \\ a_{21} & a_{22} & \cdots & a_{2n} \\ \vdots & \vdots & \ddots & \vdots \\ a_{n1} & a_{n2} & \cdots & a_{nn} \end{bmatrix} = \begin{bmatrix} 1 & \frac{w_1}{w_2} & \cdots & \frac{w_1}{w_n} \\ \frac{w_2}{w_1} & 1 & \cdots & \frac{w_2}{w_n} \\ \vdots & \vdots & \ddots & \vdots \\ \frac{w_n}{w_1} & \frac{w_n}{w_2} & \cdots & 1 \end{bmatrix} \quad (1)$$

2. Calculate the geometrical mean ($\overline{W_i}$) of each row of the judgment matrix using the product square root method.

$$\overline{W_i} = \left(\prod_{j=1}^{n} a_{ij} \right)^{\frac{1}{n}} \quad i,j = 1,2,\cdots,n \quad (2)$$

3. Normalize the geometrical mean of each row to get the eigenvectors (W_i).

$$W_i = \frac{\overline{W_i}}{\sum_{j=1}^{n} \overline{w_j}} \quad i,j = 1,2,\cdots,n \quad (3)$$

4. Calculate the maximum eigenvalue (λ_{max}) of the judgment matrix.

$$\lambda_{max} = \frac{1}{n} \sum_{i=1}^{n} \frac{\left(\sum_{j=1}^{n} a_{ij} W_j \right)}{W_i} \quad i,j = 1,2,\cdots,n \quad (4)$$

5. Calculate the consistency index (CI) and the consistency ratio (CR).

$$CI = \frac{\lambda_{max} - n}{n - 1} \quad (5)$$

When $n > 2$, CR represents the consistency of the matrix, RI values are shown in Table 3.

$$CR = \frac{CI}{RI} \quad (6)$$

Table 3. Average random consistency index.

n	1	2	3	4	5	6	7	8	9	10
RI	0	0	0.58	0.90	1.12	1.24	1.32	1.41	1.45	1.49

If $CR < 0.1$, the judgment matrix of the index meets the requirements of the consistency test.

2.4. The Calculation of the Intensity of Factors and SWOT Strategic Quadrilateral

The magnitude of the factor's effect is intensity, and its actual level is the estimated strength, then *intensity* = *estimated strength* × *weight*. The estimated strength of each factor is represented by 0–5 points, S, O are represented by positive values, W, T are represented by negative values, the greater the absolute value, the greater the intensity.

The four variables of S, W, O, and T total intensity are each semi-axis, forming a four semi-dimensional coordinate system. Draw the velocity values S', W', O', and T' on the corresponding semi-axes of the coordinate system to obtain a strategic quadrilateral.

2.5. The Calculation of the Strategic Vector (θ, ρ)

In the SWOT-AHP model, the strategic azimuth angle θ is used to judge the strategic type, and the strategic intensity coefficient ρ is used to judge the strategic intensity. In the polar coordinates of the strategic type and strategic intensity spectrum, the coordinates (θ, ρ) form a strategic vector with θ as the azimuth angle and ρ as the polar diameter.

Calculate the strategic azimuth θ, the center of gravity coordinate is:

$$P(X, Y) = P\left(\frac{\sum xi}{4}, \frac{\sum yi}{4}\right) \tag{7}$$

The strategic azimuth is:

$$\theta = \arctan\frac{Y}{X} \quad (0 \le \theta \le \pi) \tag{8}$$

Among them, xi and yi are the coordinates of S', W', O', T' in the strategic quadrilateral, respectively.

Calculate the strategic strength coefficient ρ.

The strategic positive intensity is:

$$U = O' \times S' \tag{9}$$

The strategic negative intensity is:

$$V = T' \times W' \tag{10}$$

The strategic intensity coefficient is defined as:

$$\rho = \frac{U}{U+V} \tag{11}$$

The value range of ρ is $[0, 1]$, and the size of ρ indicates the intensity of the strategic type.

3. Results

3.1. AHP Weights and the Intensities of Factors

The results obtained in Tables 4 and 5 show that opportunities are the most important consideration, followed by strengths, weaknesses, and threats. Under the strength category, construction of a leading sports nation was rated as the most important factor, followed by an increased awareness of exercise, time freedom, low cost, and convenience. Under weakness, less theoretical research and insufficient professional talents were rated as the most important factors, followed by limited space leads to fewer sports methods and monotonous and boring form of exercise. Under opportunity, the rapid development of intelligent sports was rated as the most important factor, followed by support provided by the government and the stable development of the sports industry. Under threat, fading enthusiasm for home-based exercise after the epidemic was rated as the most important factor, followed by easy to slack at home and noise.

Table 4. Comparison matrix and weights of SWOT groups and factors.

SWOT Group	Comparison Matrix	Factor Weight	Maximum Eigenvalue (λ_{max})	Consistency Index (CI)	Consistency Ratio (CR)
Strengths (S)	$\begin{bmatrix} 1 & 2 & 4 & 5 \\ 1/2 & 1 & 3 & 4 \\ 1/4 & 1/3 & 1 & 2 \\ 1/5 & 1/4 & 1/2 & 1 \end{bmatrix}$	WS1 = 0.4915 WS2 = 0.3059 WS3 = 0.1249 WS4 = 0.0777	4.0484	0.0161	0.0179
Weaknesses (W)	$\begin{bmatrix} 1 & 2 & 1/4 \\ 1/2 & 1 & 1/3 \\ 4 & 3 & 1 \end{bmatrix}$	WW1 = 0.2184 WW2 = 0.1515 WW3 = 0.6301	3.1078	0.0539	0.0929
Opportunities (O)	$\begin{bmatrix} 1 & 3 & 1/4 \\ 1/3 & 1 & 1/6 \\ 4 & 6 & 1 \end{bmatrix}$	WO1 = 0.2176 WO2 = 0.0914 WO3 = 0.6909	3.0536	0.0268	0.0462
Threats (T)	$\begin{bmatrix} 1 & 1/3 & 1/4 \\ 3 & 1 & 1/2 \\ 4 & 2 & 1 \end{bmatrix}$	WT1 = 0.1220 WT2 = 0.3196 WT3 = 0.5584	3.0183	0.00915	0.0158

CR < 0.1, pass the consistency check.

Table 5. The intensities of groups and factors.

SWOT Group	Factor Weight	Estimated Strength	Factor Intensity	Total Intensity
Strengths (S)	W_{S1} = 0.4915 W_{S2} = 0.3059 W_{S3} = 0.1249 W_{S4} = 0.0777	5 4 3 2	2.4575 1.2236 0.3747 0.1554	$\sum Si = 4.2112$
Weaknesses (W)	W_{W1} = 0.2184 W_{W2} = 0.1515 W_{W3} = 0.6301	−3 −2 −4	−0.6552 −0.3030 −2.5204	$\sum Wi = -3.4786$
Opportunities (O)	W_{O1} = 0.2176 W_{O2} = 0.0914 W_{O3} = 0.6909	3 2 5	0.6528 0.1828 3.4545	$\sum Oi = 4.2901$
Threats (T)	W_{T1} = 0.1220 W_{T2} = 0.3196 W_{T3} = 0.5584	−1 −3 −4	−0.1220 −0.9588 −2.2336	$\sum Ti = -3.3144$

3.2. SWOT Strategic Quadrilateral

The strategic quadrilateral (Figure 2) was drawn based on the calculation results of the total intensities of each group. The results are shown in Table 5:

$$\sum Oi = 4.2901 > \sum Si = 4.2112 > \sum Wi = -3.4786 > \sum Ti = -3.3144. \tag{12}$$

3.3. Strategic Vector (θ, ρ)

The center of gravity coordinate is: $(0.1832, 0.2439)$.
The strategic azimuth is: $\theta = \arctan\left(\frac{0.2439}{0.1832}\right) \approx 53.09° (0 \leq \theta \leq \pi)$.
The strategic positive intensity is: $U = 18.0665$
The strategic negative intensity is: $V = 11.5295$
The strategic strength coefficient is: $\rho = 0.6104$

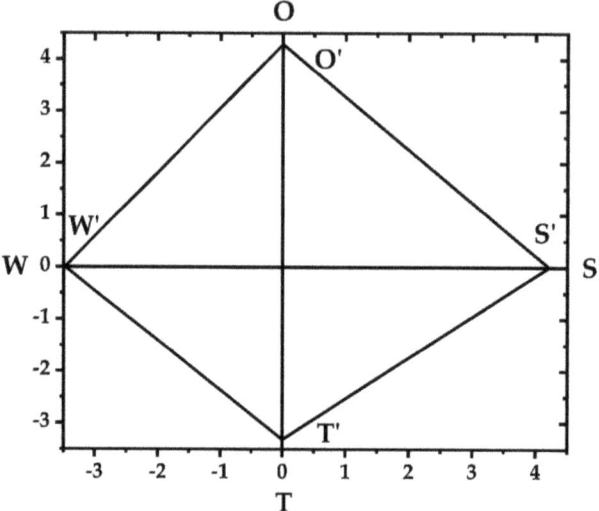

Figure 2. SWOT strategic quadrilateral.

It can be seen from Figure 3 that the coordinates are $(\theta, \rho) = (53.09°, 0.6104)$, indicating that the development of home-based exercise has a greater opportunity and its inherent advantages are also obvious.

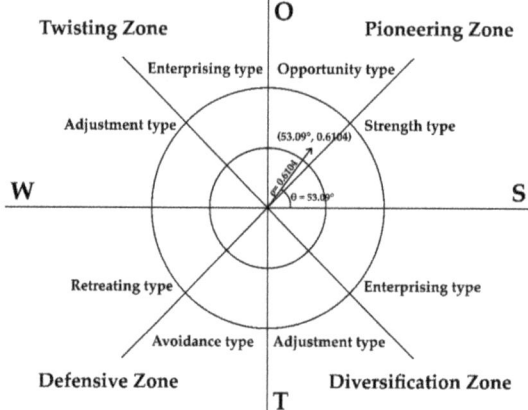

Figure 3. Strategic type and strategic intensity diagrams.

4. Discussion

The results of this study show that opportunities and strengths are more important than weaknesses and threats. It is concluded that home-based exercise in China should adopt the type of SO development strategy that combines internal advantages and external opportunities. When developing the home-based exercise with its featured advantages, its shortcomings should also be improved at the same time. The implementation focus of the development strategy of home-based exercise in China are as follows.

First, in the strength group, the construction of a leading sports nation is the highest rated factor, and under opportunity, support provided by the government has a high importance. With the support of various policies [57–59] and the stable development of

China's sports industry [67,68], the environment of sports in China will get better and better. It is necessary to seize this hard-won opportunity to improve the development of home-based exercise. Home-based exercise should be further promoted to the public with its unique strengths and it will become more popular in the future.

Second, in the opportunity group, the rapid development of intelligent sports is the highest rated factor. With the development of economy and technology in recent years, intelligent sports facilities are also constantly updated [62–66,69–71]. During the COVID-19 epidemic, various intelligent sports facilities also effectively encouraged people's physical activities [72]. In the future, the home will become an important scene for the use of sports equipment. Home-based exercise will advance the development of intelligent sports, and the rapid development of intelligent sports can also propagate the home-based exercise development.

Third, in the weakness group, less theoretical research and insufficient professional talents have a relatively high importance. Home-based exercise hardly attracted attention in the past and few people have conducted targeted research on it. It is still used as a means of rehabilitation after illness or after surgery, rather than as general exercise methods for comprehensive analysis and research [73]. However, during the epidemic, more and more people realized the necessity of home-base exercise and used it as a daily approach to keep healthy and improve mental well-being [74]. Therefore, scholars and researchers should be encouraged to actively carry out empirical research on the home-based exercise, enrich and improve the theoretical system, and fill in academic gaps.

Fourth, under threat, fading enthusiasm for home-based exercise after the epidemic was the highest rated factor. The rapid rise of home-based exercise is mainly due to the epidemic which prevents people from participating in outdoor sports [2,72,74,75]. However, at present, the epidemic prevention and control situation in China is promising, and sports venues are gradually opening up, resulting in a decrease in the number of home-based exercisers. If home-based exercise and outdoor sports are combined and developed in coordination, a new pattern of sports for all will form.

Finally, the lower rated factors in weakness and threat groups also cannot be ignored. As mobile sports apps become more practical, the number of people studying online sports courses is also increasing [76–78]. Traditional online sports courses are mainly based on physical exercise such as muscle strength and flexibility training, which is pretty boring for people. Changes in the form of courses can be made in order to increase the joy of taking courses, which can increase people's enthusiasm for participating in home-based exercise.

5. Conclusions

The COVID-19 epidemic has a great impact on all walks of life, but for home-based exercise, it is a golden opportunity for development. This article uses the SWOT-AHP hybrid model to conduct empirical research on the development of home-based exercise in China. The results indicate that strengths and opportunities have a greater influence on the development of home-based exercise than weaknesses and threats in the four dimensions of SWOT analysis. With the support of the various policies issued by governments and the rapid development of intelligent sports, home-based exercise should grasp the external development opportunities and choose the SO development strategic type that combines internal advantages and external opportunities. However, home-based exercise still has disadvantages such as limited space, low interest, and potential disturbance to the people. However, these problems can be solved with the development of science and technology. Home-based exercise will eventually form a culture and be thoroughly integrated into the lives of people.

The limitation of this study is the limited number of experts participating in the SWOT analysis and the limited SWOT factors, and the conclusions obtained may have deviations within an acceptable range. Future research will involve more experts in different fields for further analysis. The opinions of experts in different fields can be compared. The SWOT factors will be expanded, and the SWOT analysis can be combined with different MCDA methods for a comparative analysis to obtain more reliable data. Due to the bright future of intelligent sports facilities, research on their application in different sports will also be conducted in the future.

Author Contributions: Conceptualization, H.L. and X.C.; methodology, H.L.; software, H.L.; validation, H.L. and X.C.; formal analysis, H.L.; investigation, H.L. and X.C.; resources, H.L. and X.C.; data curation, H.L.; writing—original draft preparation, H.L.; writing—review and editing, X.C. and Y.F.; visualization, X.C.; supervision, X.C.; project administration, X.C.; funding acquisition, X.C. All authors have read and agreed to the published version of the manuscript.

Funding: This study is supported by "The Fundamental Research Funds for the Central Universities".

Institutional Review Board Statement: Not applicable.

Informed Consent Statement: Not applicable.

Conflicts of Interest: The authors declare no conflict of interest.

References

1. Liu, Q.; Zhou, Y.; Xie, X.; Xue, Q.; Zhu, K.; Wan, Z.; Wu, H.; Zhang, J.; Song, R. The prevalence of behavioral problems among school-aged children in home quarantine during the COVID-19 pandemic in china. *J. Affect. Disord.* **2021**, *279*, 412–416. [CrossRef] [PubMed]
2. Maher, J.P.; Hevel, D.J.; Reifsteck, E.J.; Drollette, E.S. Physical activity is positively associated with college students' positive affect regardless of stressful life events during the COVID-19 pandemic. *Psychol. Sport Exerc.* **2021**, *52*, 101826. [CrossRef]
3. Amatori, S.; Donati Zeppa, S.; Preti, A.; Gervasi, M.; Gobbi, E.; Ferrini, F.; Rocchi, M.B.L.; Baldari, C.; Perroni, F.; Piccoli, G.; et al. Dietary Habits and Psychological States during COVID-19 Home Isolation in Italian College Students: The Role of Physical Exercise. *Nutrients* **2020**, *12*, 3660. [CrossRef]
4. Meyer, S.M.; Landry, M.J.; Gustat, J.; Lemon, S.C.; Webster, C.A. Physical distancing physical inactivity. *Transl. Behav. Med.* **2021**. [CrossRef] [PubMed]
5. Tunay, V.B. Hospital-based versus home-based proprioceptive and strengthening exercise programs in knee osteoarthritis. *Acta Orthop. Traumatol. Turc.* **2010**, *44*, 270–277. [CrossRef] [PubMed]
6. Chen, B.; Hu, N.; Tan, J.H. Efficacy of home-based exercise programme on physical function after hip fracture: A systematic review and meta-analysis of randomised controlled trials. *Int. Wound J.* **2019**, *17*, 45–54. [CrossRef]
7. Büker, N.; Şavkın, R.; Ök, N. Comparison of Supervised Exercise and Home Exercise after Ankle Fracture. *J. Foot Ankle Surg.* **2019**, *58*, 822–827. [CrossRef] [PubMed]
8. Brewer, B.W.; Cornelius, A.E.; Van Raalte, J.L.; Tennen, H.; Armeli, S. Predictors of adherence to home rehabilitation exercises following anterior cruciate ligament reconstruction. *Rehabil. Psychol.* **2013**, *58*, 64–72. [CrossRef]
9. Ay, S.; Evcik, D.; Kutsal, Y.G.; Toraman, F.; Okumuş, M.; Eyigör, S.; Şahin, N. Compliance to home-based exercise therapy in elderly patients with knee osteoarthritis. *Turk. J. Phys. Med. Rehabil.* **2016**, *62*, 323–328. [CrossRef]
10. Anwer, S.; Alghadir, A.; Brismée, J.-M. Effect of Home Exercise Program in Patients with Knee Osteoarthritis. *J. Geriatric Physical Therapy* **2016**, *39*, 38–48. [CrossRef]
11. McDermott, M.M.; Polonsky, T.S. Home-Based Exercise A Therapeutic Option for Peripheral Artery Disease. *Circulation* **2016**, *134*, 1127–1129. [CrossRef] [PubMed]
12. Ohkubo, T.; Hozawa, A.; Nagatomi, R.; Fujita, K.; Sauvaget, C.; Watanabe, Y.; Anzai, Y.; Tamagawa, A.; Tsuji, I.; Imai, Y.; et al Effects of exercise training on home blood pressure values in older adults: A randomized controlled trial. *J. Hypertens.* **2001**, *19*, 1045–1052. [CrossRef] [PubMed]
13. Hwang, R.; Marwick, T. Efficacy of home-based exercise programmes for people with chronic heart failure: A meta-analysis. *Eur. J. Cardiovasc. Prev. Rehabil.* **2009**, *16*, 527–535. [CrossRef] [PubMed]
14. Wu, S.-K.; Lin, Y.-W.; Chen, C.-L.; Tsai, S.-W. Cardiac Rehabilitation vs. Home Exercise After Coronary Artery Bypass Graft Surgery. *Am. J. Phys. Med. Rehabil.* **2006**, *85*, 711–717. [CrossRef]
15. Babu, V.; Paul, N. Sudden deaths following the unexpected demise of a popular politician in India. *Int. J. Cardiol.* **2010**, *145*, 266–267. [CrossRef]
16. Besnier, F.; Gayda, M.; Nigam, A.; Juneau, M.; Bherer, L. Cardiac Rehabilitation During Quarantine in COVID-19 Pandemic: Challenges for Center-Based Programs. *Arch. Phys. Med. Rehabil.* **2020**, *101*, 1835–1838. [CrossRef]
17. Liu, X.; Li, P.; Li, J.; Xiao, L.; Li, N.; Lu, Y.; Wang, Z.; Su, J.; Wang, Z.; Shan, C.; et al. Home-Based Prescribed Pulmonary Exercise in Patients with Stable Chronic Obstructive Pulmonary Disease. *J. Vis. Exp.* **2019**. [CrossRef] [PubMed]
18. Behnke, M.; Taube, C.; Kirsten, D.; Lehnigk, B.; JÖRres, R.A.; Magnussen, H. Home-based exercise is capable of preserving hospital-based improvements in severe chronic obstructive pulmonary disease. *Respir. Med.* **2000**, *94*, 1184–1191. [CrossRef]
19. Aytekin, E.; Caglar, N.S.; Ozgonenel, L.; Tutun, S.; Demiryontar, D.Y.; Demir, S.E. Home-based exercise therapy in patients with ankylosing spondylitis: Effects on pain, mobility, disease activity, quality of life, and respiratory functions. *Clin. Rheumatol.* **2011**, *31*, 91–97. [CrossRef]

20. Wonders, K.Y.; Whisler, G.; Loy, H.; Holt, B.; Bohachek, K.; Wise, R. Ten weeks of home-based exercise attenuates symptoms of chemotherapy-induced peripheral neuropathy in breast cancer patients. *Health Psychol. Res.* **2013**, *1*, 149–152. [CrossRef]
21. Kiechle, M.; Friese, K.; Felberbaum, R. Bewegungsmangel, ungesunde Ernährung und Übergewicht. *Der Gynäkologe* **2019**, *52*, 480–481. [CrossRef]
22. Lopez, C.; Jones, J.; Alibhai, S.M.H.; Santa Mina, D. What Is the "Home" in Home-Based Exercise? The Need to Define Independent Exercise for Survivors of Cancer. *J. Clin. Oncol.* **2018**, *36*, 926–927. [CrossRef] [PubMed]
23. Kim, J.Y.; Lee, M.K.; Lee, D.H.; Kang, D.W.; Min, J.H.; Lee, J.W.; Chu, S.H.; Cho, M.S.; Kim, N.K.; Jeon, J.Y. Effects of a 12-week home-based exercise program on quality of life, psychological health, and the level of physical activity in colorectal cancer survivors: A randomized controlled trial. *Supportive Care Cancer* **2018**, *27*, 2933–2940. [CrossRef] [PubMed]
24. Schuch, F.B.; Vancampfort, D.; Richards, J.; Rosenbaum, S.; Ward, P.B.; Stubbs, B. Exercise as a treatment for depression: A meta-analysis adjusting for publication bias. *J. Psychiatr. Res.* **2016**, *77*, 42–51. [CrossRef] [PubMed]
25. Luan, X.; Tian, X.; Zhang, H.; Huang, R.; Li, N.; Chen, P.; Wang, R. Exercise as a prescription for patients with various diseases. *J. Sport Health Sci.* **2019**, *8*, 422–441. [CrossRef] [PubMed]
26. Harvey, S.B.; Øverland, S.; Hatch, S.L.; Wessely, S.; Mykletun, A.; Hotopf, M. Exercise and the Prevention of Depression: Results of the HUNT Cohort Study. *Am. J. Psychiatry* **2018**, *175*, 28–36. [CrossRef] [PubMed]
27. Stanton, R.; Reaburn, P. Exercise and the treatment of depression: A review of the exercise program variables. *J. Sci. Med. Sport* **2014**, *17*, 177–182. [CrossRef]
28. Flynn, A.; Allen, N.E.; Dennis, S.; Canning, C.G.; Preston, E. Home-based prescribed exercise improves balance-related activities in people with Parkinson's disease and has benefits similar to centre-based exercise: A systematic review. *J. Physiother.* **2019**, *65*, 189–199. [CrossRef]
29. Pu, B.; Zhang, L.; Tang, Z.; Qiu, Y. The Relationship between Health Consciousness and Home-Based Exercise in China during the COVID-19 Pandemic. *Int. J. Environ. Res. Public Health* **2020**, *17*, 5693. [CrossRef]
30. Mao, H.Y.; Hsu, H.C.; Lee, S.D. Gender differences in related influential factors of regular exercise behavior among people in Taiwan in 2007: A cross-sectional study. *PLoS ONE* **2020**, *15*, e0228191. [CrossRef]
31. Molanorouzi, K.; Khoo, S.; Morris, T. Motives for adult participation in physical activity: Type of activity, age, and gender. *BMC Public Health* **2015**, *15*, 66. [CrossRef]
32. Bennie, J.A.; De Cocker, K.; Smith, J.J.; Wiesner, G.H. The epidemiology of muscle-strengthening exercise in Europe: A 28-country comparison including 280,605 adults. *PLoS ONE* **2020**, *15*, e0242220. [CrossRef] [PubMed]
33. Ghazinoory, S.; Abdi, M.; Azadegan-Mehr, M. Swot Methodology: A State-of-the-Art Review for the Past, a Framework for the Future/Ssgg Metodologija: Praeities Ir Ateities AnalizÈ. *J. Bus. Econ. Manag.* **2011**, *12*, 24–48. [CrossRef]
34. Helms, M.M.; Nixon, J. Exploring SWOT analysis—Where are we now? *J. Strategy Manag.* **2010**, *3*, 215–251. [CrossRef]
35. Chang, H.-H.; Huang, W.-C. Application of a quantification SWOT analytical method. *Math. Comput. Model.* **2006**, *43*, 158–169. [CrossRef]
36. Sałabun, W.; Wątróbski, J.; Shekhovtsov, A. Are MCDA Methods Benchmarkable? A Comparative Study of TOPSIS, VIKOR, COPRAS, and PROMETHEE II Methods. *Symmetry* **2020**, *12*, 1549. [CrossRef]
37. Zyoud, S.H.; Fuchs-Hanusch, D. A bibliometric-based survey on AHP and TOPSIS techniques. *Expert Syst. Appl.* **2017**, *78*, 158–181. [CrossRef]
38. Kim, Y.-J.; Park, J. A Sustainable Development Strategy for the Uzbekistan Textile Industry: The Results of a SWOT-AHP Analysis. *Sustainability* **2019**, *11*, 4613. [CrossRef]
39. Lee, S.; Walsh, P. SWOT and AHP hybrid model for sport marketing outsourcing using a case of intercollegiate sport. *Sport Manag. Rev.* **2011**, *14*, 361–369. [CrossRef]
40. Saaty, T.L. Decision making with the analytic hierarchy process. *Int. J. Serv. Sci.* **2008**, *1*, 83–98. [CrossRef]
41. Saaty, T.L. *The Analytic Hierarchy Process*; McGraw-Hill: New York, NY, USA, 1980.
42. Subramanian, N.; Ramanathan, R. A review of applications of Analytic Hierarchy Process in operations management. *Int. J. Prod. Econ.* **2012**, *138*, 215–241. [CrossRef]
43. Liberatore, M.J.; Nydick, R.L. The analytic hierarchy process in medical and health care decision making: A literature review. *Eur. J. Oper. Res.* **2008**, *189*, 194–207. [CrossRef]
44. Mustafa, M.A.; Albahar, J.F. Project risk assessment using the analytic hierarchy process. *IEEE Trans. Eng. Manag.* **1991**, *38*, 46–52. [CrossRef]
45. Vaidya, O.S.; Kumar, S. Analytic hierarchy process: An overview of applications. *Eur. J. Oper. Res.* **2006**, *169*, 1–29. [CrossRef]
46. Ishizaka, A.; Labib, A. Review of the main developments in the analytic hierarchy process. *Expert Syst. Appl.* **2011**. [CrossRef]
47. Sałabun, W.; Ziemba, P.; Wątróbski, J. The Rank Reversals Paradox in Management Decisions: The Comparison of the AHP and COMET Methods. In *Intelligent Decision Technologies*; Springer: Cham, Switzerland, 2016; Volume 2016, pp. 181–191. [CrossRef]
48. Gong, T.; Yan, H. An Improvement Research of SWOT Method Based on Analytic Hierarchy Process. *Appl. Mech. Mater.* **2012**, *263–266*, 2287–2290. [CrossRef]
49. Abdel-Basset, M.; Mohamed, M.; Smarandache, F. An Extension of Neutrosophic AHP–SWOT Analysis for Strategic Planning and Decision-Making. *Symmetry* **2018**, *10*, 116. [CrossRef]
50. Ho, W. Integrated analytic hierarchy process and its applications—A literature review. *Eur. J. Oper. Res.* **2008**, *186*, 211–228. [CrossRef]
51. Marttunen, M.; Lienert, J.; Belton, V. Structuring problems for Multi-Criteria Decision Analysis in practice: A literature review of method combinations. *Eur. J. Oper. Res.* **2017**, *263*, 1–17. [CrossRef]

52. Yuan, J.; Xie, H.; Yang, D.; Xiahou, X.; Skibniewski, M.J.; Huang, W. Strategy formulation for the sustainable development of smart cities: A case study of Nanjing, China. *Int. J. Strateg. Prop. Manag.* **2020**, *24*, 379–399. [CrossRef]
53. Liu, R.; Wang, Y.; Qian, Z. Hybrid SWOT-AHP Analysis of Strategic Decisions of Coastal Tourism: A Case Study of Shandong Peninsula Blue Economic Zone. *J. Coast. Res.* **2019**, *94*. [CrossRef]
54. Liu, F.H.; Wang, M.J.; Han, Y.G. The Development Strategy of China's Wushu Sanda Based on SWOT-AHP Model. *China Sport Sci. Technol.* **2016**, *52*, 27–34. [CrossRef]
55. Liu, Y.; Liu, X.; Liang, Z. Evaluation of Henan Sports Tourism Resources Based on AHP and Fuzzy Mathematics. *Areal Res. Dev* **2012**, *31*, 108–111.
56. Kim, J. Environment Analysis Strategy for Revitalizing Cultural Sports. *J. Korea Entertain. Ind. Assoc.* **2018**, *12*, 191–201. [CrossRef]
57. Committee, C.C.; Council, S. The Central Committee of the Communist Party of China and the State Council issued the "Outline of the 'Healthy China 2030' Plan". Available online: http://www.gov.cn/xinwen/2016-10/25/content_5124174.htm (accessed on 25 October 2016).
58. Office of the State Council. Notice of the General Office of the State Council on Issuing the Outline for Building a Leading Sports Nation. Available online: http://www.gov.cn/zhengce/content/2019-09/02/content_5426485.htm (accessed on 2 September 2019).
59. General Office of the State Sports General Administration. Notice of the General Office of the State Sports General Administration on Vigorously Promoting Scientific Home-based Exercise Methods. Available online: http://www.sport.gov.cn/n316/n336/c941798/content.htm (accessed on 30 January 2020).
60. Research i. 2014–2021 China's Online Sports Goods Market Scale and Forecast. Available online: https://data.iimedia.cn/data-classification/detail/13209702.html (accessed on 10 July 2020).
61. Research i. 2012–2022 China's Sports Industry Output Value and Forecast. Available online: https://data.iimedia.cn/data-classification/detail/13002939.html (accessed on 2 July 2019).
62. Ma, H.; Pang, X. Research and Analysis of Sport Medical Data Processing Algorithms Based on Deep Learning and Internet of Things. *IEEE Access* **2019**, *7*, 118839–118849. [CrossRef]
63. Xiao, N.; Yu, W.; Han, X. Wearable heart rate monitoring intelligent sports bracelet based on Internet of things. *Measurement* **2020**, *164*. [CrossRef]
64. Tao, S. Sports Equipment Based on High-Tech Materials. *Appl. Mech. Mater.* **2013**, *340*, 378–381. [CrossRef]
65. Qiu, Y.-H.; Kai, H.; Luo, X.-J. Application of Computer Virtual Reality Technology in Modern Sports. In Proceedings of the 2013 Third International Conference on Intelligent System Design and Engineering Applications, Hong Kong, China, 16–18 January 2013; pp. 362–364.
66. Wang, S.-Y.; Zhou, Y. Study on the Application of VR Technology in Sport Reality Shows. In Proceedings of the 2018 1st International Cognitive Cities Conference (IC3), Okinawa, Japan, 7–9 August 2018; pp. 200–201.
67. Zhang, H.-L.; Zhang, H.-J.; Guo, X.-T. Research on the future development prospects of sports products industry under the mode of e-commerce and internet of things. *Inf. Syst. E-Bus. Manag.* **2020**, *18*, 511–525. [CrossRef]
68. Zhuo, L.; Guan, X.; Ye, S. Quantitative Evaluation and Prediction Analysis of the Healthy and Sustainable Development of China's Sports Industry. *Sustainability* **2020**, *12*, 2184. [CrossRef]
69. Jiang, W. Application of Plastic Composites in Sports Facilities and Fitness Equipment. *China Plast. Ind.* **2019**, *47*, 152–155.
70. Duarte-Rojo, A.; Bloomer, P.M.; Rogers, R.J.; Hassan, M.A.; Dunn, M.A.; Tevar, A.D.; Vivis, S.L.; Bataller, R.; Hughes, C.B.; Ferrando, A.A.; et al. Introducing EL-FIT (Exercise and Liver FITness): A Smartphone App to Prehabilitate and Monitor Liver Transplant Candidates. *Liver Transplant.* **2020**. [CrossRef] [PubMed]
71. McConville, R.; Archer, G.; Craddock, I.; Kozlowski, M.; Piechocki, R.; Pope, J.; Santos-Rodriguez, R. Vesta: A digital health analytics platform for a smart home in a box. *Future Gener. Comput. Syst.* **2021**, *114*, 106–119. [CrossRef]
72. Fearnbach, S.N.; Flanagan, E.W.; Hochsmann, C.; Beyl, R.A.; Altazan, A.D.; Martin, C.K.; Redman, L.M. Factors Protecting against a Decline in Physical Activity during the COVID-19 Pandemic. *Med. Sci. Sports Exerc.* **2021**. [CrossRef] [PubMed]
73. Loellgen, H.; Zupet, P.; Bachl, N.; Debruyne, A. Physical Activity, Exercise Prescription for Health and Home-Based Rehabilitation. *Sustainability* **2020**, *12*, 230. [CrossRef]
74. Puyat, J.H.; Ahmad, H.; Avina-Galindo, A.M.; Kazanjian, A.; Gupta, A.; Ellis, U.; Ashe, M.C.; Vila-Rodriguez, F.; Halli, P.; Salmon A.; et al. A rapid review of home-based activities that can promote mental wellness during the COVID-19 pandemic. *PLoS ONE* **2020**, *15*. [CrossRef]
75. Lippi, G.; Henry, B.M.; Bovo, C.; Sanchis-Gomar, F. Health risks and potential remedies during prolonged lockdowns for coronavirus disease 2019 (COVID-19). *Diagnosis* **2020**, *7*, 85–90. [CrossRef] [PubMed]
76. Garcia-Fernandez, J.; Galvez-Ruiz, P.; Grimaldi-Puyana, M.; Angosto, S.; Fernandez-Gavira, J.; Bohorquez, M.R. The Promotion of Physical Activity from Digital Services: Influence of E-Lifestyles on Intention to Use Fitness Apps. *Int. J. Environ. Res. Public Health* **2020**, *17*, 6839. [CrossRef]
77. Bitrian, P.; Buil, I.; Catalan, S. Gamification in sport apps: The determinants of users' motivation. *Eur. J. Manag. Bus. Econ.* **2020**, *29*, 365–381. [CrossRef]
78. Vega-Ramirez, L.; Notario, R.O.; Avalos-Ramos, M.A. The Relevance of Mobile Applications in the Learning of Physical Education. *Educ. Sci.* **2020**, *10*, 329. [CrossRef]

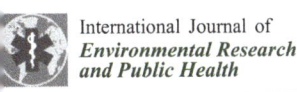

Article

Ball Impact Position in Recreational Male Padel Players: Implications for Training and Injury Management

Bernardino Javier Sánchez-Alcaraz [1], Rafael Martínez-Gallego [2], Salvador Llana [2], Goran Vučković [3], Diego Muñoz [4,*], Javier Courel-Ibáñez [1], Alejandro Sánchez-Pay [1] and Jesús Ramón-Llin [5]

1. Department of Physical Activity and Sport, Faculty of Sport Sciences, University of Murcia. C/ Argentina, s/n, 30720 San Javier, Spain; bjavier.sanchez@um.es (B.J.S.-A.); courel@um.es (J.C.-I.); aspay@um.es (A.S.-P.)
2. Department of Physical Education and Sport, Faculty of Sport Sciences, University of Valencia, Av. Blasco Ibáñez, 13, 46010 Valencia, Spain; rafael.martinez-gallego@uv.es (R.M.-G.); salvador.llana@uv.es (S.L.)
3. Faculty of Sport, University of Ljubljana, Gortanova ul. 22, 1000 Ljubljana, Slovenia; goran.vuckovic@fsp.uni-lj.si
4. Department of Musical, Plastic and Corporal Expression, Faculty of Sport Sciences, University of Extremadura, Av. de la Universidad, s/n, 10003 Cáceres, Spain
5. Department of Musical, Plastic and Corporal Expression, Faculty of Education, University of Valencia, Av. dels Tarongers, 4, 46022 Valencia, Spain; jesus.ramon@uv.es
* Correspondence: diegomun@unex.es; Tel.: +34-927-257-460

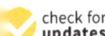

Citation: Sánchez-Alcaraz, B.J.; Martínez-Gallego, R.; Llana, S.; Vuckovic, G.; Muñoz, D.; Courel-Ibáñez, J.; Sánchez-Pay, A.; Ramón-Llin, J. Ball Impact Position in Recreational Male Padel Players: Implications for Training and Injury Management. *Int. J. Environ. Res. Public Health* **2021**, *18*, 435. https://doi.org/10.3390/ijerph18020435

Received: 26 November 2020
Accepted: 5 January 2021
Published: 7 January 2021

Publisher's Note: MDPI stays neutral with regard to jurisdictional claims in published maps and institutional affiliations.

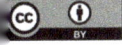

Copyright: © 2021 by the authors. Licensee MDPI, Basel, Switzerland. This article is an open access article distributed under the terms and conditions of the Creative Commons Attribution (CC BY) license (https://creativecommons.org/licenses/by/4.0/).

Abstract: Racket sports such as padel are characterized by the repetition of unilateral gestures, which can lead to negative adaptations like asymmetries or overuse musculoskeletal injuries. The purpose of this study was to determine the differences in ball impact positions (i.e., forward or backward of the center of gravity) in nine stroke types in a sample of forty-eight recreational male padel players. The sample included 14,478 shots corresponding to 18 matches from six tournaments. Forty-eight male padel players were classified into two groups according to their level: trained ($n = 24$) and novice ($n = 24$). Type of stroke and ball impact position were registered using a computerized motion tracking video system. The ball impact position was computed from the distance (cm) between the coordinates of the ball and the player's center of gravity. Results show that trained players hit the ball in a more backward position (from 11 to 25 cm, compared to novice) in serve and offensive strokes (volleys, trays, and smashes) but used more forward strokes (from 7 to 32 cm, compared to novice) in defensive shots (groundstrokes, wall strokes, and lobs). Because the current differential variables are trainable and demonstrated to be of relevance for performance, the findings of this study may assist padel coaches in designing proper training plans to improve effectiveness and to prevent musculoskeletal injuries regarding the type of stroke and ball impact position. Such knowledge may constitute a very important factor affecting technique, biomechanics, and injury management in padel players of different competitive levels.

Keywords: racket sports; overuse injury; biomechanics; game actions

1. Introduction

Racket sports such as padel are characterized by a solid game structure with little variety of actions that are constantly repeated in a very short period of time [1–3]. Particularly in padel, each player performs ~4–6 strokes per rally, for a total of ~300 hits per game [4,5], varying among just four big types of shots: volleys, smashes, serves, and groundstrokes [2,6]. This massive repetition of specific unilateral swinging gestures is a determining factor for suffering from strength imbalances [7,8] and overuse musculoskeletal injuries in the upper limb [9]. Elbow and shoulder injuries are related to improper technique and biomechanics patterns, such as an incorrect impact point location [10,11]. This notion is corroborated by electromyography-based studies, finding that highly trained players experienced a lower vibration on the forehand and wrist during a groundstroke compared to novice players [12,13]. Thus, hitting mechanics and ball impact are fundamental to preventing elbow injuries in racket sports. This is interesting since technique and stance are modifiable with proper training [14].

During a padel game, players are required to continuously perform quick changes of direction—frontal, lateral, diagonal displacements, and turns—predominantly to the same side [2,6,15]. This unilateral nature of padel has been shown to produce asymmetries between the dominant and non-dominant side after regular practice [7]. The identification of these negative adaptations is essential to assist coaches and practitioners in the need of including preventive strengthening and balance exercises in their training routines to minimize the risk of pain, injuries, and abandonment of the practice. This is particularly important in padel due to the growing number of amateur practitioners worldwide, being mainly middle-aged people between 35 and 55 years [16,17]. State-of-the-art in padel includes available literature concerning temporal structure [3,18–20], players' movements and distance covered on the court [6,15,21], game technical–tactical dynamics [1,2,22–24], fitness status [7,25,26], and injuries [11,27,28]. However, little is known about fundamental motor skills such as the ball impact position [29].

Hitting the ball earlier (forward impact) or later (backward impact) in the stroke can produce changes in a shot's velocity, direction, or accuracy [30]. In addition to affecting performance, hitting the ball chronically in a dangerous impact point may increase the risk of elbow and shoulder pain and discomfort, eventually leading to injury [10,11]. For instance, in padel, overhead actions such as smashes and trays are of relevance for winning the game [2]. To be effective, the smash implies a high velocity joint rotation to hit at the maximum speed and hitting the ball in a pronounced lumbar extension stance. This particular position may alarmingly increase the probability of suffering an injury in padel if hitting the ball in a backward stance.

Stroke types in racket sports such as padel have four different phases of motion: racket preparation, acceleration, impact point, and follow through [31]. When investigating the production of high energy in the padel strokes and their contribution to injury etiology, the kinetic chain concept of motion cannot be ignored [32,33]. Kinetic chains describe the course and route of energy flow during a padel stroke. Thereby, musculoskeletal joints involved during the hit, such us the knee, shoulder, and elbow, are integrated in the task of absorbing, generating, and transmitting energy from one joint to another, completing a cycle of energy from the ground to the ball at impact with the padel racket [33]. The optimal functioning of this process is essential to avoiding overloaded injury when energy transfer throughout joints is not well coordinated, especially during the ball impact point [14,34].

The effective use of joint biomechanics can vary among players with different experience levels. Highly trained players are shown to be more efficient at adapting the kinetic chain to reduce the impact forces transmitted to upper extremity joints. In turn, the absence of efficient technique in recreational padel players often leads to an excessive and uncoordinated use of strength that does not translate into increasing the speed of the ball, but to overloading the joint and an increased risk of injury [35,36]. Thus, developing an optimal stroke technique during one's formative and recreational stages can importantly contribute to minimizing the risk of suffering an injury by reducing the loads placed on body joints.

Evidence supports important health-related quality of life benefits in padel's regular practitioners [25]. Padel is played in pairs using tennis' rules and scoring system but is played inside an enclosed synthetic glass and metal court with small dimensions (10×20 m). One main characteristic of padel is that the ball can rebound on the side and back walls, which results in an enhanced game rhythm and more frequent actions, without increased physical intensity compared to similar racket sports [2,6]. Padel practice has important advantages compared to other racket sports that make it a powerful tool for health promotion, namely: High technical skills are not required to start practicing, the long duration of rallies increases people's enjoyment, it can be played outdoors, and its equipment is cheap [3,37,38]. Hence, padel seems to play an important role in promoting physical habits among adults. However, considering the potential rise of chronic pain that may eventually lead to injury and abandonment of the practice [10,11], recreational players should consider preventive strategies such as adopting a proper technique from the beginning of their practice.

Because better knowledge of ball impact position has important implications for training and injury management, there is a need for examining players' ball impact position in padel. Therefore, the aim of this study was to determine the differences in ball impact positions (i.e., forward or backward of the center of gravity) in nine stroke types in a sample of forty-eight recreational male padel players of two different levels: highly trained (1st regional category) and novice (3rd regional category).

2. Materials and Methods

2.1. Sample and Procedures

The sample included 14,478 shots corresponding to 18 matches (six finals and twelve semi-finals) from a total of six tournaments. Forty-eight male padel players (mean ± SD age: 31.2 ± 7.3 years; height: 181.3 ± 4.1 cm) volunteered to participate. Players were classified in two groups according to their levels of competition: highly trained (1st category of regional padel tournaments; $n = 24$) and novice (3rd category of regional padel tournaments, $n = 24$). Tournament organizers and padel players provided written consent for the recording of matches, according to the ethics board of the local university (ID: 154/2020). The matches were played following the official game regulations [39].

Matches were filmed using two digital Bosch Dinion Model IP 455 video cameras (Bosch, Munich, Germany) at 25 frames per second, placed over the courts at 6 m from the center and over the service line. Players' and balls' coordinates were analyzed using a computerized motion tracking system (SAGIT/Squash) [21,40] that uses computer vision methods on video captured via fixed cameras located above the court (Figure 1). The SAGIT/Squash tracking system has been specifically designed for racket sports analysis. In addition, the software allows the use of position inputs to track ball location. A separate input system was designed to allow the operator to watch the video from the overhead camera while highlighting the ball position on the court via a touch sensitive interface. The techniques for transferring video images into the tracker has been well documented [41]. Similarly, the reliability for the resultant calculations of player and ball position on court has been shown to be acceptable for analysis purposes [42]. Video analysis of technical actions (i.e., stroke types) was conducted by systematic observation using LINCE software [43]. This free-access software allows the creation of a coding tool synchronized with the video, and the resulting data file can be exported in Excel. Two observers, graduates in Physical Activity and Sports Sciences and padel coaches with more than 10 years' experience, were specifically trained for this task. The training focused on the clear identification of the variables and the use of the software. At the end of the training process, each observer analyzed the same sample sets in order to calculate the inter-observer reliability by means of Cohen's kappa, obtaining a very high level of agreement ($k > 0.81$) [44].

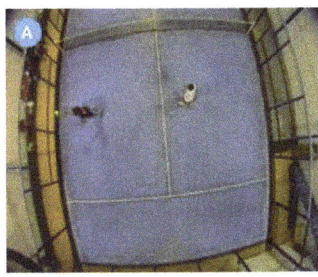 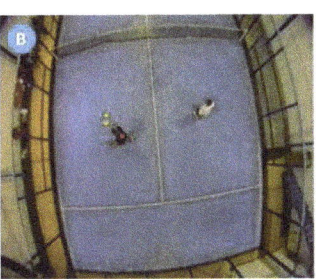 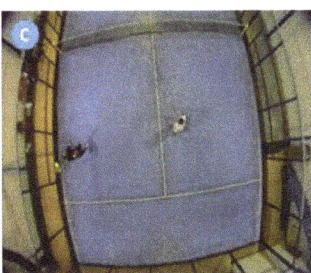

Figure 1. Example of aligned (**A**), forward (**B**), and backward (**C**) ball impact positions.

2.2. Variables Collected

Padel strokes were classified in nine different types [2]: Serve (first and second serve), groundstroke (forehand or backhand direct shot), backwall (forehand or backhand after a rebound on the back wall), lateral wall (forehand or backhand after a rebound on the lateral wall), double wall (forehand or backhand after a bounce on two walls of the court) lob (stroke made with a high trajectory with the aim of overcoming the opponents that are at the net), smash (shot without a bounce that was made by the dominant side of the player hitting the ball with the arm outstretched, over the head, with a flat or topspin effect), tray (stroke without a bounce that was made by the dominant side of the player, hitting the ball at an intermediate height between the volley and the smash and with a slice effect), and volley (stroke without a bounce that was made by hitting the ball at head height with either a forehand or backhand). These technical gestures were coded through LINCE software video analysis. The ball impact position was calculated from the distance (cm) between the coordinates of the ball and the player's center of gravity through SAGIT software. An example of aligned, forward, and backward ball impact positions are depicted in Figure 1

2.3. Data Analysis

The normal distribution of the sample was verified using the Kolmogorov–Smirnov test. Levene's test was used to test for equality of variances. Then, Student's t-test was applied to compare the distribution of means between homogenous groups, and the Welch–Satterthwaite robust test was applied when unequal variances existed. The level of significance was set at $p < 0.05$. Effect sizes (ES) were estimated by calculating the 95% confidence intervals for Cohen's d, interpreted as small (0.20), medium (0.50), and large (0.80) [45]. The chi-square test and adjusted standardized residuals (ASR) were used to identify differences in the stroke type distribution between groups of players. The Crammér's V effect size was interpreted as small, medium, and large according to degrees of freedom [46]. Statistical calculations were performed using a custom Microsoft Excel spreadsheet and SPSS v.24 (IBM Corp., Armonk, NY, USA). Figures were designed using GraphPad Prism 6.0 (GraphPad Software Inc., San Diego, CA, USA).

3. Results

Figure 2 shows the distribution of stroke types regarding the level of the players Overall, the most common strokes types were volleys, serves, groundstrokes, and backwalls Lobs accounted for less than two out of ten strokes. There were particular differences in the use of strokes among highly trained and novice players ($X^2_{(8)} = 515.264$, $p < 0.001$ $V = 0.19$), with novices using more services (ASR = 8.9), groundstrokes (ASR = 13.0), and lobs (ASR = 4.9), but the highly trained players using more volleys (ASR = 14.3), wall strokes (ASR from 1.9 to 7.2), and smashes (ASR = 6.7).

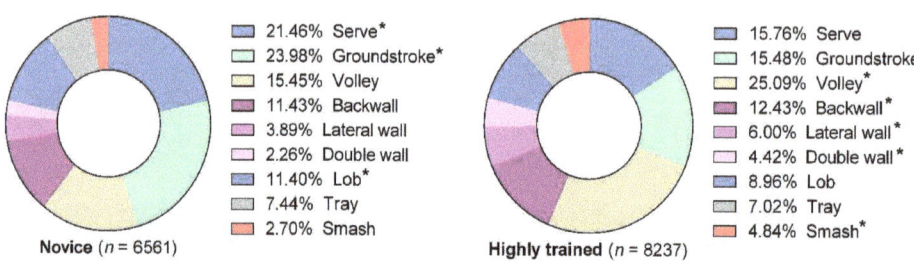

Figure 2. Stroke type distribution between highly trained and novice padel players. Asterisks indicated a significantly greater prevalence in a given group compared to the other ($p < 0.05$).

The ball impact position importantly varied among highly trained and novice players (Table 1, Figure 3). Overall, highly trained players hit the ball in a more backward position (from 11 to 25 cm back compared to novice) in serve, volley, tray, and smash strokes. In turn, they performed more forward strokes (from 7 to 32 cm forward compared to novice) in groundstrokes, wall strokes, and lobs. The greatest differences were found in backwall, tray, volley, and double wall strokes (ES > 0.50).

Table 1. Mean differences in the ball impact position (m) between highly trained and novice padel players in different stroke types.

Stroke Type	Highly Trained (n = 8237)	Novice (n = 6561)	Mean Difference	Mean Difference (95% CI)		Effect Size	p-Value
				Lower	Upper		
Serve	0.52 (0.28)	0.69 (0.25)	−0.11	−0.13	−0.09	0.42	<0.001 *
Groundstroke	0.64 (0.32)	0.57 (0.34)	0.07	0.05	0.10	−0.23	<0.001 *
Volley	0.38 (0.26)	0.51 (0.26)	−0.14	−0.15	−0.12	0.52	<0.001 *
Tray	−0.01 (0.34)	0.24 (0.31)	−0.25	−0.29	−0.21	0.76	<0.001 *
Smash	0.45 (0.44)	0.60 (0.30)	−0.15	−0.22	−0.08	0.40	<0.001 *
Backwall	0.43 (0.41)	0.11 (0.35)	0.32	0.28	0.35	−0.83	<0.001 *
Lob	0.65 (0.32)	0.59 (0.38)	0.06	0.03	0.10	−0.18	0.001 *
Lateral wall	0.73 (0.38)	0.61 (0.37)	0.13	0.07	0.19	−0.35	<0.001 *
Double wall	0.49 (0.43)	0.26 (0.44)	0.24	0.15	0.32	−0.54	<0.001 *

ES = Cohen's d effect size. * Significant mean differences between groups ($p < 0.05$).

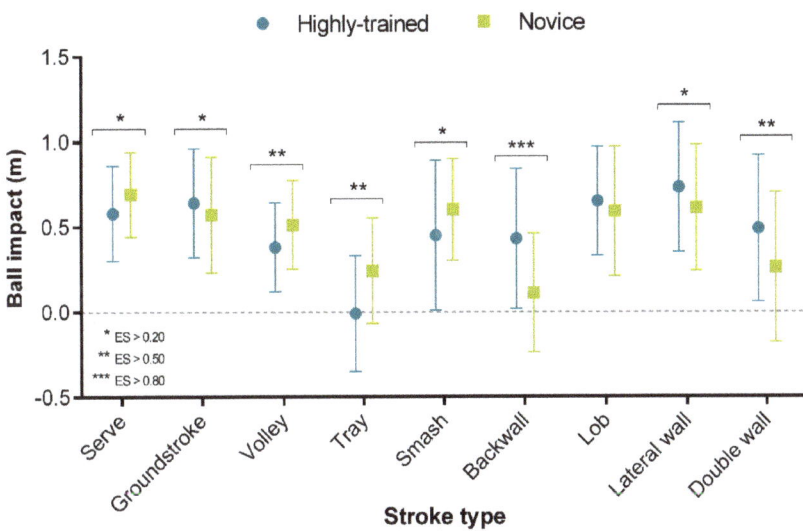

Figure 3. Differences in ball impact position (y-axis, in m) and different stroke types (x-axis) between highly trained and novice padel players (markers). Data from 14,798 strokes. Asterisks indicate significant mean differences ($p < 0.05$) at small, middle, and large effect size (ES).

4. Discussion

The aim of this study was to determine the differences in ball impact positions (i.e., forward or backward of the center of gravity) in nine padel stroke types according to players' level. The results show that the most-used strokes in padel were volleys, serves, and groundstrokes (novice: 21.46% serves, 23.98% groundstrokes, and 15.45% volleys; highly trained: 15.76% serves, 15.48% groundstrokes, and 25.09% volleys). Similar results have been reporter by previous studies that have quantified the distribution of padel strokes [2,4,47]. There were particular differences in the use of strokes among highly trained and novice players, with novices using more services (21.46%), groundstrokes (23.98%), and lobs (11.40%), but the highly trained players using more volleys (25.09%), wall strokes (22.85%), and smashes (4.84%) (Figure 1). The tactical dynamics of better players might account for these differences due to their positioning and movement when approaching the net, increasing the time spent at the net and enhancing scoring options [1,2,23]. Thus, a recent study indicated that the winning pairs performed a significantly higher percentage of smashes and volleys and a lower number of groundstrokes, walls strokes, and lobs than the losers [47]. This is important given that overhead strokes, such us smashes and volleys, imply high velocities of glenohumeral joint rotation, which is related to a higher prevalence of shoulder injuries in highly trained padel players [11,48]. In light of the current results, conditioning programs in padel should include core stabilization, kinetic chain integration, and functional strengthening (eccentric and isometric) exercises to both prevent injuries and increase performance [28]. Interestingly, our findings showed a very high percentage of serves (>15%) in both, highly trained and novice players. This is logical because the point starts with this stroke, but it suggests that coaches include serve and volley exercises, given that the serving pair has a significant advantage in rallies, which lasted until shot 7 in women and shot 12 in men [24].

One of the main contributions of this study is the analysis of the ball impact position in padel and its relationship with players' level. Our results show that ball impact positions in padel were < 0.80 m forward of the player's center of gravity. However, ball impact position importantly varied among highly trained and novice players (Table 1, Figure 3). Overall, highly trained players hit the ball in a more backward position (from 11 to 25 cm back compared to novices) in serve and attacking shots (volleys, trays, and smashes). In turn, they performed more forward strokes (from 7 to 32 cm forward compared to novices) in defensive shots (groundstrokes, wall strokes, and lobs). The more forward impact position in groundstrokes and wall strokes for highly trained players could be attributed to their technical superiority, hitting the ball quickly after the bounce, which allowed them not only to increase the pace of the game but also to anticipate the recovery movements of the opposition. However, a more backward impact position permitted more skilled players to do a longer impact point in the attacking shots (volleys, trays, and smashes), increasing the mechanical impulse during the acceleration of the shots. Taking into account that the joint lesions in padel are located mainly in the elbow (lateral epicondylitis) [11,28] and that there is evidence that this injury occurs predominately in recreational players as a consequence of improper technique (hitting the ball in a backward point) [9,10,49], these findings could help coaches to work on novice players' biomechanics patterns (i.e., backhand and backhand volleys, trays, or wall strokes), with the aim to hit the ball more forward in defensive groundstrokes. On the other hand, from a tactical point of view, these results could provide important information to develop the ability to anticipate an opponent's shots, since ball impact position is related to shot direction in racket sports [50]. Players could use this information to guide their actions or movements on court more efficiently and productively [30,50,51].

It is worth mentioning that the video system employed (SAGIT/Squash) allowed us to determine players' and ball position with high accuracy by employing low-cost and accessible equipment such as a video camera and specific PC software. Nonetheless, although effective for research purposes, these methods may be impractical for real training and competition contexts in which coaches and players require instant feedback to better perform. In this sense, wearable GPS tracking technology is rapidly evolving and providing essential information for practice, such as match activity and external load [52]. In addition, portable inertial motion systems (IMU) are emerging as an alternative to expensive 3D systems to examine angular kinematics and identify biomechanical profiles in racket sports [53]. Although this technology is extremely useful for tracking players' actions and movements, they cannot provide information about ball position. Certainly, recent auto-tracking methods such as Hawkeye or FoXTENN provide this information; however, their high costs make them inaccessible for most coaches and clubs. Thus, despite being time consuming and having the practical disadvantage of wearable devices, video systems are to date one of the best alternatives to effectively examine the interaction between the players and the ball.

The current study adds novel insights into the growing body of knowledge of padel training and assessment, providing for the first time an analysis of ball impact position in nine stroke types and its relationship with players' level. Such knowledge may constitute a very important factor affecting technique, biomechanics, and injury management in padel players. However, some limitations to the study should be noted. First, we did not take into account the ball height above the floor and the court zone in players' impacts. Future research should also consider these two variables using a tracking system and their relationship with some of the performance indicators in padel, such as shot type, effectiveness, and direction [47,54,55]. Second, players' musculoskeletal injuries were not analyzed. It would be interesting to study the relationship between technique and biomechanics patterns and injury epidemiology in adolescent padel players. Finally, future studies could repeat these analyses to compare the differences in ball impact position in professional and female padel players.

5. Conclusions

This study reports new contributions on game analysis indicators in padel and could help players and coaches detect factors related to injury. The most common stroke types were volleys, serves, groundstrokes, and backwalls. Highly trained players used more volleys, wall strokes, and smashes, but novices used more services, groundstrokes, and lobs. This implies special attention to upper body power and strength in padel conditioning sessions to prevent injuries in advanced players. Although ball impact position in padel is between 0 to 0.8 m forward of the player's center of gravity, there are important differences according to players' level. Highly trained players hit the ball in a more backward position in serve and offensive shots (volleys, trays, and smashes), and they performed more forward strokes in defensive shots (groundstrokes, wall strokes, and lobs). The findings of this study will allow padel coaches to enhance the quality and accuracy of training programs based on specific match activity and technical–tactical demands and according to stroke distribution and players' level. Finally, backhand strokes could be less invasive regarding injuries. In this sense, training exercises should propose a continuous change of strokes and situations (groundstrokes and volleys or smashes) to prevent overuse musculoskeletal injuries.

Author Contributions: Conceptualization, J.R.-L., B.J.S.-A., G.V., and D.M.; methodology, B.J.S.-A., J.C.-I., J.R.-L., A.S.-P., and D.M.; software, B.J.S.-A., G.V., S.L., and R.M.-G.; validation, B.J.S.-A., R.M.-G., J.R.-L., S.L., and G.V.; formal analysis, B.J.S.-A., J.C.-I., and A.S.-P.; investigation, B.J.S.-A., J.C.-I., R.M.-G., J.R.-L., A.S.-P., and D.M.; resources, B.J.S.-A., J.R.-L., S.L., A.S.-P., and D.M.; data curation, B.J.S.-A., J.R.-L., A.S.-P., J.C.-I., S.L., and D.M.; writing—original draft preparation, B.J.S.-A., J.C.-I., J.R.-L., and D.M.; writing—review and editing, B.J.S.-A., R.M.-G., J.R.-L., A.S.-P., and D.M.; visualization, B.J.S.-A., R.M.-G., J.R.-L., A.S.-P., and D.M.; supervision, B.J.S.-A., J.R.-L., A.S.-P., J.C.-I., and D.M. All authors have read and agreed to the published version of the manuscript.

Funding: This research received no external funding.

Institutional Review Board Statement: The study was conducted according to the guidelines of the Declaration of Helsinki, and approved by the Ethics Committee of University of Extremadura (ID: 154/2020, data of approval: 25 September 2020).

Informed Consent Statement: Informed consent was obtained from all subjects involved in the study.

Data Availability Statement: The data presented in this study are available on request from the corresponding author. The data are not publicly available due to privacy.

Conflicts of Interest: The authors declare no conflict of interest.

References

1. Courel-Ibáñez, J.; Alcaraz-Martínez, B.J.S. The role of hand dominance in padel: Performance profiles of professional players. *Motricidade* **2018**, *14*, 33–41. [CrossRef]
2. Courel-Ibáñez, J.; Sánchez-Alcaraz, B.J.; Muñoz Marín, D. Exploring Game Dynamics in Padel: Implications for Assessment and Training. *J. Strength Cond. Res.* **2019**, *33*, 1971–1977. [CrossRef]
3. Courel-Ibáñez, J.; Sánchez-Alcaraz, B.J.; Cañas, J. Game performance and length of rally in professional padel player. *J. Hum. Kinet.* **2017**, *55*, 161–169. [CrossRef]
4. Torres-Luque, G.; Ramirez, A.; Cabello-Manrique, D.; Nikolaidis, P.T.; Alvero-Cruz, J.R. Match analysis of elite players during paddle tennis competition. *Int. J. Perform. Anal. Sport* **2015**, *15*, 1135–1144. [CrossRef]
5. Sánchez-Alcaraz, B.J. Game actions and temporal structure diferences between male and female professional paddle players. *Acción Mot.* **2014**, *12*, 17–22.
6. Priego, J.I.; Melis, J.O.; Llana-Belloch, S.; Pérezsoriano, P.; García, J.C.G.; Almenara, M.S.; Priego Quesada, J.I.; Olaso Melis, J. Llana Belloch, S.; Pérez Soriano, P.; et al. Padel: A Quantitative study of the shots and movements in the high-performance. *J. Hum. Sport Exerc.* **2013**, *8*, 925–931. [CrossRef]
7. Courel-Ibáñez, J.; Herrera-Gálvez, J.J. Fitness testing in padel: Performance differences according to players' competitive level. *Sci. Sport.* **2020**, *35*, e11–e19. [CrossRef]
8. Sanchis-Moysi, J.; Idoate, F.; Izquierdo, M.; Calbet, J.A.; Dorado, C. The hypertrophy of the lateral abdominal wall and quadratus lumborum is sport-specific: An MRI segmental study in professional tennis and soccer players. *Sport. Biomech.* **2013**, *12*, 54–67. [CrossRef] [PubMed]
9. Abrams, G.; Renstrom, P.; Safran, M. Epidemiology of musculoskeletal injury in the tennis player. *Br. J. Sports Med.* **2012**, *46*, 492–498. [CrossRef] [PubMed]
10. Gruchow, H.; Pelletier, D. An epidemiologic study of tennis elbow. Incidence, recurrence and effectiveness of prevention strategies. *Am. J. Sport. Sci. Med.* **1979**, *7*, 234–238. [CrossRef]
11. Castillo-Lozano, R.; Casuso-Holgado, M.J. A comparison musculoskeletal injuries among junior and senior paddle-tennis players. *Sci. Sports* **2015**, *30*, 268–274. [CrossRef]
12. Giangarra, C.; Conroy, B.; Jobe, F. Electromyographic and cinematographic analysis of elbow function in tennis players using single- and double-handed backhand strokes. *Am. J. Sport. Sci. Med.* **1993**, *21*, 394–399. [CrossRef] [PubMed]
13. Hennig, E.; Rosenbaum, D.; Milani, T. Transfer of tennis racket vibrations onto the human forearm. *Med. Sci. Sport. Exerc.* **1992**, *24*, 1134–1140. [CrossRef]
14. Reid, M.; Elliott, B.; Crespo, M. Mechanics and learning practices Associated with the Tennis forehand: A review. *J. Sport. Sci Med.* **2013**, *12*, 225–231.
15. Ramón-Llín, J.; Guzmán, J.; Llana, S.; Vuckovic, G.; Muñoz, D.; Sánchez-Alcaraz, B.J. Analysis of distance covered in padel based on level of play and number of points per match. *Retos* **2021**, *39*, 205–209.
16. Courel-Ibáñez, J.; Sánchez-Alcaraz, B.J.; García, S.; Echegaray, M. Evolution of padel in spain according to practitioners' gender and age. *Cult. Cienc. y Deport.* **2017**, *12*, 39–46. [CrossRef]
17. International Padel Federation. List of FIP Associated Countries. Available online: https://www.padelfip.com/es/ (accessed on 31 December 2020).
18. García-Benítez, S.; Courel-Ibáñez, J.; Pérez-Bilbao, T.; Felipe, J.L. Game responses during young padel match play: Age and sex comparisons. *J. Strength Cond. Res.* **2018**, *32*, 1144–1149. [CrossRef]
19. Sañudo, B.; De Hoyo, M.; Carrasco, L. Structural characteristics and physiological demands of the paddle competition. *Apunt. Educ. Física y Deport.* **2008**, *94*, 23–28.
20. Courel-Ibáñez, J.; Sánchez-Alcaraz, B.J. Effect of situational variables on points in elite padel players. *Apunt. Educ. Fis. y Deport* **2017**, *127*, 68–74.
21. Ramón-Llin, J.; Guzmán, J.F.; Belloch, S.L.; Vučković, G.; James, N. Comparison of distance covered in paddle in the serve team according to performance level. *J. Hum. Sport Exerc.* **2013**, *8*, S738–S742. [CrossRef]
22. Muñoz, D.; Sánchez-Alcaraz, B.J.; Courel-Ibáñez, J.; Diaz, J.; Julian, A.; Munoz, J. Differences in winning the net zone in padel between professional and advance players. *J. Sport Health Res.* **2017**, *9*, 223–231.
23. Courel-Ibáñez, J.; Sánchez-Alcaraz, B.J.; Cañas, J. Effectiveness at the net as a predictor of final match outcome in professional padel players. *Int. J. Perform. Anal. Sport* **2015**, *15*, 632–640. [CrossRef]
24. Sánchez-Alcaraz, B.J.; Muñoz, D.; Pradas, F.; Ramón-Llin, J.; Cañas, J.; Sánchez-Pay, A. Analysis of Serve and Serve-Return Strategies in Elite Male and Female Padel. *Appl. Sci.* **2020**, *10*, 6693. [CrossRef]
25. Courel-Ibáñez, J.; Cordero, J.C.; Muñoz, D.; Sánchez-Alcaraz, B.J.; Grijota, F.J.; Robles, M.C. Fitness benefits of padel practice in middle-aged adult women. *Sci. Sport.* **2018**, *33*, 291–298. [CrossRef]
26. Sánchez-Muñoz, C.; Muros, J.J.; Cañas, J.; Courel-Ibáñez, J.; Sánchez-Alcaraz, B.J.B.J.; Zabala, M. Anthropometric and physical fitness profiles of world-class male padel players. *Int. J. Environ. Res. Public Health* **2020**, *17*, 508. [CrossRef]
27. Sánchez Alcaraz-Martínez, B.J.; Courel-Ibáñez, J.; Díaz García, J.; Muñoz Marín, D. Descriptive study about injuries in padel. Relationship with gender, age, players' level and injuries location. *Rev. Andaluza Med. del Deport.* **2019**, *12*, 29–34.
28. Castillo-Lozano, R.; Casuso-Holgado, M.J. Incidence of musculoskeletal sport injuries in a sample of male and female recreational paddle-tennis players. *J. Sports Med. Phys. Fitness* **2017**, *57*, 816–821.

29. Sánchez-Alcaraz Martínez, B.J.; Courel-Ibáñez, J.; Cañas, J. Temporal structure, court movements and game actions in padel: A systematic review. *Retos* **2018**, *33*, 308–312.
30. Shim, J.; Carlton, L.G.; Kwon, Y.-H. Perception of Kinematic Characteristics of Tennis Strokes for Anticipating Stroke Type and Direction. *Res. Q. Exerc. Sport* **2006**, *77*, 326–339. [CrossRef]
31. Fernandez, A.; León-Prados, J.A. Technical and tactical assessment tool for padel. *Rev. Int. Med. y Ciencias la Act. Fis. y del Deport.* **2017**, *17*, 693–714.
32. Elliott, B. Biomechanics and tennis. *Brithis J. Sport. Med.* **2006**, *40*, 392–396. [CrossRef] [PubMed]
33. Chung, K.C.; Lark, M.E. Upper Extremity Injuries in Tennis Players: Diagnosis, Treatment, and Management. *Hand Clin.* **2017**, *33*, 175–186. [CrossRef] [PubMed]
34. Elliott, B.; Flesig, G.; Nicholls, R.; Escamilla, R. Technique effects on upper limb loading in the tennis serve. *J. Sci. Med. Sport* **2003**, *6*, 76–87. [CrossRef]
35. Wei, S.H.; Chiang, J.Y.; Shiang, T.Y.; Chang, H.Y. Comparison of shock transmission and forearm electromyography between experienced and recreational tennis players during backhand strokes. *Clin. J. Sport Med.* **2006**, *16*, 129–135. [CrossRef]
36. Lo, K.H.; Hsieh, Y.C. Comparison of ball-and-racket impact force in two-handed backhand stroke stances for different-skill-level tennis players. *J. Sports Sci. Med.* **2016**, *15*, 301–307.
37. Sánchez-Alcaraz, B.J.; Courel-Ibáñez, J.; Cañas, J. Groundstroke accuracy assessment in padel players according to their level of play. *RICYDE Rev. Int. Ciencias del Deport.* **2016**, *12*, 324–333. [CrossRef]
38. Courel-Ibáñez, J.; Sánchez-Alcaraz, B.J.; Muñoz, D.; Grijota, F.J.; Chaparro, R.; Díaz, J. Gender reasons for practicing paddle tennis. *Apunt. Educ. Fis. y Deport.* **2018**, *133*, 116–125.
39. FIP—International Padel Federation (Ed.) *Rules of Padel*; Lausanne, Switzerland, 2020.
40. Ramón-Llin, J.; Guzmán, J.F.; Llana, S.; Martínez-Gallego, R.; James, N.; Vučković, G. The effect of the return of serve on the server pair's movement parameters and rally outcome in padel using cluster analysis. *Front. Psychol.* **2019**, *10*, 1–8. [CrossRef]
41. Vučković, G.; Perš, J.; James, N.; Hughes, M. Tactical use of the T area in Squash by players of differing standard. *J. Sport. Sci.* **2009**, *27*, 863–871. [CrossRef]
42. Vučković, G.; Perš, J.; James, N.; Hughes, M. Measurement error associated with the Sagit/squash computer tracking software. *Eur. J. Sport Sci.* **2010**, *10*, 129–140. [CrossRef]
43. Gabin, B.; Camerino, O.; Anguera, M.T.; Castañer, M. Lince: Multiplatform sport analysis software. *Proc. Soc. Behav. Sci.* **2012**, *46*, 4692–4694. [CrossRef]
44. Altman, D.G. *Practical Statistics for Medical Research*; Chapman & Hall: London, UK, 1991; ISBN 0412276305.
45. Cohen, J. *Statistical Power Anaylsis for the Behavioral Sciences*, 2nd ed.; Lawrence Erlbaum: Hillsdale, MI, USA, 1988; ISBN 0805802835.
46. Cohen, J. Quantitative methods in psychology: A power primer. *Psychol. Bull.* **1992**, *112*, 155–159. [CrossRef] [PubMed]
47. Ramón-llin, J.; Guzmán, J.; Martínez-Gallego, R.; Muñoz, D.; Sánchez-Pay, A.; Sánchez-Alcaraz, B.J. Stroke Analysis in Padel According to Match Outcome and Game Side on Court. *Int. J. Environ. Res. Public Health* **2020**, *17*, 7838. [CrossRef] [PubMed]
48. Fernandez-Fernandez, J.; Sanz-Rivas, D.; Sanchez-Muñoz, C.; Pluim, B.M.; Tiemessen, I.; Mendez-Villanueva, A. A comparison of the activity profile and physiological demands between advanced and recreational veteran tennis players. *J. Strength Cond. Res.* **2009**, *23*, 604–610. [CrossRef] [PubMed]
49. Jayanthi, N.; Sallay, R.; Hunker, P. Skill level related injuries in competition tennis players. *Med. Sci. Tennis* **2005**, *10*, 12–15.
50. Abernethy, B.; Gill, D.P.; Parks, S.L.; Packer, S.T. Expertise and the perception of kinematic and situational probability information. *Perception* **2001**, *30*, 233–252. [CrossRef]
51. Shim, J.; Carlton, L.G.; Chow, J.W.; Chae, W. The use of anticipatory visual cues by highly skilled tennis players. *J. Mot. Behav.* **2005**, *37*, 164–175. [CrossRef]
52. Fernández-Elías, V.E.; Courel-Ibáñez, J.; Pérez-López, A.; Jodra, P.; Moreno-Pérez, V.; Del Coso, J.; López-Samanes, Á. Acute Beetroot Juice Supplementation Does Not Improve Match-Play Activity in Professional Tennis Players. *J. Am. Coll. Nutr.* **2020**. [CrossRef]
53. Delgado-García, G.; Vanrenterghem, J.; Ruiz-Malagón, E.J.; Molina-García, P.; Courel-Ibáñez, J.; Soto-Hermoso, V.M. IMU gyroscopes are a valid alternative to 3D optical motion capture system for angular kinematics analysis in tennis. *Proc. Inst. Mech. Eng. Part. P J. Sport. Eng. Technol.* **2020**, 175433712096544. [CrossRef]
54. Sánchez-Alcaraz, B.J.; Jiménez, V.; Muñoz, D.; Ramón-Llín, J. Effectiveness and distribution of attacking strokes to finish the point in professional padel. *Rev. Int. Med. y Ciencias la Act. Fis. y del Deport.* **2021**, in press.
55. Sánchez-Alcaraz, B.J.; Courel-Ibáñez, J.; Muñoz, D.; Infantes, P.; Sáez de Zuramán, F.; Sánchez-Pay, A. Analysis of the attack actions in professional padel. *Apunt. Educ. Física y Deport.* **2020**, *142*, 29–34. [CrossRef]

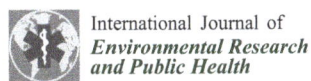

Article

Correlations between Basal Trace Minerals and Hormones in Middle and Long-Distance High-Level Male Runners

Javier Alves [1], Gema Barrientos [1,*], Víctor Toro [2], Francisco Javier Grijota [2], Diego Muñoz [2] and Marcos Maynar [2]

1. Department of Sport Science, Faculty of Education, Pontifical University of Salamanca, C/Henry Collet, 52–70, CP, 37007 Salamanca, Spain; fjalvesva@upsa.es
2. Department of Physiology, Faculty of Sports Science Faculty, University of Extremadura, University Avenue, s/n CP, 10003 Cáceres, Spain; vtororom@alumnos.unex.es (V.T.); fgrijota@nebrija.es (F.J.G.); diegomun@unex.es (D.M.); mmaynar@unex.es (M.M.)
* Correspondence: gbarrientosvi@upsa.es; Tel.: +34-923-125-027

Received: 19 November 2020; Accepted: 16 December 2020; Published: 17 December 2020

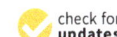

Abstract: Several essential trace minerals play an important role in the endocrine system; however, toxic trace minerals have a disruptive effect. The aim of this research was to determine basal concentrations and the possible correlations between trace minerals in plasma and several plasma hormones in runners. Sixty high-level male endurance runners (21 ± 3 years; 1.77 ± 0.05 m; 64.97 ± 7.36 kg) participated in the present study. Plasma hormones were analyzed using an enzyme-linked immunosorbent assay (ELISA) and plasma trace minerals were analyzed with inductively coupled plasma mass spectrometry (ICP-MS). Correlations and simple linear regression were used to assess the association between trace minerals and hormones. Plasma testosterone concentrations were inversely correlated with manganese (r = −0.543; β = −0.410; $p < 0.01$), selenium (r = −0.292; β = −0.024; $p < 0.05$), vanadium (r = −0.406; β = −1.278; $p < 0.01$), arsenic (r = −0.336; β = −0.142; $p < 0.05$), and lead (r = −0.385; β = −0.418; $p < 0.01$). Plasma luteinizing hormone (LH) levels were positively correlated with arsenic (r = 0.298; β = 0.327; $p < 0.05$) and cesium (r = 0.305; β = 2.272; $p < 0.05$), and negatively correlated with vanadium (r = −0.303; β = −2.467; $p < 0.05$). Moreover, cortisol concentrations showed significant positive correlations with cadmium (r = 0.291; β = 209.01; $p < 0.05$). Finally, insulin concentrations were inversely related to vanadium (r = −0.359; β = −3.982; $p < 0.05$). In conclusion, endurance runners living in areas with high environmental levels of toxic minerals should check their concentrations of anabolic hormones.

Keywords: trace mineral; LH; testosterone; cortisol; insulin; runners

1. Introduction

Endurance runners perform high amounts of training with long aerobic exercise sessions, where they run for a long time at intensities lower than the second ventilatory threshold (VT_2); training that causes great physiological stress and induces changes and adaptations in their gonadal and cortical axis [1]. Hackney [2] reported a dysfunction in the hypothalamus-hypophyseal-testicular axis, defined as "exercise-hypogonadal male condition", which leads to low levels of chronic basal testosterone (T) in endurance athletes [3], without changes in luteinizing hormone concentrations (LH), which may indicate a testicular dysfunction [4]. Other authors, however, found normal concentrations of T and LH in endurance athletes [5,6].

Trace minerals (TM) are present in body tissues as an essential part of many physiological functions, and their deficiency or excess can lead to metabolic disorders [7]. Some of these minerals are essential for human health although they may be harmful in high concentrations; other minerals to which we are exposed are considered toxic for health [8]. The main exposure sources to TM is diet and air [8]. Significant interactions have been observed between TM levels and the endocrine system since TM influence the metabolism of hormones and vice versa, so changes in hormone concentrations could affect the metabolism and redistribution of TM [9].

Essential TM such as copper (Cu), selenium (Se), and zinc (Zn) have been found to play a fundamental role in the regulation of testicular function, in the spermatogenesis process, and the production of androgens [7]. Moreover, an inverse correlation has been reported between molybdenum (Mo) and T in subjects with Zn deficiency [10] and in animals an excess of manganese (Mn) concentrations has been found to negatively impact the function of Leydig cells [11].

On the other hand, toxic minerals are considered disruptors of hormonal metabolism; the adverse effects of arsenic (As), cadmium (Cd), lead (Pb), and mercury (Hg) on testicular function have been widely reported to interfere in T levels [12,13].

Cortisol (C) is a catabolic hormone regulated by the hypothalamus-hypophysis-adrenal axis that facilitates the mobilization of substrates during exercise to improve athletic performance [14], and its concentrations can be kept high up to 48 h after exhaustive long-term exercise, interfering with the recovery process [1]. Few studies relating TM with this hormone were found; Soria et al. found that increases in C concentrations in trained athletes positively correlated with increases in Zn and Se levels, which suggests that it occurs because of the participation of these elements in the prevention of oxidative stress [15].

Insulin (I) is considered an anabolic hormone related to blood glucose control, energy balance, and the metabolism of carbohydrate, fat, and protein [16]. A decrease in plasma I concentrations has been observed during exercise, followed by an increase in I synthesis at the end of exercise, to promote glycogen repletion through lower glucose production and utilization and an increase in fat oxidation [17]. Insulin and its relationship with TM have been widely studied in metabolic diseases such as diabetes; for example, by Soria et al. [15], although this study found no correlation between I and initial plasma concentrations of Se, Zn, Mn, and cobalt (Co) in trained triathletes. In another study, Tubek [18] reported a positive correlation with Zn, which would support the hypothesis that this mineral is necessary for the synthesis, accumulation, and release of insulin [19].

Research has reported on the relationship between energy intake and the synthesis of anabolic hormones [20,21]. High-level endurance runners in training periods with an intake below 45 calories per day per kg of fat-free mass (FFM) had decreases in LH and T hormones [22]. As mentioned above, significant interactions have been observed between TM concentrations and the endocrine system. It is known that TM have biological implications for endocrine processes [23], and a large number of studies examine these relationships in animals or healthy subjects; however, few studies have examined the relationship between hormones and TM in athletes [9,15].

Previous studies by our research group reported significant differences in plasma TM concentrations between sedentary subjects and endurance runners. Runners had higher plasma concentrations of Mn, Mo, chrome (Cr), nickel (Ni), and rubidium (Rb) and lower concentrations of Se and Zn [24–26]. Higher plasma concentrations of toxic TM, such as beryllium (Be), cesium (Cs), Pb, and Cd, were also found in runners [27].

Therefore, the objectives of the study were (i) to check basal concentrations of hormones (testosterone, LH, cortisol, and insulin) and TM in highly trained endurance athletes, and (ii) to study the possible relationships between trace minerals and hormone metabolism, since hormones play a fundamental role in runners' energy metabolism, recovery, and performance.

2. Materials and Methods

2.1. Participants

Sixty male endurance runners (21 ± 3 years old; height 1.77 ± 0.05 m) took part in the study. They had a personal best in modalities of 3:37.79–4:08.24 for 1500 m and 13:11.01 and 15:16.78 for 5000 m.

The criteria for the selection of participants in our study were: to be runners who had been living in the same region for at least three years, at a latitude of 39°28′35.36″ N, to have trained regularly and six days a week during the previous six years, and to have participated in national and international track and field and cross-country competitions in that period. None of the subjects had taken regular medication, anti-inflammatory medications, or TM supplementation for 3 months prior to the study. All runners were previously informed about the purpose of the study and signed their voluntary informed consent. This research was conducted under the Helsinki Declaration ethical guidelines, updated at the World Medical Assembly in Fortaleza in 2013 for research with human participants, and the protocol was approved by the Ethics Committee of the University of Extremadura (52/2012).

The participants' characteristics are summarized in Table 1.

Table 1. Anthropometric and body composition values in the runners.

Parameters	Runners	Ranges
Height (m)	1.77 ± 0.05	1.55–1.88
Body mass (kg)	64.97 ± 7.36	49.7–78.1
Fat mass (kg)	5.35 ± 1.01	3.45–7.87
Fat mass (%)	8.20 ± 1.06	7.12–1.06
Fat-free mass (FFM) (kg)	59.77 ± 6.57	42.13–71.64
$\Sigma 6$ skinfold (mm)	45.61 ± 9.71	35.98–53.21

2.2. Nutritional Evaluation

The runners were following a similar diet. All subjects were trained to complete a nutritional questionnaire, on two pre-assigned weekdays and one weekend day. Runners indicated quantity (in grams) of every food consumed. Then, their dietary intakes were analyzed using different food composition tables [8,28,29].

2.3. Training Characteristics

Runners' training routines were monitored (some runners did double sessions), performing an average distance between 80 and 155 km per week during the sport season (75–85% aerobic running and 15–25% high intensity running). The kilometers that runners trained with an intensity higher than VT_2 according to the three-phase model [30] were identified as high intensity. Additionally, they trained one-two weekly sessions of resistance training depending on the period of the season.

2.4. Anthropometric Measurements

The anthropometric measurements were obtained at the same time (09:00–10:00 a.m.) in equal conditions and were carried out by an accredited operator in kinanthropometric techniques Level 1. Runners did not perform intense training 72 h before the sampling. Fat mass and fat-free mass content were calculated from the sum of 6 skinfolds ($\Sigma 6$) (abdominal, tricipital, suprailiac, subscapularis, thigh, and calf), in accordance with the International Society for the Advancement of Kinanthropometry recommendations [31]. Skinfold thicknesses were measured with a Harpenden caliper (Holtain Skinfold Caliper, Crosswell, Crymych, UK). Body fat percentage was calculated according to Jackson and Pollock [32]. Body weight was measured to the nearest 0.01 kg using a digital scale (Seca 769, Hamburg, Germany) and body height was measured to the nearest 0.1 cm using a wall-mounted stadiometer (Seca©, Hamburg, Germany).

2.5. Sample Collection

After the anthropometric measurements, 10 mL of venous blood was drawn from each runner. Then, the samples were collected into tubes (previously washed with diluted nitric acid) with ethylenediaminetetraacetic acid.

Later, samples were centrifuged to isolate the plasma which was deposited into an Eppendorf tube (previously washed with diluted nitric acid) and conserved at −80 °C until biochemical analysis.

2.6. Sample Determination

In order to determine the concentration of trace minerals, analyses were performed using inductively coupled plasma mass spectrometry (ICP-MS) following the method described by Maynar et al. [24].

The decomposition of the organic matrix was achieved by heating it for 10 h at 90 °C after adding 0.8 mL HNO_3 and 0.4 mL H_2O_2 to 2 mL of plasma samples. The samples were then dried at 200 °C on a hot plate. Sample reconstitution was carried out by adding 0.5 mL of nitric acid, 10 µL of indium (In) (10 mg/L) as an internal standard, and ultrapure water to complete 10 mL. Digested solutions were analyzed with an ICP-MS Nexion model 300D (PerkinElmer, Inc., Shelton, CT, USA). Three replicates were analyzed per sample. The values of the standard materials of each element (10 µg/L) used for quality controls were in accordance with intra and inter-assay coefficient variations of less than 5%.

The hormone quantification was conducted using enzyme-linked immunosorbent assay (ELISA) with an ER-500 (Sinnowa, Germany), using the commercial tests for insulin, cortisol, testosterone, and luteinizing hormone from CisRadioquímica, SA (Madrid, Spain). Hormonal analyses were performed in duplicate by the same technician. Coefficients of variation (between and within) were less than 10% for all biochemical analyses.

2.7. Statistical Evaluations

Statistical analyses were performed with IBM SPSS 21 for Windows (IBM Co., Armonk, NY, USA). The results are expressed as x ± s, where "x" represents mean values and "s" the standard deviation. A Kolmogorov–Smirnov test was used to analyze the normality of the distribution of variables, and the homogeneity of the variances was analyzed with the Levene's test. A simple linear regression model was used to determine associations between TM concentrations and plasma hormone concentrations. Pearson's correlation coefficient (r), the β coefficients, and determination coefficients (R^2) were calculated. Strength of linear association was established according to Chan [33]. A $p < 0.05$ was considered statistically significant.

3. Results

Table 2 presents data on the nutritional intake of all athletes per day.

Nutritional intakes were adequate for the athletic performance of the runners in our study [34]. Energy availability (EA) is defined as dietary energy intake minus exercise energy expenditure/FFM. For healthy young adults, an appropriate energy balance is associated with ≥45 calories per day per kg of FFM [21].

Tables 3 and 4 show the plasma values of trace minerals and plasma hormones, respectively. LH (7.94 ± 2.95 mIU/mL), insulin (7.31 ± 4.03 mIU/mL), testosterone (6.52 ± 1.14 ng/mL), and cortisol (95.81 ± 33.85 ng/mL) for all runners participating in the study.

The correlation coefficients and simple linear regressions are shown in Table 5.

Plasma LH levels were positively correlated with As (r = 0.298; β = 0.327; $p < 0.05$) and cesium (Cs) (r = 0.305; β = 2.272; $p < 0.05$), and negatively related with V (r = −0.303; β = −2.467; $p < 0.05$). Finally, insulin concentrations were inversely correlated to V (r = −0.359; β = −3.982; $p < 0.05$).

Plasma testosterone concentrations were inversely associated with Mn (r = −0.543; β = −0.410; $p < 0.01$), Se (r = −0.292; β = −0.024; $p < 0.05$), vanadium (V) (r = −0.406; β = −1.278; $p < 0.01$),

As (r = −0.336; β = −0.142; $p < 0.05$), and Pb (r = −0.385; β = −0.418; $p < 0.01$). On the other hand, cortisol levels showed significant positive correlations with Cd (r = 0.291; β = 209.01; $p < 0.05$).

Table 2. Energy, macronutrients, and trace minerals in the runners.

Parameters, Recommended Intake	Intake
Energy (kcal/d)	2885.62 ± 649.28
HC (g/kg/d)	5.70 ± 1.31
Proteins (g/kg/d)	1.79 ± 1.57
Lipids (g/kg/d)	1.67 ± 1.48
EA (kcal/kg FFM/day)	46.63 ± 4.49
Arsenic (12–300 mg/d)	16.92 ± 80.20
Boron (0.75–1.35 mg/d)	1.34 ± 1.48
Beryllium (<50 µg/d)	9.71 ± 9.02
Cadmium (<70 µg/d)	23.33 ± 15.39
Cobalt (200–300 µg/d)	295.94 ± 215.07
Copper (2000–3000 µg/d)	1676.06 ± 566.89
Lithium (180–550 µg/d)	367.03 ± 396.86
Manganese (2500–5000 µg/d)	3378.13 ± 1440.05
Molybdenum (75–400 µg/d)	309.02 ± 182.03
Lead (<400 µg/d)	209.48 ± 141.81
Rubidium (1.5–7 mg/d)	3.896 ± 4.712
Selenium (50–200 µg/d)	76.54 ± 44.96
Strontium (1000–2300 µg/d)	1889.02 ± 1782.25
Vanadium (10–70 µg/d)	25.52 ± 29.31
Zinc (10–15 mg/d)	11.12 ± 3.68

Table 3. Trace mineral concentrations in the runners.

Trace Minerals	Runners	Range
Arsenic (µg/L)	2.35 ± 2.70	0.23–12.00
Boron (µg/L)	8.63 ± 10.96	0–60.58
Beryllium (µg/L))	0.07 ± 0.03	0–0.14
Cadmium (µg/L)	0.07 ± 0.05	0.01–0.23
Cesium (µg/L)	0.69 ± 0.40	0.31–1.87
Cobalt (µg/L)	0.68 ± 0.10	0.47–0.88
Copper (µg/L)	693.16 ± 132.53	454.9–937.01
Lithium (µg/L)	1.38 ± 0.79	0.36–4.72
Manganese (µg/L)	2.06 ± 1.49	0.19–5.46
Molybdenum (µg/L)	0.62 ± 0.59	0.1–3.33
Lead (µg/L)	0.96 ± 1.07	0.01–4.94
Rubidium (µg/L)	138.49 ± 22.98	98.8–185.98
Selenium (µg/L)	96.5 ± 13.8	69.7–124.1
Strontium (µg/L)	26.24 ± 8.12	14.83–47.47
Vanadium (µg/L)	0.29 ± 0.37	0–1.78
Zinc (µg/L)	792.20 ± 143.91	539.52–1210.95

Table 4. Plasma hormonal concentrations in runners.

Hormones	Runners	Ranges
LH (mIU/mL)	7.94 ± 2.95	2.94–16.03
Insulin (µIU/mL)	7.31 ± 4.03	1.39–18.91
Testosterone (ng/mL)	6.52 ± 1.14	4.13–9.94
Cortisol (ng/mL)	95.81 ± 33.85	42.40–170.92

Table 5. Correlations and simple linear regressions between trace minerals and hormones.

		LH (mIU/mL)				Insulin (µIU/mL)				Testosterone (ng/mL)				Cortisol (ng/mL)		
	r	β (95% CI)	R^2	p	r	β (95% CI)	R^2	p	r	β (95% CI)	R^2	p	r	β (95% CI)	R^2	p
As	0.298	0.327 (0.01/0.63)	0.089	0.040	−0.015			0.917	−0.336	−0.142 (−0.26/−0.02)	0.113	0.020	−0.082			0.580
B	−0.142			0.335	0.007			0.963	−0.105			0.476	−0.084			0.571
Be	−0.075			0.613	0.237			0.104	0.080			0.589	−0.266			0.068
Cd	0.095			0.521	−0.135			0.362	−0.001			0.996	0.291	209.01 (4.90/413.1)	0.085	0.045
Cs	0.305	2.272 (0.16/4.38)	0.093	0.035	0.186			0.205	−0.234			0.110	−0.073			0.622
Cu	−0.099			0.502	0.020			0.894	−0.204			0.163	−0.149			0.312
Li	−0.251			0.085	−0.042			0.776	0.053			0.720	0.135			0.360
Mn	−0.226			0.122	−0.197			0.180	−0.543	−0.410 (−0.59/−0.22)	0.295	0.000	−0.268			0.066
Mo	−0.158			0.285	0.160			0.278	0.209			0.154	0.102			0.492
Pb	−0.045			0.759	−0.220			0.133	−0.385	−0.418 (−0.71/−0.12)	0.148	0.007	−0.283			0.052
Rb	−0.144			0.032	0.195			0.185	0.033			0.826	0.098			0.508
Se	0.043			0.773	0.027			0.855	−0.292	−0.024 (−0.04/−0.01)	0.085	0.044	−0.190			0.195
Sr	−0.131			0.376	−0.223			0.127	−0.229			0.117	−0.196			0.183
V	−0.303	−2.467 (−4.71/−0.16)	0.092	0.036	−0.359	−3.982 (−7.05/−0.90)	0.129	0.012	−0.406	−1.278 (−2.13/−0.425)	0.165	0.004	−0.212			0.148
Zn	0.276			0.058	0.102			0.491	0.135			0.361	0.003			0.981

LH: luteinizing hormone; As: arsenic; B: boron; Be: beryllium; Cd: cadmium; Cs: cesium; Cu: copper; Li: lithium; Mn: manganese; Mo: molybdenum; Pb: lead; Rb: rubidium; Se: selenium; Sr: strontium; V: vanadium; Zn: zinc; r: Pearson's coefficient of correlation; β: beta coefficient; CI: confidence interval; R^2: coefficient of determination; p: p-value.

4. Discussion

In our runners, energy availability, macronutrients, and TM intake from the diet were appropriate according to the recommended intakes [8,35].

Plasma Co concentrations were higher, although without negative health effects in healthy individuals [36].

Runners' plasma LH and T hormones were within normal ranges [37], although plasma T concentrations were lower than those reported in untrained males [38].

An inverse correlation was found between plasma concentration of LH and V plasma concentrations. Vanadium is considered a toxic mineral [39]. However, there are still some ambiguous assertions about its possible essentiality that require further studies in the future [40]. The correlations found in our study could be related to previous studies in rats suggesting that the nucleus of Leydig cells are a possible target of V, and its excessive accumulation could produce a transient suppression in testicular function by reducing plasma concentrations of LH and T [41]. This would be a consequence of an increase in oxidative stress in the testes as demonstrated by Chandra et al. [42], where rats receiving injections of sodium vanadate had high levels of indices of lipid peroxidation in testicular tissues compared to control tissues, caused by a decrease in the activity of antioxidant enzymes. It is known that physical training in high-level runners increases reactive oxygen species (ROS) production and the possibility of oxidative stress (OS) [43]. Therefore, the runners' antioxidant activity would not be sufficient to compensate for the production of ROS by V and accumulation of training loads.

Plasma concentration of LH had a positive correlation with plasma As concentration. Banerjee et al. [44] found that decreases in serum T concentrations were observed in animals with As poisoning. In males, As may induce gonad dysfunction through declined T synthesis [45]. In another study, Zeng et al. [46] concluded that As has an inhibitory effect on the production of T. These data could be related to the correlations found in our athletes between plasma As concentration and the plasma concentration of LH and serum T. Athletes' plasma As concentrations were within reasonable limits, and according to these correlations, we could infer that the increase in As concentration would lead to a decrease in T concentrations and this would increase plasma concentrations of LH to try to compensate for the reduction of T and increase its synthesis. More research studies on humans are needed.

A correlation was also found between LH and Cs. Previous studies have reported that chronic Cs exposure does not negatively affect steroid hormone concentrations or the correct functioning of the hypothalamus-hypophysis-testicular (HPT) axis [47]; however, with our current knowledge we cannot explain this relationship.

A negative correlation was found between Mn and total plasma T. Mn is an essential mineral in specific physiological processes, and is a compound of manganese superoxide dismutase (Mn-SOD) enzyme which neutralizes superoxide radicals during physical exercise [48]. In their study, Plumlee and Ziegler [49] indicated that a deficiency of this mineral can lead to testicular and skeletal dysfunctions, which could be linked to the dependence of testicular Leydig cells on plasma Mn for the testicular synthesis of this hormone. Lee et al. [50] showed that Mn acts on the hypothalamus inducing the secretion of LH, a hormone that controls the production of T from Leydig cells, but in this study, there was no correlation with LH although there was a correlation with T.

Another interesting positive correlation was T with plasma Se concentrations. This correlation in our athletes could be related to what was described earlier; Se would be necessary for the healthy metabolism of T and normal testicular morphology, and this could explain the presence of several selenium-proteins in male gonads [51,52]. Furthermore, Pond et al. [53] seem to indicate that alterations in spermatogenesis could be due to lack of activity of the glutathione peroxidase (GPx) enzymes. In a recent review, it was concluded that essential hormonal regulators and testicular functions can be negatively affected when there is an uncontrolled generation of ROS with respect to the antioxidant defense mechanism, as a consequence of lack of activity of the GPx enzymes, which would alter the production of T [54]. Therefore, it is essential for runners to maintain adequate Se concentrations to ensure correct activity of antioxidant enzymes as well as the synthesis of T.

A negative correlation was found between plasma T and V concentrations. As previously discussed in plasma LH concentrations, V has been reported to increase ROS generation in the body, which would induce oxidative stress, and could reduce testicular T synthesis [42]. Recently, Zwolak [55] reported the positive role of several dietary antioxidants in vanadium toxicology.

A negative correlation with As was also found with plasma T. Arsenic is a toxic TM that due to its ability to generate ROS could alter the synthesis of T [45], a relationship that was previously discussed.

Testosterone was also found to have an important negative correlation with Pb. The toxic effects of Pb have been reported to have an adverse impact on the central nervous system, liver, kidneys, and the reproductive system [56]. This correlation in our athletes could indicate that lowering serum concentrations of Pb produced an increase in T concentrations. It has been reported that Pb causes oxidative stress by generating ROS that results in critical damage to several biomolecules such as DNA, enzymes, proteins, and the membrane of lipids, as well as a decrease in antioxidant activity [57]. Increases in ROS production due to training and the toxic action of this mineral could affect the synthesis of T in runners. Darbandi et al. [54] reported the excess generation of ROS with respect to the antioxidant defense mechanism, which could alter the synthesis of T in endurance runners.

In relation to C, runners' baseline plasma concentrations were within reference ranges [58]. Cortisol increases its synthesis during training and can remain elevated up to 48 h after finishing [59]; however, our runners did not perform intense training 72 h before the sampling. We only found a positive correlation with Cd. Cadmium is an environmental toxin and an endocrine disruptor, and humans are very sensitive to its toxic effects. Recent data have shown that exposure to Cd leads to an increase in plasma levels of adrenocorticotropic hormone (ACTH) [60], a hormone secreted by the pituitary gland that controls the release of C in the adrenal gland [61]. Pérez-Cadahía et al. [62] reported positive relationships between C and Cd, that indicate that this mineral could have an implication with the catabolic processes that occur in the body, so the runner's body attempts to eliminate Cd although its concentrations are normal in order to avoid this negative effect [63]. Future studies are required to clarify this point.

With respect to I, baseline plasma concentrations of the runners were within normal ranges [58]. A negative correlation was found with plasma V concentration. Therefore, this could indicate the need for this mineral to synthetize I or for the correct functioning of this hormone. In this respect, Cam et al. [64] concluded that V enhances the effects of endogenous circulating I, and even could be used as an I supplement to avoid the insulin resistance that its exogenous chronic administration can cause [65]. More studies are needed to establish the long-term effects of V treatment and to establish doses in different groups of people [66].

The limitations of this study include that the intake of TM by the runners was obtained using a self-report questionnaire that could introduce some inaccuracies. Another limitation was that some of our assessments may be somewhat speculative and may not allow us to have a solid discussion, due to the scarcity of studies in runners.

5. Conclusions

Plasma hormone concentrations and several trace mineral concentrations in high training endurance runners were in normal ranges.

LH correlated with the plasma concentrations of vanadium, arsenic, and cesium. Testosterone reflected correlations with manganese, selenium, arsenic, lead, and vanadium concentrations. Cortisol showed a correlation with cadmium concentration, and insulin correlated with vanadium concentration.

Essential and toxic trace elements are involved in the endocrine system, and their deficiency or excess could lead to metabolic disorders in endurance runners. Our results indicate that endurance athletes living and training in places with high environmental levels of toxic minerals should check concentrations of anabolic hormones (LH and T) as they could suffer decreases in their plasma concentrations that would negatively affect sports performance.

Author Contributions: Conceptualization, M.M.; methodology, M.M.; formal analysis, M.M., F.J.G., V.T., and G.B.; data curation, M.M. and V.T.; writing—original draft preparation, J.A., G.B., and D.M.; writing—review and editing, M.M., J.A., and G.B. All authors have read and agreed to the published version of the manuscript.

Funding: This research received no external funding.

Acknowledgments: The authors gratefully acknowledge the collaboration of the athletes.

Conflicts of Interest: The authors declare no conflict of interest.

References

1. Anderson, T.; Lane, A.R.; Hackney, A.C. Cortisol and testosterone dynamics following exhaustive endurance exercise. *Eur. J. Appl. Physiol.* **2016**, *116*, 1503–1509. [CrossRef] [PubMed]
2. Hackney, A.C. Effects of endurance exercise on the reproductive system of men: The "exercise-hypogonadal male condition". *J. Endocrinol. Investig.* **2008**, *31*, 932–938. [CrossRef] [PubMed]
3. Lucía, A.; Díaz, B.; Hoyos, J.; Fernández, C.; Villa, G.; Bandrés, F.; Chicharro, J.L. Hormone levels of world class cyclists during the Tour of Spain stage race. *Br. J. Sports Med.* **2001**, *35*, 424–430. [CrossRef] [PubMed]
4. Wheeler, G.; Singh, M.; Pierce, W.; Epling, W.; Cumming, D. Endurance training decreases serum testosterone levels in men without change in luteinizing hormone pulsatile release. *J. Clin. Endocrinol. Metab.* **1991**, *72*, 422–425. [CrossRef] [PubMed]
5. Lehmann, M.; Knizia, K.; Gastmann, U.; Petersen, K.G.; Khalaf, A.N.; Bauer, S.; Kerp, L.; Keul, J. Influence of 6-week, 6 days per week, training on pituitary function in recreational athletes. *Br. J. Sports Med.* **1993**, *27*, 186–192. [CrossRef] [PubMed]
6. Tissandier, O.; Peres, G.; Fiet, J.; Piette, F. Testosterone, dehydroepiandrosterone, insulin-like growth factor 1, and insulin in sedentary and physically trained aged men. *Eur. J. Appl. Physiol.* **2001**, *85*, 177–184. [CrossRef]
7. Fayed, A.-H.A. Serum and testicular trace element concentration in rabbits at different ages. *Biol. Trace Elem. Res.* **2010**, *134*, 64–67. [CrossRef]
8. Kabata-Pendias, A.; Mukherjee, A.B. Trace elements from soil to human. *Trace Elem. Soil Hum.* **2007**, 1–550. [CrossRef]
9. Soria, M.; Gonzalez-Haro, C.; Anson, M.; Lopez-Colon, J.L.; Escanero, J.F. Plasma levels of trace elements and exercise induced stress hormones in well-trained athletes. *J. Trace Elem. Med. Biol.* **2015**, *31*, 113–119. [CrossRef]
10. Meeker, J.D.; Rossano, M.G.; Protas, B.; Padmanahban, V.; Diamond, M.P.; Puscheck, E.; Daly, D.; Paneth, N.; Wirth, J.J. Environmental exposure to metals and male reproductive hormones: Circulating testosterone is inversely associated with blood molybdenum. *Fertil. Steril.* **2010**, *93*, 130–140. [CrossRef]
11. Cheng, J.; Fu, J.; Zhou, Z. The mechanism of manganese-induced inhibition of steroidogenesis in rat primary Leydig cells. *Toxicology* **2005**, *211*, 1–11. [CrossRef] [PubMed]
12. Hsieh, F.-I.; Hwang, T.-S.; Hsieh, Y.-C.; Lo, H.-C.; Su, C.-T.; Hsu, H.-S.; Chiou, H.-Y.; Chen, C.-J. Risk of erectile dysfunction induced by arsenic exposure through well water consumption in Taiwan. *Environ. Health Perspect.* **2008**, *116*, 532–536. [CrossRef] [PubMed]
13. De Queiroz, E.K.R.; Waissmann, W. Occupational exposure and effects on the male reproductive system. *Cad. Saude Publica* **2006**, *22*, 485–493. [CrossRef]
14. Brownlee, K.K.; Moore, A.W.; Hackney, A.C. Relationship between circulating cortisol and testosterone: Influence of physical exercise. *J. Sports Sci. Med.* **2005**, *4*, 76. [PubMed]
15. Soria, M.; Anson, M.; Escanero, J.F. Correlation Analysis of Exercise-Induced Changes in Plasma Trace Element and Hormone Levels During Incremental Exercise in Well-Trained Athletes. *Biol. Trace Elem. Res.* **2016**, *170*, 55–64. [CrossRef] [PubMed]
16. Comitato, R.; Saba, A.; Turrini, A.; Arganini, C.; Virgili, F. Sex hormones and macronutrient metabolism. *Crit. Rev. Food Sci. Nutr.* **2015**, *55*, 227–241. [CrossRef]
17. Horton, T.J.; Grunwald, G.K.; Lavely, J.; Donahoo, W.T. Glucose kinetics differ between women and men, during and after exercise. *J. Appl. Physiol.* **2006**, *100*, 1883–1894. [CrossRef]
18. Tubek, S. Selected zinc metabolism parameters in relation to insulin, renin-angiotensin-aldosterone system, and blood pressure in healthy subjects. *Biol. Trace Elem. Res.* **2006**, *114*, 65–72. [CrossRef]

19. Miranda, E.R.; Dey, C.S. Effect of chromium and zinc on insulin signaling in skeletal muscle cells. *Biol. Trace Elem. Res.* **2004**, *101*, 19–36. [CrossRef]
20. De Souza, M.J.; Koltun, K.J.; Williams, N.I. The Role of Energy Availability in Reproductive Function in the Female Athlete Triad and Extension of its Effects to Men: An Initial Working Model of a Similar Syndrome in Male Athletes. *Sport. Med.* **2019**, *49*, 125–137. [CrossRef]
21. Dipla, K.; Kraemer, R.R.; Constantini, N.W.; Hackney, A.C. Relative energy deficiency in sports (RED-S): Elucidation of endocrine changes affecting the health of males and females. *Hormones* **2020**. [CrossRef] [PubMed]
22. Alves, J.; Toro, V.; Barrientos, G.; Bartolomé, I.; Muñoz, D.; Maynar, M. Hormonal Changes in High-Level Aerobic Male Athletes during a Sports Season. *Int. J. Environ. Res. Public Health* **2020**, *17*, 5833. [CrossRef] [PubMed]
23. Neve, J. Clinical implications of trace elements in endocrinology. *Biol. Trace Elem. Res.* **1992**, *32*, 173–185. [CrossRef]
24. Maynar, M.; Llerena, F.; Grijota, F.J.; Alves, J.; Robles, M.C.; Bartolomé, I.; Muñoz, D. Serum concentration of several trace metals and physical training. *J. Int. Soc. Sports Nutr.* **2017**, *14*, 19. [CrossRef] [PubMed]
25. Maynar, M.; Llerena, F.; Bartolomé, I.; Alves, J.; Robles, M.-C.; Grijota, F.-J.; Muñoz, D. Seric concentrations of copper, chromium, manganesum, nickel and selenium in aerobic, anaerobic and mixed professional sportsmen. *J. Int. Soc. Sports Nutr.* **2018**, *15*, 8. [CrossRef] [PubMed]
26. Maynar, M.; Llerena, F.; Grijota, F.J.; Pérez-Quintero, M.; Bartolomé, I.; Alves, J.; Robles, M.C.; Muñoz, D. Serum concentration of cobalt, molybdenum and zinc in aerobic, anaerobic and aerobic-anaerobic sportsmen. *J. Int. Soc. Sports Nutr.* **2018**, *15*, 1–8. [CrossRef]
27. Maynar-Mariño, M.; Llerena, F.; Bartolomé, I.; Crespo, C.; Muñoz, D.; Robles, M.-C.; Caballero, M.-J. Effect of long-term aerobic, anaerobic and aerobic-anaerobic physical training in seric toxic minerals concentrations. *J. Trace Elem. Med. Biol.* **2018**, *45*, 136–141. [CrossRef]
28. Reilly, C. *The Nutritional Trace Metals*; Blackwell Publishing Ltd.: Oxford, UK, 2004.
29. Moreiras, O. *Tablas de Composición de Alimentos*, 16th ed.; Pirámide: Madrid, Spain, 2013.
30. Skinner, J.S.; Mclellan, T.H.; McLellan, T.H. The Transition from Aerobic to Anaerobic Metabolism. *Res. Q. Exerc. Sport* **1980**, *51*, 234–248. [CrossRef]
31. Eston, R.G.; Reilly, T. *Kinanthropometry and Exercise Physiology Laboratory Manual: Tests, Procedures, and Data*; Routledge: London, UK, 2001; ISBN 9780415251860.
32. Jackson, A.S.; Pollock, M.L. Practical Assessment of Body Composition. *Phys. Sportsmed.* **1985**, *13*, 76–90. [CrossRef]
33. Chan, Y. Biostatistics 104: Correlational analysis. *Singap. Med. J.* **2003**, *44*, 614–619.
34. Rodriguez, N.R.; DiMarco, N.M.; Langley, S. Position of the American Dietetic Association, Dietitians of Canada, and the American College of Sports Medicine: Nutrition and athletic performance. *J. Am. Diet. Assoc.* **2009**, *109*, 509–527. [PubMed]
35. Potgieter, S. Sport nutrition: A review of the latest guidelines for exercise and sport nutrition from the American College of Sport Nutrition, the International Olympic Committee and the International Society for Sports Nutrition. *S. Afr. J. Clin. Nutr.* **2013**, *26*, 6–16. [CrossRef]
36. Leyssens, L.; Vinck, B.; Van Der Straeten, C.; Wuyts, F.; Maes, L. Cobalt toxicity in humans—A review of the potential sources and systemic health effects. *Toxicology* **2017**, *387*, 43–56. [CrossRef] [PubMed]
37. Hackney, A.C.; Lane, A.R. Exercise and the Regulation of Endocrine Hormones. In *Progress in Molecular Biology and Translational Science*; Academic Press: Cambridge, MA, USA, 2015; Volume 135, pp. 293–311.
38. Hackney, A.C.; Sinning, W.E.; Bruot, B.C. Reproductive Hormonal Profiles of Endurance-Trained and Untrained Males. *Med. Sci. Sports Exerc.* **1988**, *20*, 60–65. [CrossRef]
39. Imtiaz, M.; Rizwan, M.S.; Xiong, S.; Li, H.; Ashraf, M.; Shahzad, S.M.; Shahzad, M.; Rizwan, M.; Tu, S. Vanadium, recent advancements and research prospects: A review. *Environ. Int.* **2015**, *80*, 79–88. [CrossRef]
40. Kowalski, S.; Wyrzykowski, D.; Inkielewicz-Stępniak, I. molecules Molecular and Cellular Mechanisms of Cytotoxic Activity of Vanadium Compounds against Cancer Cells. *Molecules* **2020**, *25*, 1757. [CrossRef]
41. Chandra, A.K.; Ghosh, R.; Chatterjee, A.; Sarkar, M. Vanadium-induced testicular toxicity and its prevention by oral supplementation of zinc sulphate. *Toxicol. Mech. Methods* **2007**, *17*, 175–187. [CrossRef]
42. Chandra, A.K.; Ghosh, R.; Chatterjee, A.; Sarkar, M. Protection against vanadium-induced testicular toxicity by testosterone propionate in rats. *Toxicol. Mech. Methods* **2010**, *20*, 306–315. [CrossRef]

43. Powers, S.K.; Hamilton, K. Antioxidants and exercise. *Clin. Sports Med.* **1999**, *18*, 525–536. [CrossRef]
44. Banerjee, P.; Bhattacharyya, S.S.; Pathak, S.; Boujedaini, N.; Belon, P.; Khuda-Bukhsh, A.R. Evidences of protective potentials of microdoses of ultra-high diluted arsenic trioxide in mice receiving repeated injections of arsenic trioxide. *Evid. Based Complement. Altern. Med.* **2011**, *2011*. [CrossRef]
45. Kim, J.-M.; Kim, Y.-J. Arsenic Toxicity in Male Reproduction and Development. *Dev. Reprod.* **2015**, *19*, 167–180. [CrossRef] [PubMed]
46. Zeng, Q.; Yi, H.; Huang, L.; An, Q.; Wang, H. Reduced testosterone and Ddx3y expression caused by long-term exposure to arsenic and its effect on spermatogenesis in mice. *Environ. Toxicol. Pharmacol.* **2018**, *63*, 84–91. [CrossRef] [PubMed]
47. Grignard, E.; Guéguen, Y.; Grison, S.; Dublineau, I.; Gourmelon, P.; Souidi, M. Testicular steroidogenesis is not altered by 137 cesium Chernobyl fallout, following in utero or post-natal chronic exposure. *C. R. Biol.* **2010**, *333*, 416–423. [CrossRef] [PubMed]
48. Michalke, B.; Halbach, S.; Nischwitz, V. Speciation and toxicological relevance of manganese in humans. *J. Environ. Monit.* **2007**, *9*, 650–656. [CrossRef]
49. Plumlee, G.S.; Ziegler, T.L.; Lollar, B.S. The medical geochemistry of dusts, soils, and other earth materials. *Environ. Geochem.* **2003**, *9*, 263–310.
50. Lee, B.; Pine, M.; Johnson, L.; Rettori, V.; Hiney, J.K.; Les Dees, W. Manganese acts centrally to activate reproductive hormone secretion and pubertal development in male rats. *Reprod. Toxicol.* **2006**, *22*, 580–585. [CrossRef]
51. Behne, D.; Weiler, H.; Kyriakopoulos, A. Effects of selenium deficiency on testicular morphology and function in rats. *Reproduction* **1996**, *106*, 291–297. [CrossRef]
52. Rayman, M.P. Selenium and human health. *Lancet* **2012**, *379*, 1256–1268. [CrossRef]
53. Pond, F.R.; Tripp, M.J.; Wu, A.S.H.; Whanger, P.D.; Schmitz, J.A. Incorporation of selenium-75 into semen and reproductive tissues of bulls and rams. *Reproduction* **1983**, *69*, 411–418. [CrossRef]
54. Darbandi, M.; Darbandi, S.; Agarwal, A.; Sengupta, P.; Durairajanayagam, D.; Henkel, R.; Sadeghi, M.R. Reactive oxygen species and male reproductive hormones. *Reprod. Biol. Endocrinol.* **2018**, *16*, 1–14. [CrossRef]
55. Zwolak, I. Protective Effects of Dietary Antioxidants against Vanadium-Induced Toxicity: A Review. *Oxid. Med. Cell. Longev.* **2020**, *2020*. [CrossRef] [PubMed]
56. Bellinger, D.C. Lead. *Pediatrics* **2004**, *113*, 1016–1022. [CrossRef] [PubMed]
57. Flora, G.; Gupta, D.; Tiwari, A. Toxicity of lead: A review with recent updates. *Interdiscip. Toxicol.* **2012**, *5*, 47–58. [CrossRef] [PubMed]
58. Viru, A.M.; Hackney, A.C.; Välja, E.; Karelson, K.; Janson, T.; Viru, M. Influence of prolonged continuous exercise on hormone responses to subsequent exercise in humans. *Eur. J. Appl. Physiol.* **2001**, *85*, 578–585. [CrossRef]
59. Viru, A.; Viru, M. Cortisol—Essential adaptation hormone in exercise. *Int. J. Sports Med.* **2004**, *25*, 461–464. [CrossRef]
60. Lafuente, A.; Cano, P.; Esquifino, A.I. Are cadmium effects on plasma gonadotropins, prolactin, ACTH, GH and TSH levels, dose-dependent? *Biometals* **2003**, *16*, 243–250. [CrossRef]
61. Hackney, A.C. Stress and the neuroendocrine system: The role of exercise as a stressor and modifier of stress. *Expert Rev. Endocrinol. Metab.* **2006**, *1*, 783–792. [CrossRef]
62. Pérez-Cadahía, B.; Laffon, B.; Porta, M.; Lafuente, A.; Cabaleiro, T.; López, T.; Caride, A.; Pumarega, J.; Romero, A.; Pásaro, E.; et al. Relationship between blood concentrations of heavy metals and cytogenetic and endocrine parameters among subjects involved in cleaning coastal areas affected by the 'Prestige' tanker oil spill. *Chemosphere* **2008**, *71*, 447–455. [CrossRef]
63. Llerena, F.; Maynar, M.; Barrientos, G.; Palomo, R.; Robles, M.C.; Caballero, M.J. Comparison of urine toxic metals concentrations in athletes and in sedentary subjects living in the same area of Extremadura (Spain). *Eur. J. Appl. Physiol.* **2012**, *112*, 3027–3031. [CrossRef]
64. Cam, M.C.; Brownsey, R.W.; McNeill, J.H. Mechanisms of vanadium action: Insulin-mimetic or insulin-enhancing agent? *Can. J. Physiol. Pharmacol.* **2000**, *78*, 829–847. [CrossRef]

65. Jakusch, T.; Pessoa, J.C.; Kiss, T. The speciation of vanadium in human serum. *Coord. Chem. Rev.* **2011**, *255*, 2218–2226. [CrossRef]
66. Gruzewska, K.; Michno, A.; Pawelczyk, T.; Bielarczyk, H. Essentiality and toxicity of vanadium supplements in health and pathology. *J. Physiol. Pharmacol.* **2014**, *65*, 603–611. [PubMed]

Publisher's Note: MDPI stays neutral with regard to jurisdictional claims in published maps and institutional affiliations.

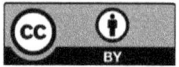

© 2020 by the authors. Licensee MDPI, Basel, Switzerland. This article is an open access article distributed under the terms and conditions of the Creative Commons Attribution (CC BY) license (http://creativecommons.org/licenses/by/4.0/).

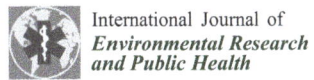

Article

Stroke Analysis in Padel According to Match Outcome and Game Side on Court

Jesús Ramón-Llin [1], José Guzmán [2], Rafael Martínez-Gallego [2], Diego Muñoz [3], Alejandro Sánchez-Pay [4,*] and Bernardino J. Sánchez-Alcaraz [4]

1. Department of Musical, Plastic and Corporal Expression, University of Valencia, 46010 Valencia, Spain; jesus.ramon@uv.es
2. Department of Physical Activity and Sport, Faculty of Sport Sciences, University of Valencia, 46010 Valencia, Spain; jose.f.guzman@uv.es (J.G.); rafael.martinez-gallego@uv.es (R.M.-G.)
3. Department of Musical, Plastic and Corporal Expression, Faculty of Sport Sciences, University of Extremadura, 10003 Cáceres, Spain; diegomun@unex.es
4. Department of Physical Activity and Sport, Faculty of Sport Sciences, University of Murcia, 30720 San Javier, Spain; bjavier.sanchez@um.es
* Correspondence: aspay@um.es; Tel.: +34-868-88-92-97

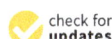

Received: 25 September 2020; Accepted: 23 October 2020; Published: 26 October 2020

Abstract: The aim of this study was to analyze the distribution of padel strokes, their effectiveness, direction, and court zone, comparing between the winning and losing pairs in the match and the playing side of the players. The sample included 8441 strokes corresponding to 1055 points out of a total of nine padel matches in the First National Category. The variables analyzed were type of stroke, court area, effectiveness and directions of the strokes, match outcome, and game side. Matches were analyzed through systematic observation. The results showed that the winning pair made a significantly higher percentage of winners, and cross-court smashes and volleys from the offensive zone. In addition, players on the left side executed a higher percentage of cross-court and winning shots than the players on the right side. Such knowledge may constitute a useful guide in the design of appropriate game strategies and specific training sessions based on the shots that will help players to win the match according to the role of the player and depending on their game side.

Keywords: performance analysis; racquet sports; professional sport; game actions

1. Introduction

Padel is a relatively new sport [1], which is practiced in pairs (2 vs. 2) on a 20 × 10 m court, surrounded by walls or glass and metal fences, which allow the bounce of the ball, and is scored like tennis [2]. It is characterized as a sport with an average duration of efforts between 10–15 s per point [3,4], different technical-tactical actions, and high-intensity movements from the players in different directions, which require continuous decision making [5]. In recent years, there have been numerous studies on padel that have evaluated parameters related to performance analysis [6], with the aim of extracting relevant data from spontaneous behaviors and in real contexts of competition [7]. These investigations provide objective information on real game situations [8], which is vital for planning specific and effective training [9], designing strategies for better performance, and improving decision making and feedback, according to the behavior of the players during the game [10].

These investigations have been based on those variables or indicators that contribute to success in competition and that are common in racquet sports [11]. In this respect, studies carried out with professional padel players have determined that, from a tactical point of view, there are two basic game positions: The attack position, which is when the pair plays close to the net, and the defense position, which is where the pair plays at the baseline of the court [12,13]. This approach has been confirmed by different studies that concluded that there is a greater probability of winning the point when occupying positions close to the net [14,15]. These investigations have shown that more than 80% of the padel winning points are made from the attack position, using different strokes such as volleys (20–25%), the tray, and the smash (12–18%) [16–18]. On the other hand, players in defensive positions perform other types of strokes, among which the lob predominates, with the aim of forcing the attacking pair to move backwards to hit the ball in positions further away from the net or sending them to the baseline in order to reach the offensive position [19].

Therefore, the players constantly try to get a position close to the net, for which they use different behaviors and technical-tactical actions, which define different styles of play [20,21]. The distribution of the different types of stroke, their trajectories, and their efficacy stand out among these behaviors [16,22,23]. The results of the studies have shown that these variables may differ depending on the gender, laterality, or level of the players [17,24]. Particularly in padel, the optimal use of the space is essential to enhance performance and increase scoring rate [20]. Results reveal a solid structure of padel game dynamics depending on game side on court. Left-side players seems to be more effective using smashes but made more errors when hitting the ball after bouncing on the wall; in turn, right-side players made more lobs and committed fewer errors [20]. This seems to indicate a specialization of left-sided as 'scorers' and right-sided as 'defenders' [25]. In this sense, a better knowledge on players' profiles regarding playing side (right or left) is required to set optimal training plans and goals. However, there is a lack of studies that identify the different actions that players perform comparing winners and losers in the match or the side of the court on which the padel player plays. Knowledge of these parameters will help to achieve greater specialization in training sessions, prioritizing those actions that will enable success in the match, and differentiating according to the side of the player depending on the court. In this sense, we hypothesized that paddle players will have different tactical and technical actions according to position and performance. Therefore, the main aim of this study was to analyze the distribution of the different strokes, their effectiveness, direction, and hitting area, and to compare these data according to the final result of the match and the playing side of each player.

2. Materials and Methods

2.1. Sample and Variables

The sample included 8441 shots corresponding to 1055 points from nine matches (three finals and six semifinals) from a total of three top national tournaments (First National Category). A total of 24 male padel players (mean (SD) age: 31.18 (7.27) years; height: 181.3 (4.1) cm) performed the matches.

The matches were played following the official game regulations [2]. The ethics board of the local university reviewed and approved the study (ethic code: 154/2020). The following variables were analyzed:

- Type of stroke: The technical actions of hitting were analysed distinguishing between [14] serve (first or second serve), volleys (stroke without a bounce that is made by hitting the ball at head height, with either a forehand or backhand), tray (stroke without a bounce that is made by the dominant side of the player, hitting the ball at an intermediate height between the volley and the smash and with a slice effect), smash (shot without a bounce that is made by the dominant side of the player, hitting the ball with the arm outstretched, over the head, with a flat or topspin effect), ground stroke (forehand or backhand direct shot), back-wall stroke (forehand or backhand after a rebound on the back wall), side-wall stroke (forehand or backhand after a rebound on the side wall), double-wall stroke (forehand or backhand after a bounce on two walls of the court, depending on the bounce order (side and back wall or back and side wall)), lob (stroke made with a high trajectory with the aim of overcoming the opponents that are at the net), and wall boast (forehand or backhand hitting the ball against the wall of the court itself).

- Court area: Two areas were distinguished, the net area (offensive area) and the baseline area (defensive area). The line that delimited both areas was located on the visual reference on the horizontal-side fence of the court, four meters from the net (Figure 1), following a previous proposal [10,26].
- Stroke direction: Direction was divided between two possible options, down the line and cross court (Figure 1).
- Stroke effectiveness: The stroke effectiveness classification distinguished between continuity (shot causing the point to continue), winner (the player wins the point with a direct stroke), and error (the player loses the point by missing the shot) [7].
- Playing side: The player on the left and right sides of the game was distinguished in each pair (Figure 1).

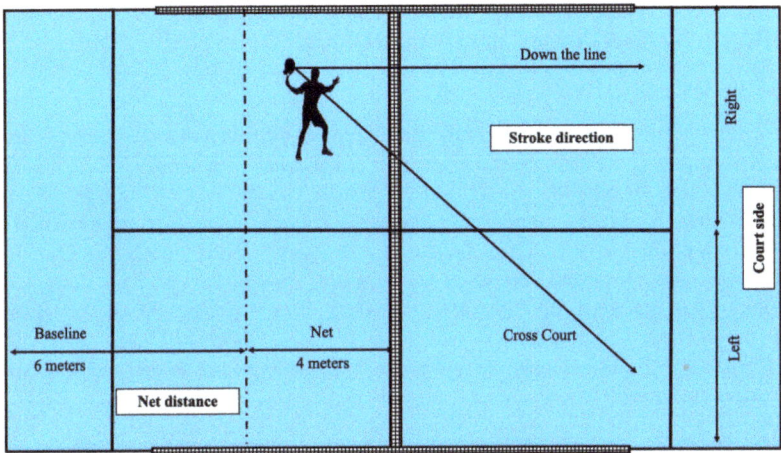

Figure 1. Net distance (baseline and net), playing side (right and left), and stroke trajectory (down the line or cross court).

2.2. Procedure

Firstly, informed consent was requested from tournament organizers and athletes for the recording of matches. Two digital Bosch Dinion Model IP 455 video cameras (Bosch, Munich, Germany) were used to film the matches (25 frames per second), sagittally placed over the courts at 6 m from the center and over the service line. The techniques for transferring video images into Tracker were identical to SAGIT/Squash, i.e., automatic processing with operator supervision, which has been well documented [27]. This software allows to track the movements of the players automatically. Similarly, the reliability for the resultant calculations of distance and speed for each player and positions on court has been shown to be acceptable for analysis purposes [28]. The data were recorded through systematic observation, using specific software for video analysis: LINCE software [29]. The Kinovea software (V.08.26, www.kinovea.org, Bordeaux, France) was used to place a visual grid over the video image for court side, net distance, and stroke direction. Two observers, graduates in Physical Activity and Sports Sciences, and padel coaches, with more than 10 years of experience in the sport, were specifically trained for this task. The training focused on the clear identification of the variables and the use of the observational instrument software (Lince and Kinovea). At the end of the training process, each observer analyzed the same two sets in order to calculate the inter-observer reliability with the Multirater Kappa Free [30], obtaining values above 0.80. To ensure the consistency of the data, intra-observer reliability was evaluated at the end of the observation process, obtaining minimum values of 0.80. The kappa values showed the degree of agreement as very high (>0.80) [31].

2.3. Data Analysis

The data were obtained via the visual analysis of matches. These data were entered onto a spreadsheet (Microsoft Excel) for processing purposes. From the spreadsheet, the data were exported to the IBM SPSS 25.0 statistical package for Macintosh (IBM Corp: Armonk, NY, USA) for analysis. Firstly, a descriptive exploration of the data obtained was carried out and frequency (n) and percentage (%) were calculated. Subsequently, the Kolmogorov–Smirnov tests were performed for the study of normality and the Levene test for the homogeneity of variances. A comparison was made of the statistics on the type of strokes, efficiency, and direction according to match outcome and the playing side using Pearson's chi-square test. In the variables of type of stroke and effectiveness of the stroke subsequent Z tests were carried out to compare column proportions, adjusting the values of $p < 0.05$ according to Bonferroni. The associations among the categories of the variables was performed with corrected standardized residuals (CSR). The effect size was calculated from Crammer's V [32]. The Crammer's V effect size was interpreted as small, medium, and large according to degrees of freedom [33]. A significance level of $p < 0.05$ was established.

3. Results

Table 1 shows the descriptive results of the distribution of the different strokes, their effectiveness, and direction, comparing the winning and losing pair of the match. The type of hitting performed by both pairs showed significant differences according to match outcome ($\chi^2 = 77.19$; $gl = 11$; $p < 0.001$; $V = 0.096$). The winners made a significantly higher percentage of smashes and trays and a lower number of side-wall shots, side and back wall, and wall boast than the losers. The effectiveness of the stroke also showed significant differences among pairs ($\chi^2 = 16.579$; $gl = 2$; $p < 0.001$; $V = 0.044$), with the winning pair making a higher percentage of winners than the losers. Moreover, regarding the direction of the shots, significant differences were found between winners and losers ($\chi^2 = 7.306$; $gl = 1$; $p = 0.007$; $V = 0.033$), with the winning pair in the match performing a higher percentage of cross-court shots than down the line.

Table 1. Type of stroke, effectiveness, and direction according to match outcome.

	Winning			Losing			Sig.
	N	%	CSR	N	%	CSR	
Type of stroke							
Serve	490	11.6	−1.1	525	12.5	1.1	
Volley	1133	26.8	2.0	1056	25.0	−2.0	
Tray	368	8.7a	4.1	255	6.0b	−4.1	
Smash	246	5.8a	3.8	185	4.4b	−3.8	
Ground stroke	655	15.5	−0.8	653	15.5	0.8	
Back wall	528	12.5	−0.6	540	12.8	0.6	<0.001
Side wall	209	4.9a	−3.4	272	6.5b	3.4	
Side and back wall	86	2.0a	−2.1	112	2.7b	2.1	
Back and side wall	79	1.9	−2.9	106	2.5	2.9	
Lob	378	8.9	−1.8	391	9.3	1.8	
Wall boast	53	1.2a	−3.5	121	2.9b	3.5	
Effectiveness of stroke							
Continuity	3671	86.9	−2.3	3716	88.1	2.3	
Winner	236	5.6a	4.3	158	3.7b	−4.3	<0.001
Error	318	7.5	−1.2	342	8.1	1.2	
Direction							
Down the line	1464	34.7	−2.0	1580	37.5	2.0	0.007
Cross court	2761	65.3	2.0	2636	62.5	−2.0	

Note: N = frequency; % = percentage; CSR = Corrected Standardized Residuals; a,b = indicate significant differences in the Z tests for comparison of column proportions from $p < 0.05$ adjusted according to Bonferroni.

The results relative to the distribution of the strokes according to the area of the court are shown in Figure 2. The area of the court where the shots were made was significantly different according to match outcome (χ^2 = 31.145; gl = 1; $p < 0.001$; V = 0.060). Thus, the winning players made a higher percentage of shots in offensive areas (41.2%) than the losing players (35.3%).

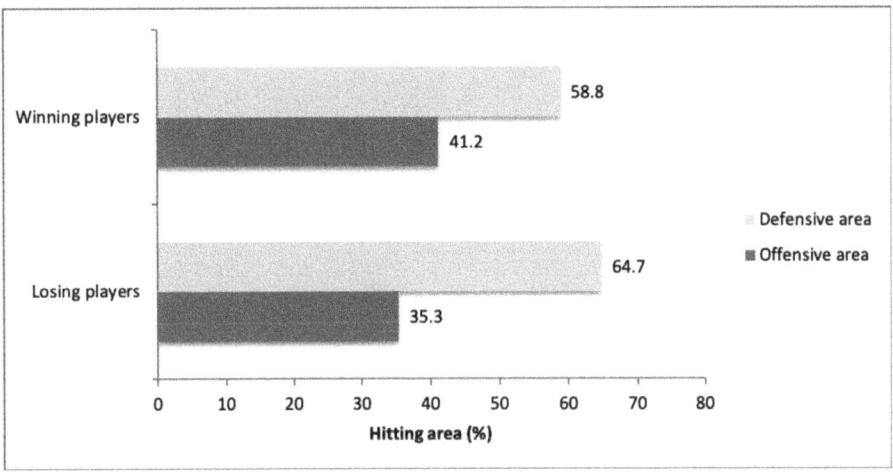

Figure 2. Distribution of the percentage of defensive and offensive shots performed by the winning and losing pairs.

Table 2 shows the descriptive results of the distribution of the different strokes, their effectiveness, and direction, depending on the playing side. The player on the left side made a significantly higher number of hits than the player on the right side (χ^2 = 42.588; gl = 1; $p < 0.001$). The playing side of the players also showed significant differences in the type of stroke (χ^2 = 57.895; gl = 11; $p < 0.001$; V = 0.084). Thus, the players on the left side performed a higher percentage of trays, smashes, side-wall, and wall boast shots than the players on the right side. In addition, differences were found in the effectiveness of these strokes depending on the side of the court (χ^2 = 17.375; gl = 2; $p < 0.001$; V = 0.045). The players on the left side made a significantly higher percentage of winners and a lower percentage of errors than the players on the right side. Finally, significant differences were also found in the shot directions (χ^2 = 13.878; gl = 1; $p < 0.001$; V = 0.043) with the players on the left side making a higher percentage of cross-court and fewer down-the-line shots than the players on the right side.

The results related to the direction of the strokes in each court area are shown in Figure 3. The area of the court where the strokes were made significantly influenced the direction of the strokes made by the padel players (χ^2 = 29.415; gl = 1; $p < 0.001$; V = 0.058). Thus, when the players hit in offensive positions, close to the net, they made a higher percentage of cross-court shots (67.5%) than when they were positioned at the baseline of the court (61.7%).

Table 2. Differences in the number and type of strokes, their effectiveness, and direction depending on the playing side of the court.

	Right Side Player			Left Side Player			Sig.
	N	%	CSR	N	%	CSR	
Participation							
Number of shots	3934	46.60	−4.1	4507	53.40	4.1	<0.001
Type of stroke							
Serve	480	12.2	1.1	536	11.9	−1.1	
Volley	1078	27.4	3.5	1111	24.7	−3.5	
Tray	266	6.8a	−1.6	357	7.9b	1.6	
Smash	148	3.8a	−4.2	282	6.3b	4.2	
Ground stroke	634	16.1	1.6	674	15.0	−1.6	
Back wall	524	13.3	0.3	544	12.1	−0.3	<0.001
Side wall	198	5.0a	−1.2	283	6.3b	1.2	
Side and back wall	86	2.2	−0.2	112	2.5	0.2	
Back and side wall	75	1.9	−1.0	110	2.4	1.0	
Lob	380	9.7	1.1	389	8.6	−1.1	
Wall boast	65	1.7a	−0.2	109	2.4b	0.2	
Effectiveness of stroke							
Continuity	3484	88.6	0.8	3904	86.6	−0.8	
Winner	143	3.6	−3.2	250	5.5	3.2	<0.001
Error	307	7.8	1.9	353	7.8	−1.9	
Direction							
Down the line	1501	38.1	2.3	1543	34.2	−2.3	<0.001
Cross court	2433	61.9	−2.3	2964	65.8	2.3	

Note: N = frequency; % = percentage; CSR = Corrected Standardized Residuals; a,b = indicate significant differences in the Z tests for comparison of column proportions from $p < 0.05$ adjusted according to Bonferroni.

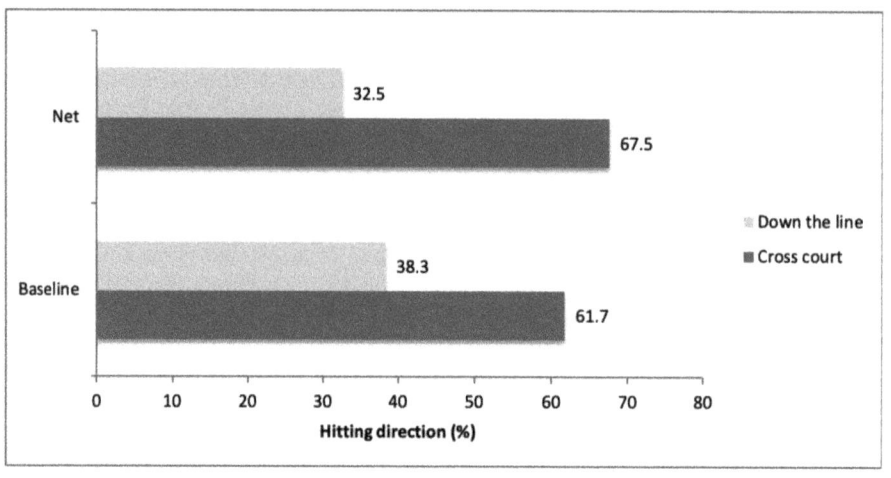

Figure 3. Distribution of the percentage of down-the-line and cross-court shots according to the court area.

4. Discussion

The aim of the present study was to analyze the distribution of the different strokes, their effectiveness, direction, and hitting area, and compare them according to the final result of the match and the playing side of each padel player. The results showed that the most-used strokes by the players were volleys, ground strokes, and back-wall strokes, results similar to those of other studies that have quantified the distribution of padel strokes [16–18,23]. However, these results may be especially relevant when analyzed according to the result of the match, since they would show the strokes that are most used to win a padel match. In this regard, the results of this study indicated that the winning pairs perform a significantly higher percentage of smashes and volleys and a lower number of ground strokes, walls strokes, and lobs than the losers.

Considering the area of the court where the stroke is made, the results showed that the winning players made a significantly higher percentage of shots in positions close to the net, results that confirm the data already provided by similar studies [10,14]. Additionally, the winning pairs performed a higher percentage of cross-court shots than the losing pairs. These results confirm the importance of cross-court shots in professional padel [34,35]. The use of cross-court shots would send the ball toward the side of the court that could cause the ball to rebound off the metal fence, the side wall, or the corner between the back wall and the side wall, increasing the opponent's uncertainty and the chance of their making mistakes.

Thus, the results of this study also showed that the players who lost the match made a higher percentage of shots after the rebound on the side wall or double wall, confirming the data from other studies that observed that the players on the baseline perform a greater number of strokes at the corners of the court [14]. Thus, it seems that varying the directions of the shots and hitting the ball to the corners of the court have been two of the fundamental tactical principles to achieve success in racket sports [5,19,36]. Considering the effectiveness of the stroke, the winning pairs achieved a higher percentage of winners (5.6%) and a lower percentage of errors (7.5%) than the losers, which has been corroborated in other studies [10], and indicated that most of the winners were made through smashes and trays in areas close to the net [14,34]. However, deeper analysis and complementary variable collection is encouraged for a more relevant advance in this knowledge.

One of the main contributions of this study is the distribution of strokes regarding the side of the court on which the player is playing. The results showed that the left-side player performs more strokes than the right-side player, and there are even differences in the distribution of strokes. In this regard, the left-side players made a significantly higher percentage of trays and smashes than the players on the right side (Table 2). The smash seems to be the stroke with the highest percentage of efficiency in padel at the professional level [37]. The data from this study confirm a greater specialization of the players on the left side in the winners, which would define them as having a more offensive style of play. These results could be related, also, to the laterality of the players, since, in pairs with two right-handed players, the player on the left side is the one who would perform the most power smashes, being able to hit the ball with his dominant arm in the central area of the court [20]. So, if the pair of players included two right-handed players, the one on the right side has the paddle near the side wall, which sometimes constitutes a limiting factor when returning a ball. However, a game combination including a left-handed players on the right side allows both players defending the center line in better conditions (i.e., both using quick and balanced forehand strokes) and making easy the use of overhead strokes for returning balls near the side wall [19,20,25]. Their greater participation would be directly related to the ability to finish points. In addition, the results obtained showed a higher percentage of the use of cross-court shots in the players on the left side, trajectories that have shown greater effectiveness in this study.

The results of this study present some limitations that must be considered when interpreting them. In the first place, the laterality of the players has not been taken into account, a variable that could influence the distribution, trajectory, or effectiveness of the strokes [20]. Furthermore, the research sample has only evaluated high-level male players, so it is proposed that future studies compare these data in other categories such as women or young players. Finally, stroke effectiveness distinguished winners, errors, and continuity, but continuity could mean different realities, from easy balls to very difficult balls, so it would be recommended to separate in future studies.

5. Conclusions

This study presents new contributions on game analysis indicators in national padel level. The data show that the winning pairs in padel execute a higher percentage of volleys, trays, and smashes, predominantly cross court and with fewer errors. Moreover, the player on the left side of the court makes more total shots per match and a significantly higher percentage of smashes and cross-court shots than the player on the right side. These data have an important practical application, since they will allow padel coaches and sports technicians to design exercises by selecting those strokes and directions that will lead to success in the match, adapting the tasks specifically to the two players in the pair, differentiating between the right- and left-side players' style of play. The findings of this study suggest that coaches should consider teaching cross-court volleys and smashes from a tactical perspective, because controlling the net game seems to be a key factor in national padel that may distinguish the best players.

Author Contributions: Conceptualization, J.R.-L., B.J.S.-A., and D.M.; methodology, B.J.S.-A., J.G., J.R.-L., A.S.-P., and D.M.; software, B.J.S.-A. and R.M.-G.; validation, B.J.S.-A., R.M.-G., J.R.L., and D.M.; formal analysis, B.J.S.-A. and A.S.-P; investigation, B.J.S.-A., J.G., R.M.-G., J.R.-L., A.S.-P., and D.M; resources, B.J.S.-A., J.R.-L., A.S.-P., and D.M.; data curation, B.J.S.-A., J.R.-L., A.S.-P., and D.M; writing—Original draft preparation, B.J.S.-A., J.G., R.M.-G., and D.M; writing—Review and editing, B.J.S.-A., R.M.-G., J.R.-L., A.S.-P., and D.M; visualization, B.J.S.-A., R.M.-G., J.R.L., A.S.-P., and D.M; supervision, B.J.S.-A., J.R.-L., A.S.-P., and D.M. All authors have read and agreed to the published version of the manuscript.

Funding: This research received no external funding.

Conflicts of Interest: The authors declare no conflict of interest.

References

1. Sánchez-Alcaraz, B.J. History of padel. *Mater. Para. Hist. Deport.* **2013**, *11*, 57–60. (In Spanish)
2. International Padel Federation. *Rules of Padel*; International Padel Federation: Lausanne, France, 2020.
3. Muñoz, D.; García, A.; Grijota, F.J.; Díaz, J.; Sánchez, I.B.; Muñoz, J. Influence of set duration on time variables in paddle tennis matches. *Apunt. Educ. Física Deport.* **2016**, *123*, 69–75. (In Spanish)
4. Sánchez-Alcaraz, B.J. Game actions and temporal structure diferences between male and female professional paddle players. *Acción. Mot.* **2014**, *12*, 17–22. (In Spanish)
5. Ramón-Llin, J.; Guzmán, J.F.; Llana, S.; Martínez-Gallego, R.; James, N.; Vučković, G. The Effect of the Return of Serve on the Server Pair's Movement Parameters and Rally Outcome in Padel Using Cluster Analysis. *Front. Psychol.* **2019**, *10*, 1194. [CrossRef]
6. Sánchez-Alcaraz, B.J.; Cañas, J.; Courel-Ibáñez, J. Analysis of scientific research in padel. *Agon. Int. J. Sport. Sci.* **2015**, *5*, 44–54.
7. Courel-Ibáñez, J.; Sánchez-Alcaraz, B.J. Effect of situational variables on points in elite padel players. *Apunt. Educ. Física Deport.* **2017**, *127*, 68–74. (In Spanish)
8. McGarry, T. *Routledge Handbook of Sports Performance Analysis*; Informa UK Limited: Colchester, UK, 2013.
9. Martínez, B.J.S.-A.; Courel-Ibáñez, J.; Cañas, J. Temporal structure, court movements and game actions in padel: A systematic review. *Retos* **2017**, *33*, 308–312. [CrossRef]
10. Courel-Ibáñez, J.; Sánchez-Alcaraz, J.B.; Cañas, J. Effectiveness at the net as a predictor of final match outcome in professional padel players. *Int. J. Perform. Anal. Sport* **2015**, *15*, 632–640. [CrossRef]
11. Hughes, M.D.; Bartlett, R.M. The use of performance indicators in performance analysis. *J. Sports Sci.* **2002**, *20*, 739–754. [CrossRef]
12. Ramón-Llin, J.; Guzmán, J.F.; Llana, S.; James, N.; Vučković, G. Analysis of padel rally characteristics for three competitive levels. *Kinesiol. Slov.* **2017**, *23*, 39–49.
13. Sánchez-Alcaraz, B.J. Padel tactic in initiation stage. *Trances. Rev. Transm. Conoc. Educ. Salud.* **2013**, *5*, 109–116. (In Spanish)
14. Courel-Ibáñez, J.; Martinez, B.J.S.-A.; Marín, D.M. Exploring Game Dynamics in Padel. *J. Strength Cond. Res.* **2019**, *33*, 1971–1977. [CrossRef]
15. Ramón-Llin, J.; Guzmán, J.; Llana, S.; Vučković, G.; James, N. Comparison of distance covered in paddle in the serve team according to performance level. *J. Hum. Sport Exerc.* **2013**, *8*, 738–742. [CrossRef]

16. Carrasco, L.; Romero, S.; Sañudo, B.; De Hoyo, M. Game analysis and energy requirements of paddle tennis competition. *Sci. Sports* **2011**, *26*, 338–344. [CrossRef]
17. García-Benítez, S.; Pérez-Bilbao, T.; Echegaray, M.; Felipe, J.L. The influence of gender on temporal structure and match activity patterns of professional padel tournaments. *Cultura* **2016**, *11*, 241–247. [CrossRef]
18. Quesada, J.I.P.; Melis, J.O.; Belloch, S.L.; Pérez-Soriano, P.; García, J.C.G.; Almenara, M.S. Padel: A quantitative study of the shots and movements in the high-performance. *J. Hum. Sport Exerc.* **2013**, *8*, 925–931. [CrossRef]
19. Muñoz, D.; Courel-Ibáñez, J.; Sánchez-Alcaraz, B.J.; Díaz, J.; Grijota, F.J.; Munoz, J. Analysis of the use and effectiveness of lobs to recover the net in the context of padel. *Retos Nuevas. Tend. Deport. Educ. Física. Recreación* **2017**, *31*, 19–22. (In Spanish)
20. Courel-Ibáñez, J.; Alcaraz-Martínez, B.J.S. The role of hand dominance in padel: Performance profiles of professional players. *Motricidade* **2018**, *14*, 33–41. [CrossRef]
21. Lupo, C.; Condello, G.; Courel-Ibáñez, J.; Gallo, C.; Conte, D.; Tessitore, A. Effect of gender and match outcome on professional padel competition. *RICYDE Rev. Int. Cienc. Deport.* **2018**, *14*, 29–41. [CrossRef]
22. Courel-Ibáñez, J.; Martínez, B.J.S.-A.; Cañas, J. Game Performance and Length of Rally in Professional Padel Players. *J. Hum. Kinet.* **2017**, *55*, 161–169. [CrossRef]
23. Sañudo, B.; De Hoyo, M.; Carrasco, L. Structural characteristics and physiological demands of the paddle competition. *Apunt. Educ. Física Deport.* **2008**, *94*, 23–28. (In Spanish)
24. Torres-Luque, G.; Ramirez, A.; Cabello-Manrique, D.; Nikolaidis, T.P.; Alvero-Cruz, J.R. Match analysis of elite players during paddle tennis competition. *Int. J. Perform. Anal. Sport* **2015**, *15*, 1135–1144. [CrossRef]
25. Courel-Ibáñez, J.; Sánchez-Alcaraz, B.J.; Marín, D.M. Exploring Game Dynamics in Padel. Implications for Assessment and Training. Available online: http://www.ncbi.nlm.nih.gov/pubmed/28723819 (accessed on 17 July 2017).
26. Ramón-Llin, J.; Guzmán, J.F. Distance to the net of padel players according to their receiving position on the court. *Rev. Int. Deport. Colect.* **2014**, *18*, 105–113. (In Spanish)
27. Vučković, G.; Perš, J.; James, N.; Hughes, M. Tactical use of the T area in squash by players of differing standard. *J. Sports Sci.* **2009**, *27*, 863–871. [CrossRef]
28. Vučković, G.; Perš, J.; James, N.; Hughes, M. Measurement error associated with the SAGIT/Squash computer tracking software. *Eur. J. Sport Sci.* **2010**, *10*, 129–140. [CrossRef]
29. Gabin, B.; Camerino, O.; Anguera, M.T.; Castañer, M. Lince: Multiplatform Sport Analysis Software. *Procedia Soc. Behav. Sci.* **2012**, *46*, 4692–4694. [CrossRef]
30. Randolph, J.J. Free-Marginal Multirater Kappa: An Alternative to Fleiss' Fixed-Marginal Multirater Kappa. Available online: https://eric.ed.gov/?id=ED490661 (accessed on 14 October 2005).
31. Altman, D.G. *Practical Statistics for Medical Research*; Chapman and Hall: London, UK, 1991.
32. Cohen, J. Statistical Power Analysis for the Behavioural Science. In *Statistical Power Anaylsis for the Behavioural Science*, 2nd ed.; Lawrence Erlbaum Associates: Mahwah, NJ, USA, 1988; ISBN 080580283.
33. Cohen, J. Quantitative methods in psychology: A power primer. *Psychol. Bull.* **1992**, *112*, 155–159. [CrossRef]
34. Sánchez-Alcaraz, B.J.; Perez-Puche, D.T.; Pradas, F.; Ramón-Llin, J.; Sánchez-Pay, A.; Muñoz, D. Analysis of Performance Parameters of the Smash in Male and Female Professional Padel. *Int. J. Environ. Res. Public Health* **2020**, *17*, 7027. [CrossRef]
35. Sánchez Alcaraz, B.J.; Muñoz, D.; Pradas, F.; Ramón-Llin, J.; Cañas, J.; Sánchez-Pay, A. Analysis of Serve and Serve-Return Strategies in Elite Male and Female Padel. *Appl. Sci.* **2020**, *10*, 6693. [CrossRef]
36. Escudero-Tena, A.; Fernández-Cortes, J.; García-Rubio, J.; Ibáñez, S.J. Use and Efficacy of the Lob to Achieve the Offensive Position in Women´s Professional Padel. Analysis of the 2018 WPT Finals. *Int. J. Environ. Res. Public Health* **2020**, *17*, 4061. [CrossRef]
37. Sánchez-Alcaraz, B.J.; Courel-Ibáñez, J.; Muñoz, D.; Infantes, P.; Sáez de Zuramán, F.; Sánchez-Pay, A. Analysis of the attack actions in professional padel. *Apunt. Educ. Física Deport.* **2020**, in press.

Publisher's Note: MDPI stays neutral with regard to jurisdictional claims in published maps and institutional affiliations.

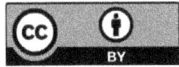

© 2020 by the authors. Licensee MDPI, Basel, Switzerland. This article is an open access article distributed under the terms and conditions of the Creative Commons Attribution (CC BY) license (http://creativecommons.org/licenses/by/4.0/).

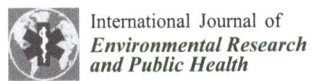

Article

Citations Network Analysis of Vision and Sport

Henrique Nascimento [1,2], Clara Martinez-Perez [2,*], Cristina Alvarez-Peregrina [2] and Miguel Ángel Sánchez-Tena [3]

1   ISEC Lisboa, Instituto de Educação e Ciência de Lisboa, 1750-179 Lisboa, Portugal; henrique.nascimento@iseclisboa.pt
2   Faculty of Biomedical and Health Science, Universidad Europea de Madrid, 28670 Madrid, Spain; cristina.alvarez@universidadeuropea.es
3   Faculty of Sport Sciences, Universidad Europea de Madrid, 28670 Madrid, Spain; miguelangel.sanchez@universidadeuropea.es
*   Correspondence: claramarperez@hotmail.com

Received: 1 October 2020; Accepted: 15 October 2020; Published: 18 October 2020

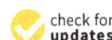

Abstract: *Background*: Sports vision is a relatively new specialty, which has attracted particular interest in recent years from trainers and athletes, who are looking at ways of improving their visual skills to attain better performance on the field of play. The objective of this study was to use citation networks to analyze the relationships between the different publications and authors, as well as to identify the different areas of research and determine the most cited publication. *Methods*: The search for publications was carried out in the Web of Science database, using the terms "sport", "vision", and "eye" for the period between 1911 and August 2020. The publication analysis was performed using the Citation Network Explorer and CiteSpace software. *Results*: In total, 635 publications and 801 citations were found across the network, with 2019 being the year with the highest number of publications. The most cited publication was published in 2002 by Williams et al. By using the clustering functionality, four groups covering the different research areas in this field were found: ocular lesion, visual training methods and efficiency, visual fixation training, and concussions. *Conclusions*: The citation network offers an objective and comprehensive analysis of the main papers on sports vision.

Keywords: sport; vision; performance

1. Introduction

Over the years, the field of ophthalmology has placed great emphasis on the idea of achieving "normal vision" (20/20). Nevertheless, there is much more to perfect vision than having normal vision. While the term "eyesight" refers to the clarity of the image in the retina, the term "vision" has a broader meaning, which encompasses the mental process of deriving meaning from what is seen. Therefore, vision is the result of visual pathway integrity, visual efficiency, and visual information processing [1,2].

Sports vision is a relatively new specialty in the field of optometry, and its objective is to improve and preserve visual function to increase sports performance. Its beginning dates back to the 18th century when the good eye began to occlude in amblyopic patients; however, concerns about athletes' vision did not emerge until the 20th century, when an optometrist began to advise a group of athletes in the United States [3]. In the 1960s, visual examinations were performed on a baseball team in the United States, and, in the 1970s, optometrist services began to be offered routinely to athletes [4]. The first time that a series of visual tests was performed was in the 1984 Olympics, which were held in Los Angeles; in the 2004 Olympics, which were held in Athens, visual tests were conducted on a large number of the athletes. In 1988, the European Academy of Sports Vision was created in Rome with the aim of training specialist technicians in sports vision [4]. These days, sports vision is considered as a very important discipline for the preparation of athletes in the United States.

Many studies have demonstrated that vision plays a vital role in good sports performance [1,2,5]. Most of the athletes and trainers that participated in these studies demonstrated that sports performance requires a wide range of perceptive, technique, psychological, and physical skills. Each sport requires a combination of visual skills, which are essential to ensure adequate sporting performance. By training these specific visual skills, athletes will exhibit better skills and effectiveness in the field of play [6]. Likewise, over the last few decades, perception has been acknowledged as a key aspect of the field of play [7–10]. The study by Spera et al. [11] evaluated and compared balance with both open and closed eyes and the strength of the lower extremities in sighted and visually impaired athletes. The results of the research showed that postural stability was different as a function of the evaluation with the eyes closed and open. Furthermore, the comparison between blind and sighted judo athletes highlighted greater difficulties with closed eyes for sighted athletes than for blind ones. In this way, they showed that vision loss significantly affects performance, especially if athletes do not have a congenital visual deficit, but rather progressively lose vision.

Burris et al. [12] concluded that visual–motor skills play an important role in sports performance; therefore, it has been suggested that sensorimotor skills could be a useful tool when examining players. Another investigation observed that elite athletes have better cognitive skills, with volleyball players demonstrating highly flexible attention and superior executive control [13–15].

Ciućmański et al. [16] demonstrated that, in terms of peripheral vision, depth perception, and the ability to visually track a moving object, footballers had better results than their nonathletic peers. This is since training focusing on developing visual perceptive abilities increased the levels of these abilities and consequently the efficiency of an athlete's perception.

Basic elements of sports vision include visual reaction time and peripheral vision [17]. Both factors significantly affect the athlete's perceptive skills, although they have fundamentally different precedents. Peripheral vision is influenced by the general functions of the human visual system. On the other hand, visual reaction time is related to information and the cognitive processes that control and regulate movement, and these are affected by the central nervous system functions and the muscular effects. Motor reaction time is the time between the signal and the completion of an action; therefore, it has both sensory and motor characteristics [18]. In this way, handball players receive most of their information through their vision, with the player having to pay attention to more than two different stimuli, for instance, an unmarked teammate or a close opponent. That is to say, optimal central–peripheral simultaneity is vital as this allows the player to take in all of the visual information about the object that their vision is focused on, as well as all that is happening around them, without having to make any ocular movement [19,20].

Sports vision training makes use of stimuli in optometric exercises such as videos, images, or stroboscopic interruptions of vision. It is based on the idea that improving visual skills through oculomotor exercises can be associated with motor actions, thereby resulting in an improved sports performance [21–23]. The study performed by Abernethy et al. [24] used generic stimuli (alphanumeric symbols, shapes, patterns, and colors) that were presented in painted graphics or objects. Participants had to answer with a simple ocular adjustment which was combined with simple motor actions such as pointing or touching objectives. In another study, sports training (university football, basketball, or throwing and catching exercises) was assessed using Nike Vapor Strobe glasses, comparing the results to those of athletes who had trained with training eyewear. Participants wearing the Strobe glasses had better results in terms of central visual field motion sensitivity and transient attention abilities than the control group. However, no differences were found in terms of their peripheral motion sensitivity or in terms of their multiple-object tracking [23]. In 2003, García Manso et al. [25] concluded that "vision constitutes a hugely important tool in sports practice and, therefore, visual education must occupy a special part in the athletes' training, primarily when the tasks to be performed are open".

Citation network analysis is used to search scientific literature on a specific subject. In other words, citations can help us find other publications that may be of interest, to demonstrate, both qualitatively and quantitatively, the relationships that exist between articles and authors through the creation of groups [26]. Furthermore, it is possible to quantify the most cited publications in each group and, likewise, we can study the development of a research area or focus the literature search on a specific subject [26–29].

Therefore, taking into consideration the increasing number of publications on sports vision, this study aimed to identify the different research areas and determine the most frequently cited publication. Likewise, it aimed to analyze the relationships between the publications and the different research groups by using the CitNetExplorer software (Ness Jan van Eck and Ludo Waltman, Centre for Science and Technology Studies (CWTS), Leiden University, Leiden, The Netherlands), which examines the development of the scientific literature in a specific research field.

2. Materials and Methods

2.1. Database

The search of publications was carried out in the Web of Science (WOS) database, using the following search terms: "sport", "vision", and "eye". These terms were selected as the study objective because they are the most common terms in all of the research fields.

As the search results had articles in common, the boolean NOT and AND operators were used, and the truncation symbol * was used to search for the singular and plural form of the terms. The first search used the terms ("sport* vision"), the second search used the terms ("sport*" AND "eye" NOT "sport* vision"), and the third search used the terms ("sport*" AND "vision" NOT "sport* vision"). Additionally, the search field was classified by topics, and the results were limited by abstract, title, and keywords. The selected timeframe was from 1911 to August 2020.

Web of Science also makes it possible to add references to your library while conducting bibliographic searches directly in external databases or library catalogs.

Several citation indexes were used in our study, namely, the Social Sciences Citation Index, the Science Citation Index Expanded, and the Emerging Sources Citation Index.

Likewise, given how certain authors and institutions cite works may vary, the CiteSpace software (Chaomei Chen, College of Computing and Informatics, Drexel University, PA, USA) was also used in order to standardize the data. The publications were searched and downloaded on 27 August 2020.

2.2. Data Analysis

The Citation Network Explorer software was used to analyze the publications, as it is a tool that allows the researcher to analyze and visualize the citation networks of scientific publications and even download these directly from Web of Science. Managing citation networks obtained in this way makes it possible for the researcher seeking to analyze a certain subject to use a citation network comprising several million publications and related citations as the starting point for a deeper analysis that will eventually yield a smaller subnetwork of 100 publications.

A quantitative analysis of the most-mentioned publications within a specific timeframe was conducted using the citation score attribute. As such, not only were the internal connections within the Web of Science database quantified, but also any external connections, meaning that other databases were considered [30].

The Citnetexplorer provides several techniques for analyzing publications citation networks. The clustering functionality is achieved using the formula developed by Van Eck in 2012 [30].

$$V(c_1, \ldots, c_n) = \sum_{i<j} \delta(c_i, c_j)(s_{ij} - \gamma). \tag{1}$$

This functionality was used to assign a group to each publication. As a result, the most related publications tended to be found in the same group as a function of citation networks [30].

Finally, the core publications were analyzed using the identifying core publications functionality. This functionality serves to identify the publications that are considered to be the core of a citation network, that is to say, publications with a minimum number of connections with other core publications, thereby allowing irrelevant publications to be eliminated. The researchers established the number of connections in the knowledge that a higher value of this parameter denoted a lower number of core publications [30]. In this way, this study considered publications that presented four or more citations in the citation network.

Additionally, the drilling down functionality was used, as it enables the researcher to conduct a deeper analysis of each of the groups at different levels.

On the other hand, CiteSpace software (5.6.R2) was used to perform scientometric analysis. This software, developed by Chen Chaomei, is based on Java language and it comprises five basic theoretical aspects: Kuhn's model of scientific revolutions, Price's scientific frontier theory, the organization of ideas, the best information foraging theory of scientific communication, and the theory of discrete and reorganized knowledge units [31,32]. A specific assessment can also be conducted within the scientometric analysis process by using certain parameter indicators. Physicist Jorge Hirsch (University of California, USA) proposed the H index, a mixed quantitative index that can provide an assessment of the level and amount of academic output produced by a certain researcher or academic institution. This index, computed by evaluating the number of citations for given papers within a journal, is used as an indicator showing that h of the N published papers have been cited at least h times. It is also used to quantify the productivity and impact of a group of researches that belong to a department, university, or country. It should be noted that, if the software yields a value of 1, this does not constitute a professional answer [33]. The parameter indicator "degree" is used to show the number of co-occurrences between authors, institutions, or countries in the knowledge graph; consequently, more communication and cooperation between them would result in a higher degree value. Likewise, the importance of nodes in the research cooperation network and the continuity of institutional research over time can also be measured by using the intermediary centrality and the half-life indicators, respectively [31].

2.3. Ethical Approval

This study was approved by the ethics committee of the General Directorate for Research and Development (DGID) of Instituto Superior de Educação e Ciências (ISEC) Lisbon, Portugal. The ethical approval number is 01/27052020.

3. Results

The first articles about sports vision were published in 1911; thus, the selected time interval was from 1911 to August 2020. In total, 635 publications and 801 citations networks were found in the search that was conducted in WOS (Figure 1). Of all the publications, 73.75% were articles, 8.85% were proceedings, 5.90% were reviews, 4.13% were congress and conference summaries, 3.24% were letters, and 2.06% were book chapters.

The number of publications about sports vision has increased significantly since 2011 (1911–2010: 34.96% of the publications; 2011–2020: 65.04% of the publications). The year 2019 had the largest number of publications, accounting for 68 publications and six citations networks (Figure 2).

Table 1 shows the 20 most cited publications in this citation network. The most cited article was the article by Williams et al. [34], which was published in November 2002, with a citation index of 28. This study analyzed the relationship among the "quiet eye" (final fixation on the target before the initiation of movement), expertise, and task complexity in a near and a far aiming task in 24 billiards players (12 professional players and 12 less skilled players). In order to do so, two experiments were established, which were based on establishing the different visual fixation time during the preparation phase of the action. They found that shorter quiet eye periods resulted in poorer performance, irrespective of participant skill level. Therefore, the authors argued that quiet eye duration represents a critical period for movement programming in the aiming response.

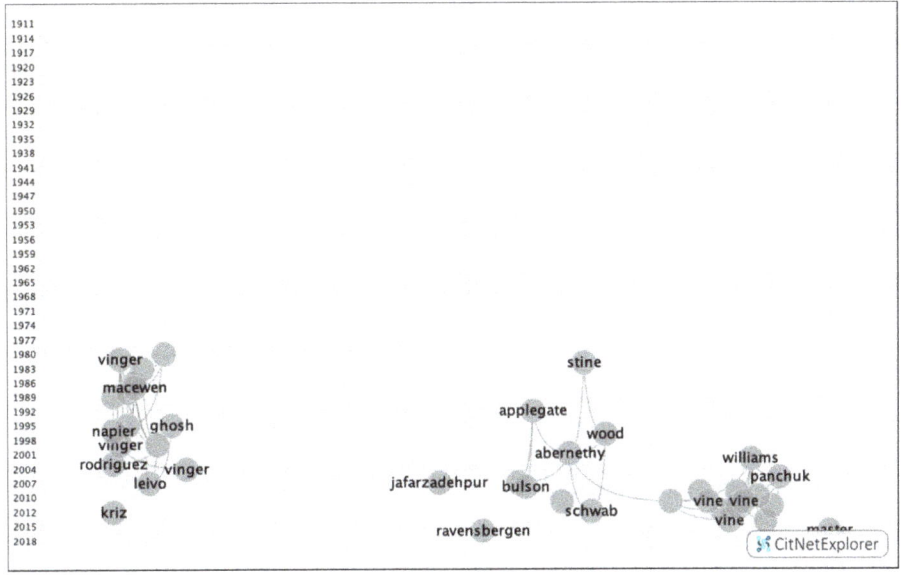

Figure 1. Citation networks on sports vision.

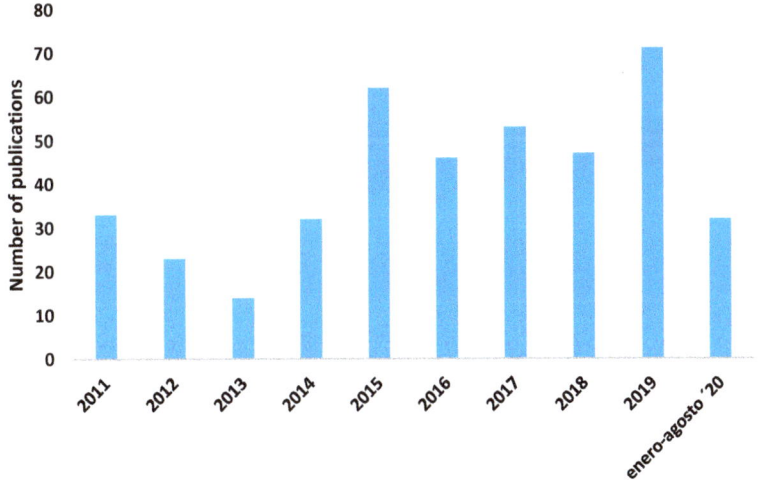

Figure 2. Number of publications per year.

Table 1. Description of the 20 most cited publications on sports vision.

Author	Title	Journal	Year	Total Number Citations	Citation Rate	h-Index
Williams et al. [34]	Quiet eye duration, expertise, and task complexity in near and far aiming tasks	J. Mot. Behav. 2002, 34, 197–207	2002	28	1.55	1
Vine et al. [35]	Quiet eye training facilitates competitive putting performance in elite golfers	Front Psychol. 2011, 8, 8	2011	21	2.33	1
MacEwen et al. [36]	Sport-associated eye injury: a casualty department survey	Br. J. Ophthalmol. 1987, 71, 701–705	1987	18	0.54	1
Vine et al. [37]	The influence of quiet eye training and pressure on attention and visuo-motor control	Acta Psychol. (Amst). 2011, 136, 340–346.	2011	17	1.89	1
Causer et al. [38]	Quiet eye duration and gun motion in elite shotgun shooting	Med. Sci. Sports Exerc. 2010, 42, 1599–1608	2010	17	1.70	1
Abernethy et al. [24]	Do generalized visual training programs for sport really work? An experimental investigation	J. Sports Sci. 2001, 19, 203–22	2001	16	0.84	1
Stine et al. [39]	Vision and sports: a review of the literature	J. Am. Optom. Assoc. 1982, 53, 627–633.	1982	16	0.42	1
Mann et al. [40]	Quiet eye and the Bereitschaftspotential: visuomotor mechanisms of expert motor performance	Cogn. Process. 2011, 12, 223–234	2011	15	1.67	1
Vickers et al. [41]	Advances in coupling perception and action: the quiet eye as a bidirectional link between gaze, attention, and action	Prog. Brain Res. 2009, 174, 279–288	2009	14	1.27	1
Panchuk et al. [42]	Gaze behaviors of goaltenders under spatial-temporal constraints	Hum. Mov. Sci. 2006, 25, 733–752	2006	14	1.00	1
Wood et al. [43]	An assessment of the efficacy of sports vision training programs	Optom. Vis. Sci. 1997, 74, 646–659.	1997	13	0.56	1
Vine et al. [44]	Quiet eye training: the acquisition, refinement and resilient performance of targeting skills	Eur. J. Sport Sci. 2014, 14 (Suppl. 1), S235–S242	2014	12	2.00	1
Causer et al. [45]	Quiet eye training in a visuomotor control task	Med. Sci. Sports Exerc. 2011, 43, 1042–1049.	2011	12	1.33	1
Vinger et al. [46]	Sports eye injuries a preventable disease	Ophthalmology 1981, 88, 108–113.	1981	12	0.31	1
Napier et al. [47]	Eye injuries in athletics and recreation	Surv. Ophthalmol. Nov.-Dec 1996, 41, 229–444.	1996	11	0.46	1
Gregory et al. [48]	Sussex Eye Hospital sports injuries	Br. J. Ophthalmol. 1986, 70, 748–750	1986	11	0.32	1
Master et al. [49]	Vision diagnoses are common after concussion in adolescents	Clin. Pediatr. (Phila) 2016, 55, 260–267	2016	10	2.50	1
Schwab et al. [50]	The impact of a sports vision training program in youth field hockey players	J. Sports Sci. Med. 2012, 11, 624–631.	2012	10	1.25	1
Vinger et al. [51]	Sports-related eye injury. A preventable problem	Surv. Ophthalmol. Jul.-Aug.1980, 25, 47–51	1980	10	0.25	1
Klostermann et al. [52]	On the interaction of attentional focus and gaze: the quiet eye inhibits focus-related performance decrements	J. Sport Exerc. Psychol. 2014, 36, 392–400	2014	9	1.50	1

The 20 most cited articles were analyzed. Five of these discussed ocular lesions associated with sport [36,47–49,52], four discussed the use of visual training for improving sports skills, 10 discussed training visual fixation skills ("quiet eye") [24,34,35,37–46,51], and the final article was about the significance of training of oculomotor movements in subjects with sports-related concussion [50].

3.1. Description of the Publications

The research on sports vision is multidisciplinary. The fields of sport science (17.09%) and ophthalmology (13.25%) (Table 2) are particularly worth mentioning. Table 3 shows the 10 journals with the largest number of publications.

Table 2. Number of publications by research area.

Category	Frequency	Centrality	Degree
Sports sciences	44	0.27	23
Psychology	33	0.10	16
Social sciences, other topics	29	0.07	10
Ophthalmology	28	0.08	10
Hospitality, leisure, sport, and tourism	25	0.01	8
Engineering	23	0.62	29
Computer science	23	0.18	23
Neurosciences and neurology	16	0.14	15
Psychology, multidisciplinary	13	0.01	8
Psychology, applied	13	0.00	6

Table 3. Top 10 journals with the most publications.

Journal	Total Publications	Impact Factor (2019)	Quartile Score	SJR (Scimago Journal & Country Rank) (2019)	Citations/Docs (2 Years)	Total Citations (2019)	Centrality	h-Index	Country
Optometry and Vision Science	12	1.46	Q1	0.89	1.789	1011	0.00	92	United States
Physician and Sports Medicine	12	1.66	Q1	0.82	1.792	407	0.00	41	United Kingdom
Frontiers in Psychology	12	2.07	Q1	0.91	2.536	17,548	0.00	95	Switzerland
Medicine and Science in Sports and Exercise	10	4.03	Q1	1.89	4.053	4257	0.00	216	United States
Eye and Contact Lens Science and Clinical Practice	9	1.52	Q2	0.74	2.099	663	0.00	54	United States
British Journal of Ophthalmology	7	3.61	Q1	1.88	4.026	3591	0.00	146	United Kingdom
Acta Ophthalmological	7	3.36	Q1	1.42	3.304	2369	0.00	82	United States
British Medical Journal	7	17.21	Q1	2.05	4.235	16,584	0.00	412	United Kingdom
Journal of Sport Exercise Psychology	7	2.24	Q1	1.20	2.013	366	0.00	93	United States
Clinical and Experimental Optometry	6	1.92	Q2	0.75	2.034	559	0.00	51	United States

As shown in Table 4, the authors with the largest number of publications on sports vision were Mann (4.27%), Balcer (2.56%), and Galetta (2.56%).

Table 4. Top 10 authors with the largest number of publications.

Author	Number of Publications	h-Index	Total Citations	Citation Average	Centrality	Degree
Mann DL	10	4	76	7.6	0.00	3
Balcer LJ	6	5	157	26.17	0.00	14
Galetta SL	6	5	157	26.17	0.00	14
Vater C	6	3	25	4.17	0.00	3
Hasanaj L	4	2	87	21.75	0.00	10
Hossner EJ	4	3	22	5.50	0.00	3
Ravensbergen RHJC	4	3	10	2.50	0.00	1
Akhand O	3	1	6	2.00	0.00	10
Allen PM	3	2	7	2.33	0.00	1
Kredel R	3	2	19	6.33	0.00	3

The United States (20.94%), England (12.82%), and China (8.97%) were the countries with the highest publication rate (Table 5).

Table 5. Publication rate depending on the country.

Country	Publications (%)	Centrality	Degree	Half-life
United States	49 (20.94%)	0.36	20	1.5
England	30 (12.82%)	0.26	15	1.5
China	21 (8.97%)	0.05	8	0.5
Australia	18 (7.69%)	0.16	12	1.5
Spain	16 (6.84%)	0.10	7	0.5
Netherlands	13 (5.56%)	0.10	6	1.5
Germany	12 (5.13%)	0.00	3	0.5
Japan	11 (4.70%)	0.01	3	2.5
Brazil	8 (3.42%)	0.04	2	1.5
Switzerland	8 (3.42%)	0.03	7	2.5

Additionally, the most used keywords were "implantation" (325 publications), "contrast sensitivity" (285 publications), and "performance" (231 publications). Table 6 shows the 30 most used keywords from the most significant publications.

3.2. Clustering Function

The clustering function identified four groups, all of which contained a significant number of articles (Figure 3). Table 7 shows the information on the citation networks for the four main groups, listed by size from the largest to the smallest.

Table 6. The most used keywords.

Keyword	Frequency	Centrality	Degree
Sport	41	0.12	21
Performance	32	0.15	27
Attention	18	0.14	27
Vision	16	0.16	29
Eye movement	14	0.02	14
Expertise	14	0.09	30
Children	14	0.11	28
Traumatic brain injury	13	0.06	26
Skill	12	0.08	22
Impact	12	0.08	19
Concussion	12	0.08	27
Injury	11	0.03	9
Eye tracking	11	0.09	15
Epidemiology	11	0.09	23
Anxiety	11	0.10	26
Movement	10	0.12	20
Saccade	9	0.08	27
Perception	9	0.11	21
Quiet eye	8	0.03	17
Visual acuity	7	0.04	16
Adolescent	7	0.09	28
Protective eyewear	6	0.09	20
Information	6	0.04	15
Gaze behavior	6	0.04	18
Eye-tracking	6	0.08	14
Eye injury	6	0.04	15
Behavior	6	0.02	11
Vision impairment	5	0.01	11
Validity	5	0.05	14
United States	5	0.01	10

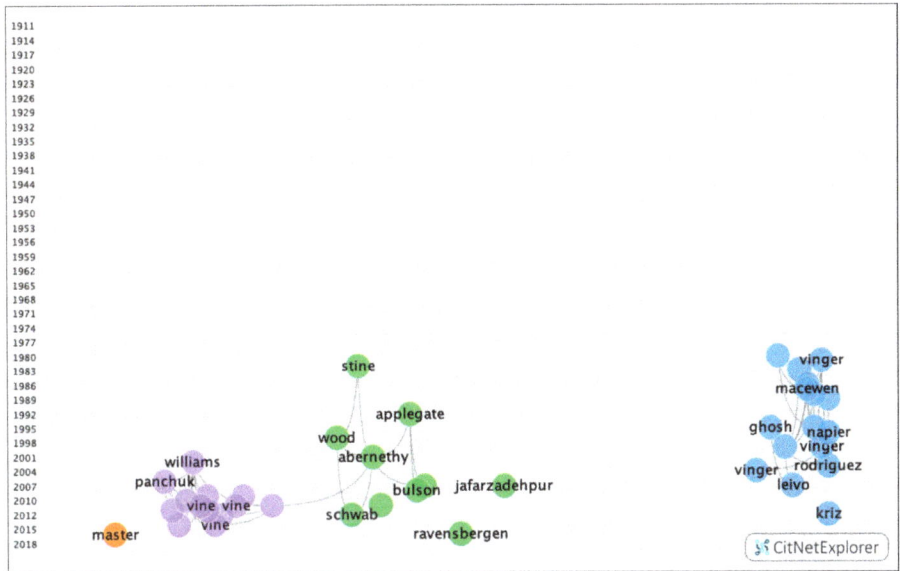

Figure 3. Clustering function in the citations network of sports vision.

Table 7. Information about citations network of the four main groups.

Main Groups	Number of Publications	Number of Citation Networks	Number of Citations, Median (Range)	Number of Publications with ≥4 Citations	Number of Publications in the 100 Most Cited Publications
Group 1	108	276	1 (0–18)	46	40
Group 2	80	203	1 (0–16)	34	30
Group 3	68	238	1 (0–28)	34	24
Group 4	28	40	0 (0–10)	0	6

In group 1, 108 publications and 276 citations were found throughout the network. The most cited publication was the article by MacEwen et al. [36], which was published in 1987 in the *British Journal of Ophthalmology*. In this study, a survey was performed with all patients presenting with sport-related ocular lesions and a total of 246 patients presented with this type of injury during an 18-month period. Football was responsible for 110 (44.7%), rugby for 24 (9.8%), squash for 19 (7.7%), badminton for 16 (6.5%), and ski for nine (3.7%), while 68 (27.6%) were caused by other sports. In total, 46 patients (18.7%) required inpatient care and 200 (81.3%) were treated as outpatients, of whom 104 required at least one follow-up appointment (42.3% of the total). The authors concluded that, with increasing time available for leisure activities, there has been a parallel increase in sport associated eye traumas. The studies in this group dealt with ocular lesions associated with sport, as well as their prevalence (Figure 4).

In group 2, 80 publications and 202 citations were found throughout the network. The most cited publication was the article by Stine et al. [39], which was published in 1982 in the *Journal of the American Optometric Association*. This article addressed two studies that demonstrated that athletes have better visual skills than non-athletes and, in turn, that better athletes have better visual abilities than poorer athletes. They also confirmed that visual skills are trainable and transferable to athletic performance, meaning that players present a larger extent of visual field, larger fields of recognition, larger motion perception fields, lower amounts of heterophoria at near and far ranges, more consistent simultaneous vision, more accurate depth perception, better dynamic vision acuity, and better ocular motility, whereby all of these visual skills can be improved with appropriate visual training. The publications in this group addressed efficiency and the different methods of visual training with the purpose of improving the visual skills of athletes, leading to better on-field performance (Figure 5).

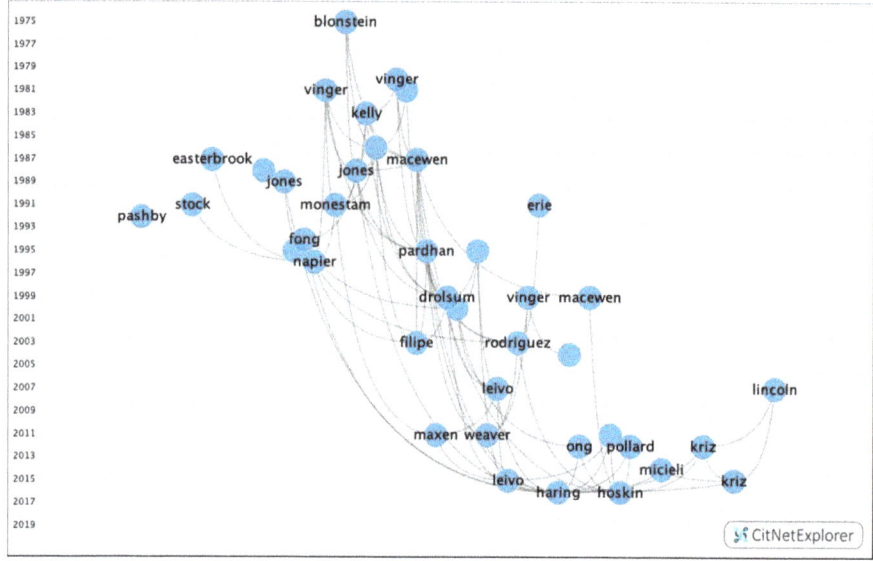

Figure 4. Citation network in group 1.

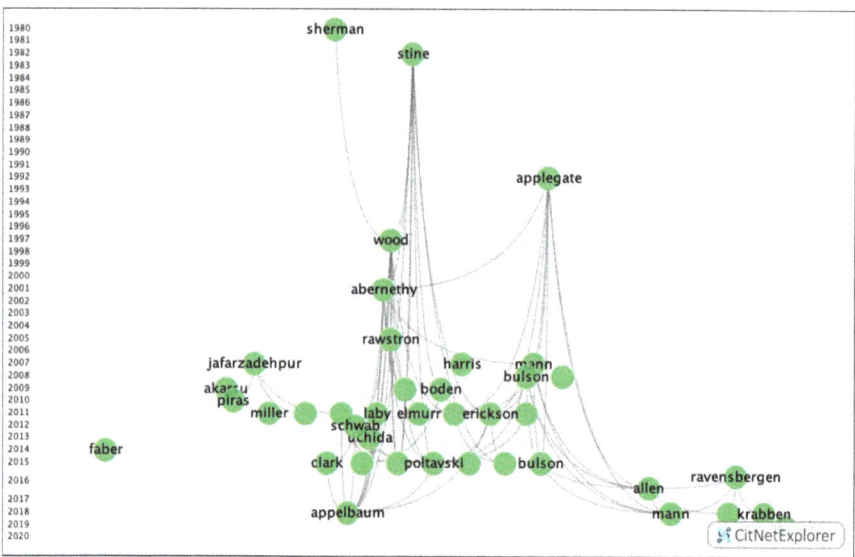

Figure 5. Citation network in group 2.

In group 3, 68 articles and 238 citations were found throughout the network. The most cited publication was the article by Williams et al. [34], which was published in 2002 in the *Journal of Motor Behavior*, which was also at the top of the list of the 20 most cited publications. The publications in this group addressed how visual fixation training (quiet eye) allows for better results to be achieved in the field (Figure 6).

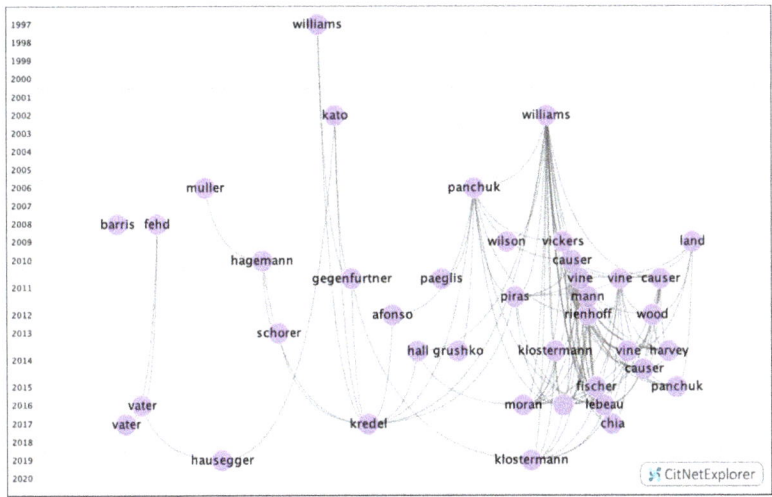

Figure 6. Citation network in group 3.

In group 4, 28 publications and 40 citations were found throughout the network. The most cited publication was the article by Master et al. [49], which was published in 2016 in *Clinical Pediatrics*. This article looked to determine the prevalence of visual impairment after concussion in adolescents. In order to do so, 100 teenagers with a mean age of 14.5 years were examined, and it was found that 69% presented with one or more of the following vision diagnoses: accommodative disorders (51%), convergence insufficiency (49%), and saccadic dysfunction (29%). Therefore, they concluded that performing a visual examination is recommended and that these visual diagnoses must be taken into account when they return to the field of play. The publications in this group addressed the importance of evaluating oculomotor movements in patients with concussions, as this type of training can help athletes who present with or who have suffered concussions (Figure 7).

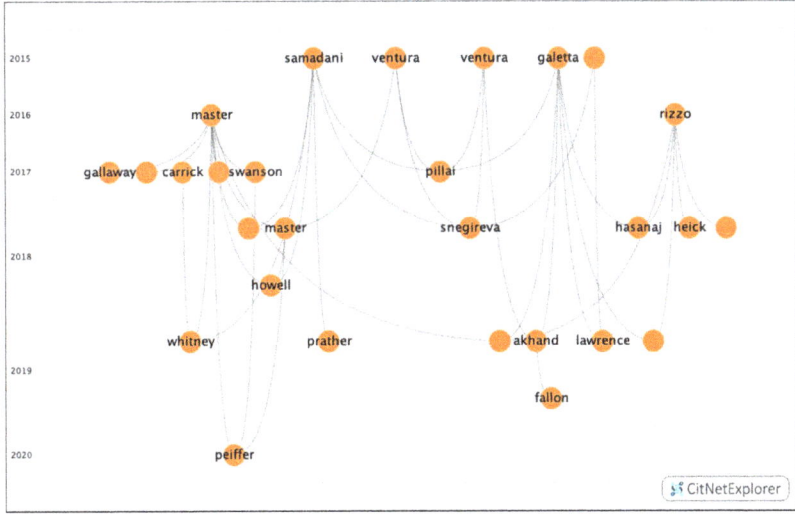

Figure 7. Citation network in group 4.

Table 8 shows a detailed description of the oldest and newest publications in the four main groups.

Table 8. Information about the oldest and most recent publications in the four main groups.

Group		Author	Title	Year	Total Citations
Group 1	Oldest	Blonstein [53]	Eye injuries in sport: with particular reference to squash rackets and badminton	1975	3
	Most recent	Toldi et al. [54]	Evaluation and management of sports-related eye injuries	2020	0
Group 2	Oldest	Sherman [55]	Overview of research information regarding vision and sports	1980	2
	Most recent	Vera et al. [56]	Basketball free-throw performance depends on the integrity of binocular vision	2020	0
Group 3	Oldest	Williams et al. [57]	Assessing cue usage in performance contexts: a comparison between eye-movement and concurrent verbal report methods	1997	3
	Most recent	Witkowski et al. [58]	Fighting left handers promote different visual perceptual strategies than right handers: the study of eye movements of foil fencers in attack and defense	2020	1
Group 4	Oldest	Galetta et al. [59]	Adding vision to concussion testing	2015	6
	Most recent	Peiffer et al. [60]	The influence of binocular vision symptoms on computerized neurocognitive testing of adolescents with concussion	2020	0

After using the drilling down functionality to analyze the relationships among the four main groups, no connections were found between them (Figure 8).

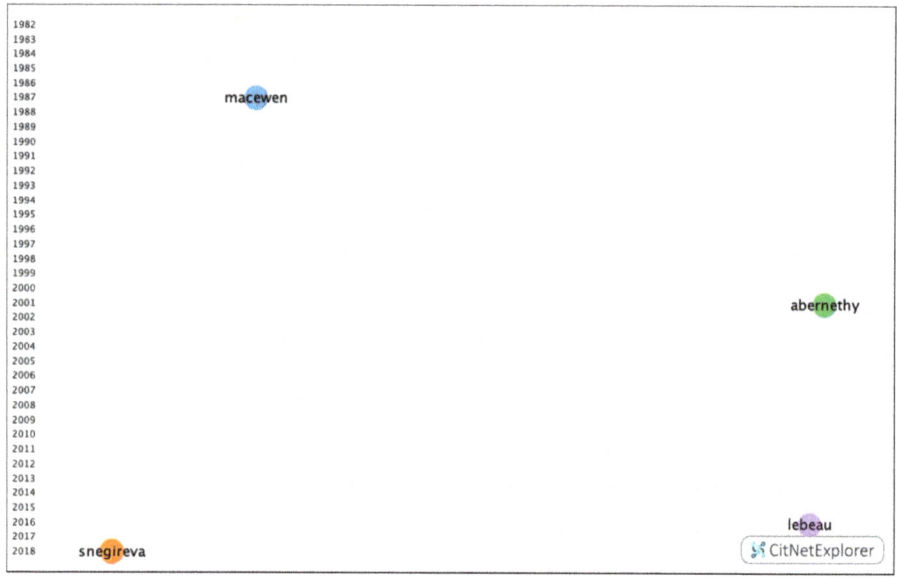

Figure 8. Connection between the four main groups.

3.2.1. Subclusters in Group 1

Four subgroups were found (Figure 9), three of which contained a significant number of publications (Table 9). The remaining group was relatively small with fewer than 12 publications and 15 citations networks.

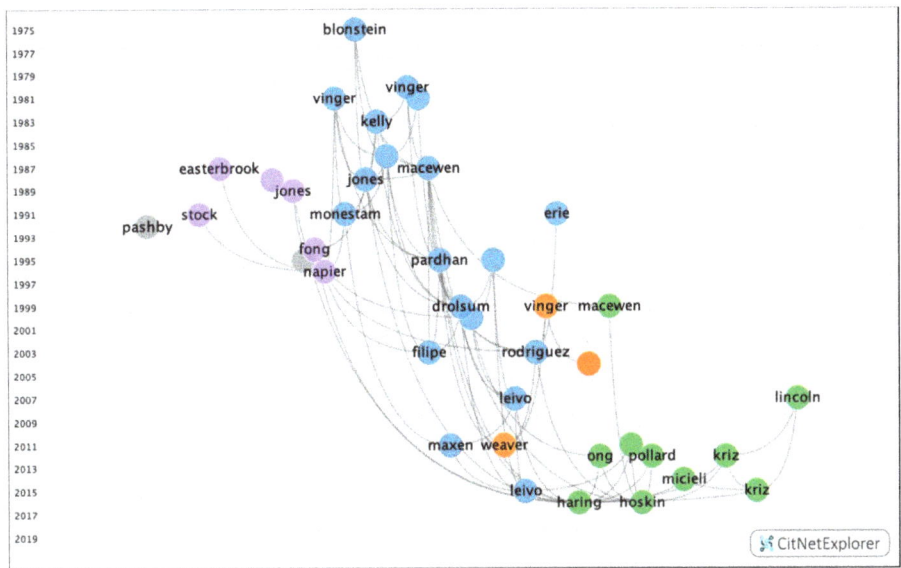

Figure 9. Citation network of subclusters in group 1.

Table 9. Main citation network groups from the subcluster in group 1.

Subcluster	1	2	3
Number of publications	40	27	16
Number of citation links	110	53	22
First publication	Blonstein et al., 1975 [53]	MacEwen et al., 1999 [62]	Vinger et al., 1983 [64]
Most cited publication	MacEwen et al., 1987 [36]	Kriz et al., 2012 [63]	Napier et al., 1996 [47]
Most recent publication	Micieli et al.; 2017 [61]	Toldi et al., 2020 [54]	Woo et al., 2006 [65]
Main keywords	Injuries, impact, prevention	Epidemiology, trauma, risk	Hockey, injuries, head
Topic of discussion	Ocular lesions associated with sport	Rates of emergency admissions for sport-related ocular lesions	Sports which present the highest risk of ocular lesion
Conclusion	Sport is becoming an increasingly significant cause of severe ocular lesions, and the promoted use of adequate ocular protection is considered to be of the utmost importance.	Ocular lesions associated with sport present a potential impact on the provision of services. It is fundamental that ophthalmologists, optometrists, and another healthcare professionals are aware of possible ocular morbidity in the case of sport traumas and the importance of providing advice on how to prevent said lesions.	The sports which are responsible for the highest number of lesions are baseball, ice hockey, and racquet sports. Specific criteria must be developed for protection glasses. Impact-resistant polycarbonate plastic lenses and frames offer optimum protection.

3.2.2. Subclusters in Group 2

Four subgroups (Figure 10) were found, of which three contained a significant number of publications (Table 10). The remaining group was relatively small with fewer than 12 publications and 13 citation networks.

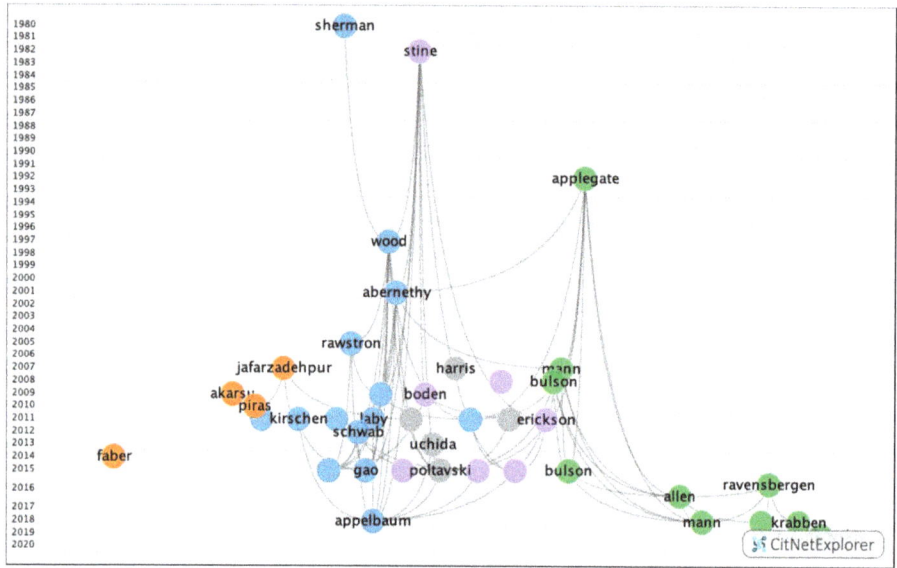

Figure 10. Citation network from the subclusters in group 2.

Table 10. Main groups of citation network of subcluster in group 2.

Subcluster	1	2	3
Number of publications	29	16	15
Number of citation links	69	40	22
First publication	Sherman, 1980 [55]	Applegate et al., 1992 [67]	Stine et al., 1982 [39]
Most cited publication	Abernethy et al., 2001 [24]	Applegate et al., 1992 [67]	Stine et al., 1982 [39]
Most recent publication	Jorge et al., 2019 [66]	Vera et al., 2020 [56]	Schumacher et al., 2019 [68]
Main keywords	Vision training, exercise, movement	Visual acuity, visual impairment, perception	Anticipation, reaction time, strategies
Topic of discussion	Evaluating the efficacy of sports vision training programs	Importance of the optimal visual acuity in the field	Comparison between the visual skills of athletes and non-athletes
Conclusion	Visual training allows for improvements to be made in terms of the visual skills of athletes, leading to greater precision in the playing field. However, there is a great controversy as to whether this training actually helps improve the on-field performance; therefore, further scientific evidence is required.	A reduction in visual acuity does not have a significant influence on sports performance. The motor–perceptual system is capable of compensating for this.	Athletes demonstrated better visual skills than non-athletes. Likewise, they presented stereopsis and a more developed visual field.

3.3. Core Publications

In Figure 11, after the analysis was performed using the core publications functionality, 114 publications with four or more citations (16.9% of the publications) and 471 citations networks were obtained.

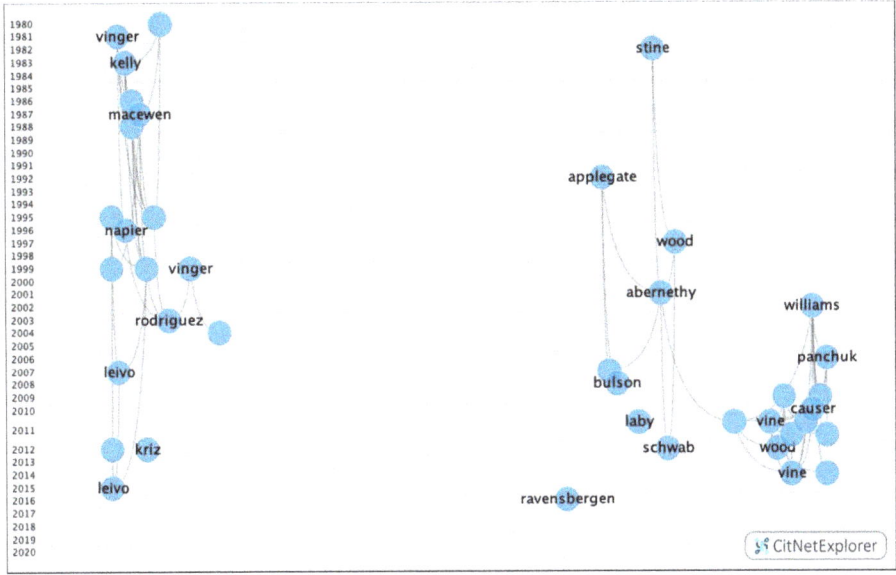

Figure 11. Core publications in the citation network about multifocal IOLs.

4. Discussion

The first publication about sports vision was published by Walker et al. [69] in 1911, just as concern for sports vision was beginning to emerge at the beginning of the 20th century. This article analyzed the importance of the dominant eye and how skills in shooting sports could be improved. However, publications on sports visions were still very limited until the mid-1990s; nonetheless, the number of papers being published was increasing and these were beginning to cover a range of topics [70]. Studies by Fullerton [71] and Winogrand [72], which were published in 1925 and 1942, respectively, demonstrated that athletes presented better visual skills than amateur athletes. Following this, a considerable number of studies analyzed the effect of visual training programs on visual skills and sports performance, with these studies modifying the experimental parameters such as stimuli or contexts [24,73]. Numerous studies have shown that visual perception skills and cognitive performance improve after a visual training program. In Clark et al.'s study [74], a team of baseball players was subjected to a visual skills training program that incorporated both traditional and technological methods. The results showed that the players' batting averages and slugging percentage were better than those recorded in the previous season. In another study, Di Noto et al. [75] used the "rapid serial visual presentation" (RSVP) method to evaluate ocular movements and visual attention. In this study, the 20 subjects were divided equally into control and experimental groups, each of which performed a pre-training RSVP assessment where the target letters, to which subjects were asked to respond by pressing a spacebar, were serially and rapidly presented. The response time to target letters, the accuracy of correctly responding to target letters, and the correct identification of the target letters in each of the 12 sessions were measured. The experimental group then performed active eye exercises, while the control group performed a task that minimized eye movements for 18.5 min. A post-training RSVP assessment was performed by both groups, and the response time, accuracy, and letter identification were compared between and within the subject groups for both pre- and post-training. Subjects who performed eye exercises were more accurate in responding to target letters separated by one distractor and in letter identification in the post-training RSVP assessment, while the latency of responses was unchanged between and within groups. This suggests that eye exercises may prove useful in enhancing cognitive performance on tasks related to attention and memory over a very brief course of training, and RSVP may be a useful measure of this efficacy. This relates to the fact that athletes and their trainers are constantly looking for ways to improve their physical and mental skills, and, due to the demanding nature of sports, visual and motor skills are often the focal point of sports training programs.

At the same time, 2019 was identified as a key year, due to the considerable number of studies that were published that year and due to the progress that was made in the research into sports vision. Hausegger et al. [76] study that suggested that gaze anchoring is functional for optimizing the use of peripheral visual information was seen to be particularly relevant. This study predicted that the height of gaze anchoring on the opponent's body would depend on the potential attacking locations that need to be monitored. To test this prediction, the authors compared high-level athletes in kung fu (Qwan Ki Do), who attack with their arms and legs, with Tae Kwon Do fighters, who attack mostly with their legs. As predicted, the results showed that Qwan Ki Do athletes anchor their gaze higher than Tae Kwon Do athletes do before and even during the first attack. Furthermore, gaze anchoring seems to depend on three factors: the particulars of the evolving situation, crucial cues, and specific visual costs (especially suppressed information pickup during saccades). Another relevant study published by Mashkovskiy et al. [77] analyzed how the degree of visual impairment influenced the outcomes in a judo team. The findings confirmed that blind athletes had fewer chances to win a judo fight given that the loss of vision functions affects movement coordination, balance, and emotional state, which are important for martial arts.

One journal with a particularly high number of publications about sports vision is *Optometry and Vision Science*, which occupies the 40th place in the ophthalmology category, and which boasts an impact factor of 1.46. Articles were published in 150 magazines in the ophthalmology topic category, which seems reasonable given that sports vision is a specialty of the field of optometry and ophthalmology. The journal with the highest impact factor was the *British Medical Journal*, 17.21. However, it is important to consider that, although the impact factor is a critical index of the journal's importance, it is not an absolute measure index. The main difference between both indexes is that the latter is based on the impact of the research results, as well as the authors' physical and intellectual contributions [78].

The countries with the largest number of published articles were the United States, England, and China. This is not surprising given that the first studies about sports vision were published in the United States and the sports vision section of the American Optometric Association, the oldest in the world, was founded in 1978. However, it is worth mentioning that the authors' institution with the highest rate of publications was "Vrije Universiteit Amsterdam", because, in recent years, both athletes and trainers have shown an increased interest in improving their visual skills, especially in competitive sports. The creation of the European Association of Sports Vision and the Sports Vision Association of the United Kingdom are also considered relevant. Equally, the upward trend in the numbers of publications from countries such as the United States or the United Kingdom has been linked to a combination of factors, for example, the fact that these are English-speaking countries or the possible connections that may exist between the different research groups within the scientific community [79,80].

Sports vision as a specialty in the ophthalmology and optometry field is constantly expanding. In recent years, research has commenced into the benefits of advanced visual training. In a study that looked to analyze the stroboscopic effects on anticipatory timing, the skills of athletes were compared before and after using the Bassin anticipation timer. The experimental group practiced with the Bassin timer wearing Nike Vapor Strobe glasses set to level 3 (100 ms clear/150 ms opaque), while the control group practiced with normal vision. The post-training assignments were administered immediately, 10 min, and 10 days after training. In comparison to the control group, the Strobe group was significantly more accurate immediately after training, and it was more likely to respond early than to respond late immediately after training and 10 min later [81]. Using low visual level tools, Deveau et al. [82], trained 19 players with the Ultimeyes app for 30 sessions of 25 min, while another

18 players did not undergo training as the control subjects. The binocular VA (visual acuity) and SC (contrast sensitivity) were tested before and after the training. Results showed improved VA and SC, and, after seven days, the VA was superior to the normal levels. In baseball, it led to a reduction in the number of strikeouts and an increase of 4–5 extra games won compared to previous years.

Vision allows muscles to respond to signals, that is, it provides information to the athlete about when and where current activity is occurring. Therefore, all athletes require good vision, in order to reduce head and body movements, analyze three-dimensional space, or clearly see an object in motion. However, depending on the sport, it is necessary that certain skills are more developed than others.

It is possible to create citation networks using the main databases such as Web of Science or Scopus. However, when conducting a systematic review of all the existing literature on a subject, their usefulness is limited, given that they do not offer a general overview of the connection between the citations of a group of publications. That is why the CitNetExplorer software was selected, as it allows the researcher to visualize, analyze, and explore the citation networks of scientific publications. As such, the CitNetExplorer offers a more detailed analysis when creating citation networks compared to other databases such as Web of Science or Scopus [30]. The main aim of this study was to analyze the existing literature on vision and sport. In order to do so, the Web of Science database was used. The Web of Science database is one of the most comprehensive databases, as its search range goes back to the year 1900. Nevertheless, it is important to take into consideration the fact that the Web of Science (WOS) only accepts international journals once they have undergone a rigorous selection process.

Therefore, once the existing bibliography was downloaded from the WOS, the CitNetExplorer and CiteSpace software allowed us to collect and analyze every available piece of literature on sports vision to date. Furthermore, by analyzing the citation networks, it was possible to obtain the connection between the fields of study and the different research groups. The clustering function was used to collect the results, and the publications were then grouped according to the relationships between the citations. The drilling down function was used to examine the existing bibliography for each group, and the core publication function was used to show the main publications, that is to say, those with a minimum number of citations. These functions, therefore, made it possible for a complete study and analysis of the research on the field of study to be conducted.

Regarding the limitations of this study, publications where title, abstract, or keywords did not contain the search terms may not have been considered. Furthermore, if we compare this study with systemic reviews, explicit and prespecified methods were used to identify, evaluate, and synthesize all the available evidence related to a clinical question. Where appropriate, systematic reviews may include a meta-analysis, that is, a statistical combination of results from two or more separate studies. Some systematic reviews compare only two interventions, in which a conventional peer-to-peer meta-analysis can be performed, while others examine the comparative effectiveness of many or all available interventions for a given condition. Therefore, the analysis of citation networks allows a broader analysis of the bibliography that exists on a given topic.

In perceptive–cognitive training, the NeuroTracker system was investigated on a football field. The precision of passes, dribbling, and shooting was compared during small-sided games in university-level football players. The experimental group was formed by nine players who trained with the NeuroTracker system for 10 sessions, while the active control group was formed by seven players who trained for 10 sessions with three-dimensional (3D) football videos, and the passive control group was formed by seven players who did not receive any training. The results indicated that there were improvements in the players' passing accuracy, but no improvements were noted in terms of dribbling and shooting between the pre- and post-sessions in the players in the NeuroTracker group, compared with those in the control groups. Moreover, the result was correlated with the players' subjective decision-making accuracy, rated after pre- and post-sessions through a visual analogue scale questionnaire. These results indicate that the training exercise with the NeuroTracker protocol could selectively improve dynamic performance skills which are important for the sports performance [83].

However, although there is an increasing interest in the training of visual skills to improve sports performance, it is not clear whether or not visual training will improve performance on the field of play. This is related to the lack of scientific evidence supporting the efficacy of vision training on sports performance, as a result of a focus on the methodology, which results in a lack of validity of the training methods [70].

In the coming years, future research will focus on developing a diverse range of training programs to continue training the visual skills that are most relevant in sport in order to improve performance on the field of play. Furthermore, sports vision techniques can also be used to evaluate or rehabilitate sports-related concussions. Additionally, the expansion of the sports vision discipline could be used as a platform to develop a closer interprofessional connection between ophthalmology and optometry. Offering eye care to athletes is a field in which the possibility of greater synergy, mutual respect, and an exchange of knowledge between professionals is possible. In addition, interaction with other related health disciplines is possible and may lead to significant discoveries.

Consequently, the number of studies being published on sports vision is on the rise, given the need for more scientific evidence to demonstrate the positive effect that visual training programs have on sports performance. Regarding citation network studies, these are more numerous, given that it is the only analysis method providing a global overview of the different research fields within a specific topic. Furthermore, the CitNetExplorer and Citespace software allow analyzing all existing research on a specific topic through detailed studies. This could change how studies in different research areas are conducted.

5. Conclusions

In conclusion, this research offered an exhaustive and objective analysis of the main articles on sports vision. In this study, it was possible to visualize, analyze, and explore the most cited articles and citation networks existing to date using the Web of Science database and the Citation Network Explorer software.

Sports vision is a relatively new specialty; therefore, more scientific evidence is required in order to confirm the benefits of visual training in the sports field. All athletes must be aware of the importance of the visual system and the impact that it can have on sports performance. In some countries such as the United States, visual training is performed on all athletes on a routine basis; however, in other countries, it remains a very much unknown specialty.

The extant bibliography shows a wide variety of tools and options in the field of visual training, from basic optometry materials to special advanced systems for sports optometry. There are infinite ways in which these visual training tools can be combined to improve results by transferring skills from the training room to the playing field. Therefore, performing multisensorial and integrated visual training is ideal as it simultaneously works the different aspects. Furthermore, performing training exercises in the field is recommended.

Author Contributions: Conceptualization, H.N., C.M.-P., C.A.-P. and M.Á.S.-T.; methodology, H.N., C.M.-P., C.A.-P. and M.Á.S.-T.; software, H.N., C.M.-P., C.A.-P. and M.Á.S.-T.; validation, H.N., C.M.-P., C.A.-P. and M.Á.S.-T.; formal analysis, H.N., C.M.-P., C.A.-P. and M.Á.S.-T.; investigation, H.N., C.M.-P., C.A.-P. and M.Á.S.-T.; resources, H.N., C.M.-P., C.A.-P. and M.Á.S.-T.; data curation, H.N., C.M.-P., C.A.-P. and M.Á.S.-T.; writing—original draft preparation, H.N., C.M.-P., C.A.-P. and M.Á.S.-T.; writing—review and editing, H.N., C.M.-P., C.A.-P. and M.Á.S.-T.; visualization, H.N., C.M.-P., C.A.-P. and M.Á.S.-T.; supervision, H.N., C.M.-P., C.A.-P. and M.Á.S.-T.; project administration, H.N., C.M.-P., C.A.-P. and M.Á.S.-T.; funding acquisition, H.N., C.M.-P., C.A.-P. and M.Á.S.-T. All authors read and agreed to the published version of the manuscript.

Funding: This research received no external funding.

Conflicts of Interest: The authors declare no conflict of interest.

References

1. Abernethy, B. Enhancing sports performance through clinical and experimental optometry. *Clin. Exp. Optom.* **1986**, *69*, 189–196. [CrossRef]
2. Abernethy, B.; Wollstein, J. Improving anticipation in racquet sports. *Sports Coach.* **1989**, *12*, 15–18.
3. García, T.; Martin, Y.; Nieto, A. Visión deportiva. In *Suplemento de la Revista Gaceta óptica nº273*; Colegio nacional de ópticos-optometristas: Madrid, Spain, 1993.
4. Morilla, R.R.G. *Libro Visión Deportiva*, 1st ed.; Wanceulen: Sevilla, Spain, 2006.
5. Blundell, N.L. The contribution of vision to the learning and performance of sports skills: Part The role of selected visual parameters. *Aust. J. Sci. Med. Sport* **1985**, *17*, 3–11.
6. Erickson, G.B. *Sports Vision: Vision Care for the Enhancement of Sports Performance*, 1st ed.; Butterworth-Heinemann: St. Louis, MO, USA, 2007.
7. Mann, D.T.; Williams, A.M.; Ward, P.; Janelle, C.M. Perceptual-Cognitive Expertise in Sport: A Meta-Analysis. *J. Sport Exerc. Psychol.* **2007**, *29*, 457–478. [CrossRef] [PubMed]
8. Savelsbergh, G.J.; Williams, A.M.; Van Der Kamp, J.; Ward, P. Visual search, anticipation and expertise in soccer goalkeepers. *J. Sports Sci.* **2002**, *20*, 279–287. [CrossRef] [PubMed]
9. Van Der Kamp, J.; Rivas, F.; Van Doorn, H.; Savelsbergh, G. Ventral and dorsal system contributions to visual anticipation in fast ball sports. *Int. J. Sport Psychol.* **2008**, *39*, 100–130.
10. Ward, P.; Williams, A.M. Perceptual and Cognitive Skill Development in Soccer: The Multidimensional Nature of Expert Performance. *J. Sport Exerc. Psychol.* **2003**, *25*, 93–111. [CrossRef]
11. Spera, R.; Belviso, I.; Sirico, F.; Palermi, S.; Massa, B.; Mazzeo, F.; Montesano, P. Jump and balance test in judo athletes with or without visual impairments. *J. Hum. Sport Exerc.* **2019**, *14*, S937–S947. [CrossRef]
12. Burris, K.; Vittetoe, K.; Ramger, B.; Suresh, S.; Tokdar, S.T.; Reiter, J.P.; Appelbaum, L.G. Sensorimotor abilities predict on-field performance in professional baseball. *Sci. Rep.* **2018**, *8*, 116. [CrossRef]
13. Fischer, L.; Baker, J.; Rienhoff, R.; Strauß, B.; Tirp, J.; Büsch, D.; Schorer, J. Perceptual-cognitive expertise of handball coaches in their young and middle adult years. *J. Sports Sci.* **2016**, *34*, 1637–1642. [CrossRef]
14. Voss, M.W.; Kramer, A.F.; Basak, C.; Prakash, R.S.; Roberts, B. Are expert athletes 'expert' in the cognitive laboratory? A meta-analytic review of cognition and sport expertise. *Appl. Cogn. Psychol.* **2009**, *24*, 812–826. [CrossRef]
15. Ealves, H.; Voss, M.W.; Boot, W.R.; Deslandes, A.C.; Ecossich, V.; Salles, J.E.; Kramer, A.F. Perceptual-Cognitive Expertise in Elite Volleyball Players. *Front. Psychol.* **2013**, *4*, 36. [CrossRef]
16. Ciućmański, B.; Wątroba, J. Training selected visual perception abilities and the efficiency footballers. In *Gry Zespołowe w Wychowaniu Fizycznym i Sporcie*, 1st ed.; Żak, S.R., Spieszny, M., Klocek, T., Eds.; Studia i Monografie nr 33 AWF: Cracow, Poland, 2005; pp. 298–303. (In Polish)
17. Planer, P.M. *Sports Vision Manual*, 1st ed.; International Academy of Sports Vision: Harrisburg, PA, USA, 1994.
18. Raczek, J. Motor Coordination abilities: Their theoretical and empirical principles, and their meaning in sport. *Sport Wyczyn.* **1991**, *5–6*, 8–19.
19. Espar, X. *Balonmano*, 1st ed.; Martínez Roca: Barcelona, Spain, 2001.
20. Quevedo, L.; Solé, J. Visión periférica: Propuesta de entrenamiento. *Apunt. Edu. Fís. Deportes* **2007**, *88*, 75–80.
21. Appelbaum, L.G.; Erickson, G. Sports vision training: A review of the state-of-the-art in digital training techniques. *Int. Rev. Sport Exerc. Psychol.* **2016**, *11*, 160–189. [CrossRef]
22. Broadbent, D.P.; Causer, J.; Williams, A.M.; Ford, P.R. Perceptual-cognitive skill training and its transfer to expert performance in the field: Future research directions. *Eur. J. Sport Sci.* **2014**, *15*, 322–331. [CrossRef] [PubMed]
23. Appelbaum, L.G.; Schroeder, J.E.; Cain, M.S.; Mitroff, S.R. Improved Visual Cognition through Stroboscopic Training. *Front. Psychol.* **2011**, *2*, 276. [CrossRef]
24. Abernethy, B.; Wood, J.M. Do generalized visual training programmes for sport really work? An experimental investigation. *J. Sports Sci.* **2001**, *19*, 203–222. [CrossRef]
25. Manso, J.M.G.; Campos, J.; Lizaur, P.; Pablo, C. *El Talento Deportivo*, 1st ed.; Gymnos: Madrid, Spain, 2003.
26. Leydesdorff, L. Can scientific journals be classified in terms of aggregated journal-journal citation relations using the Journal Citation Reports? *J. Am. Soc. Inf. Sci. Technol.* **2006**, *57*, 601–613. [CrossRef]
27. González, C.M. Análisis de citación y de redes sociales para el estudio del uso de revistas en centros de investigación. Un aporte al desarrollo de colecciones. *Ciênc. Infor.* **2009**, *38*, 46–55. [CrossRef]

28. Van Eck, N.J.; Waltman, L. Visualizing bibliometric networks. In *Measuring Scholarly Impact: Methods and Practice*, 1st ed.; Rousseau, D.R., Wolfram, D., Eds.; Springer: Cham, Switzerland, 2014; pp. 285–320.
29. Van Eck, N.J.; Waltman, L. Citation-based clustering of publications using CitNetExplorer and VOSviewer. *Science* **2017**, *111*, 1053–1070. [CrossRef] [PubMed]
30. Van Eck, N.; Nees, J.; Waltman, L. CitNetExplorer: A new software tool for analyzing and visualizing citation networks. *J. Inf.* **2014**, *8*, 802–823. [CrossRef]
31. Chen, C. CiteSpace II: Detecting and visualizing emerging trends and transient patterns in scientific literature. *J. Am. Soc. Inf. Sci. Technol.* **2006**, *57*, 359–377. [CrossRef]
32. De Solla Price, D.J. *Little Science, Big Science*, 1st ed.; Columbia University Press: New York, NY, USA, 1963.
33. Hirsch, J.E. An index to quantify an individual's scientific research output. *Proc. Natl. Acad. Sci. USA* **2005**, *102*, 16569–16572. [CrossRef] [PubMed]
34. Williams, A.M.; Singer, R.N.; Frehlich, S.G. Quiet Eye Duration, Expertise, and Task Complexity in Near and Far Aiming Tasks. *J. Mot. Behav.* **2002**, *34*, 197–207. [CrossRef] [PubMed]
35. Vine, S.J.; Moore, L.J.; Wilson, M.R. Quiet Eye Training Facilitates Competitive Putting Performance in Elite Golfers. *Front. Psychol.* **2011**, *2*, 8. [CrossRef]
36. MacEwen, C.J. Sport associated eye injury: A casualty department survey. *Br. J. Ophthalmol.* **1987**, *71*, 701–705. [CrossRef] [PubMed]
37. Vine, S.J.; Wilson, M. The influence of quiet eye training and pressure on attention and visuo-motor control. *Acta Psychol.* **2011**, *136*, 340–346. [CrossRef] [PubMed]
38. Causer, J.; Bennett, S.J.; Holmes, P.S.; Janelle, C.M.; Williams, A.M. Quiet Eye Duration and Gun Motion in Elite Shotgun Shooting. *Med. Sci. Sports Exerc.* **2010**, *42*, 1599–1608. [CrossRef]
39. Stine, C.D.; Arterburn, M.R.; Stern, N.S. Vision and sports: A review of the literature. *J. Am. Optom. Assoc.* **1982**, *53*, 627–633.
40. Mann, D.T.Y.; Coombes, S.A.; Mousseau, M.B.; Janelle, C.M. Quiet eye and the Bereitschaftspotential: Visuomotor mechanisms of expert motor performance. *Cogn. Process.* **2011**, *12*, 223–234. [CrossRef] [PubMed]
41. Vickers, J.N. Advances in Coupling Perception and Action: The Quiet Eye as a Bidirectional Link between Gaze, Attention, and Action. *Prog. Brain Res.* **2009**, *174*, 279–288. [CrossRef] [PubMed]
42. Panchuk, D.; Vickers, J. Gaze behaviors of goaltenders under spatial–temporal constraints. *Hum. Mov. Sci.* **2006**, *25*, 733–752. [CrossRef]
43. Wood, J.M.; Abernethy, B. An Assessment of the Efficacy of Sports Vision Training Programs. *Optom. Vis. Sci.* **1997**, *74*, 646–659. [CrossRef]
44. Vine, S.J.; Moore, L.J.; Wilson, M.R. Quiet eye training: The acquisition, refinement and resilient performance of targeting skills. *Eur. J. Sport Sci.* **2012**, *14*, S235–S242. [CrossRef] [PubMed]
45. Causer, J.; Holmes, P.; Williams, A.M. Quiet Eye Training in a Visuomotor Control Task. *Med. Sci. Sports Exerc.* **2011**, *43*, 1042–1049. [CrossRef]
46. Vinger, P.F. Sports Eye Injuries A Preventable Disease. *Ophthalmology* **1981**, *88*, 108–113. [CrossRef]
47. Napier, S.M.; Baker, R.S.; Sanford, D.G.; Easterbrook, M. Eye injuries in athletics and recreation. *Surv. Ophthalmol.* **1996**, *41*, 229–244. [CrossRef]
48. Gregory, P.T. Sussex Eye Hospital sports injuries. *Br. J. Ophthalmol.* **1986**, *70*, 748–750. [CrossRef]
49. Master, C.L.; Scheiman, M.; Gallaway, M.; Goodman, A.; Robinson, R.L.; Master, S.R.; Grady, M.F. Vision Diagnoses Are Common After Concussion in Adolescents. *Clin. Pediatr.* **2015**, *55*, 260–267. [CrossRef]
50. Schwab, S.; Memmert, D. The Impact of a Sports Vision Training Program in Youth Field Hockey Players. *J. Sports Sci. Med.* **2012**, *11*, 624–631. [PubMed]
51. Vinger, P.F. Sports-related eye injury. A preventable problem. *Surv. Ophthalmol.* **1980**, *25*, 47–51. [CrossRef]
52. Klostermann, A.; Kredel, R.; Hossner, E.J. On the Interaction of Attentional Focus and Gaze: The Quiet Eye Inhibits Focus-Related Performance Decrements. *J. Sport Exerc. Psychol.* **2014**, *36*, 392–400. [CrossRef] [PubMed]
53. Blonstein, J.L. Eye injuries in sport: With particular reference to squash rackets and badminton. *Practitioner* **1975**, *215*, 208–209. [PubMed]
54. Toldi, J.P.; Thomas, J.L. Evaluation and Management of Sports-Related Eye Injuries. *Curr. Sports Med. Rep.* **2020**, *19*, 29–34. [CrossRef] [PubMed]

55. Sherman, A. Overview of research information regarding vision and sports. *J. Am. Optom. Assoc.* **1980**, *51*, 661–666. [PubMed]
56. Vera, J.; Molina, R.; Cárdenas, D.; Redondo, B.; Jiménez, R. Basketball free-throws performance depends on the integrity of binocular vision. *Eur. J. Sport Sci.* **2019**, *20*, 407–414. [CrossRef]
57. Williams, A.M.; Davids, K. Assessing cue usage in performance contexts: A comparison between eye-movement and concurrent verbal report methods. *Behav. Res. Methods Instrum. Comput.* **1997**, *29*, 364–375. [CrossRef]
58. Witkowski, M.; Tomczak, E.; Łuczak, M.; Bronikowski, M.; Tomczak, M. Fighting Left Handers Promotes Different Visual Perceptual Strategies than Right Handers: The Study of Eye Movements of Foil Fencers in Attack and Defence. *BioMed. Res. Int.* **2020**, *2020*, 1–11. [CrossRef]
59. Galetta, K.M.; Morganroth, J.; Moehringer, N.; Mueller, B.; Hasanaj, L.; Webb, N.; Civitano, C.; Cardone, D.A.; Silverio, A.; Galetta, S.L.; et al. Adding Vision to Concussion Testing. *J. Neuro-Ophthalmol.* **2015**, *35*, 235–241. [CrossRef]
60. Peiffer, A.J.; Macdonald, J.; Duerson, D.; Mitchell, G.; Hartwick, A.T.E.; McDaniel, C.E. The Influence of Binocular Vision Symptoms on Computerized Neurocognitive Testing of Adolescents with Concussion. *Clin. Pediatr.* **2020**, *59*, 961–969. [CrossRef] [PubMed]
61. Micieli, J.A.; Easterbrook, M. Eye and Orbital Injuries in Sports. *Clin. Sports Med.* **2017**, *36*, 299–314. [CrossRef]
62. MacEwen, C.J.; Baines, P.S.; Desai, P. Eye injuries in children: The current picture. *Br. J. Ophthalmol.* **1999**, *83*, 933–936. [CrossRef]
63. Kriz, P.K.; Zurakowski, D.; Almquist, J.L.; Reynolds, J.; Ruggieri, D.; Collins, C.L.; D'Hemecourt, P.A.; Comstock, R.D. Eye Protection and Risk of Eye Injuries in High School Field Hockey. *Pediatrics* **2015**, *136*, 521–527. [CrossRef]
64. Vinger, P. Sports eye injuries. A model for prevention. *JAMA* **1983**, *250*, 3322–3323. [CrossRef]
65. Woo, J.H.; Sundar, G. Eye injuries in Singapore–don't risk it. Do more. A prospective study. *Ann. Acad. Med. Singap.* **2006**, *35*, 706–718. [PubMed]
66. Jorge, J.; Fernandes, P.R. Static and dynamic visual acuity and refractive errors in elite football players. *Clin. Exp. Optom.* **2018**, *102*, 51–56. [CrossRef]
67. Applegate, R.A. Set Shot Shooting Performance and Visual Acuity in Basketball. *Optom. Vis. Sci.* **1992**, *69*, 765–768. [CrossRef]
68. Schumacher, N.; Schmidt, M.; Reer, R.; Braumann, K.-M. Peripheral Vision Tests in Sports: Training Effects and Reliability of Peripheral Perception Test. *Int. J. Environ. Res. Public Health* **2019**, *16*, 5001. [CrossRef]
69. Walker, C. "EYE" in SPORT. *Br. Med. J.* **1911**, *1*, 49. [CrossRef]
70. Kirschen, D.G.; Laby, D.L. The Role of Sports Vision in Eye Care Today. *Eye Contact Lens Sci. Clin. Pr.* **2011**, *37*, 127–130. [CrossRef]
71. Fullerton, C. Eye, ear brain and muscle tests on Babe Ruth. *West. Opt. World* **1925**, *13*, 160–161.
72. Winograd, S. The Relationship of Timing and Vision to Baseball Performance. *Res. Quarterly. Am. Assoc. Health Phys. Educ. Recreat.* **1942**, *13*, 481–493. [CrossRef]
73. Maman, P.; Gaurang, S.; Sandhu, J.S. The effect of vision training on performance in tennis players. *Serb. J. Sports Sci.* **2011**, *5*, 6.
74. Clark, J.F.; Ellis, J.K.; Bench, J.; Khoury, J.; Graman, P. High-Performance Vision Training Improves Batting Statistics for University of Cincinnati Baseball Players. *PLoS ONE* **2012**, *7*, e29109. [CrossRef]
75. Di Noto, P.; Uta, S.; DeSouza, J.F.X. Eye Exercises Enhance Accuracy and Letter Recognition, but Not Reaction Time, in a Modified Rapid Serial Visual Presentation Task. *PLoS ONE* **2013**, *8*, e59244. [CrossRef] [PubMed]
76. Hausegger, T.; Vater, C.; Hossner, E.-J. Peripheral Vision in Martial Arts Experts: The Cost-Dependent Anchoring of Gaze. *J. Sport Exerc. Psychol.* **2019**, *41*, 137–145. [CrossRef] [PubMed]
77. Mashkovskiy, E.; Magomedova, A.; Achkasov, E. Degree of vision impairment influence the fight outcomes in the Paralympic judo: A 10-year retrospective analysis. *J. Sports Med. Phys. Fit.* **2019**, *59*, 376. [CrossRef]
78. Biswal, A.K. An Absolute Index (Ab-index) to Measure a Researcher's Useful Contributions and Productivity. *PLoS ONE* **2013**, *8*, e84334. [CrossRef] [PubMed]
79. Lee, M.; Wu, Y.; Tsai, C.-C. Research Trends in Science Education from 2003 to 2007: A content analysis of publications in selected journals. *Int. J. Sci. Educ.* **2009**, *31*, 1999–2020. [CrossRef]

80. Aparicio-Martínez, P.; Perea-Moreno, A.-J.; Martínez-Jiménez, P.; Redel-Macías, M.D.; Vaquero-Abellan, M.; Pagliari, C. A Bibliometric Analysis of the Health Field Regarding Social Networks and Young People. *Int. J. Environ. Res. Public Health* **2019**, *16*, 4024. [CrossRef] [PubMed]
81. Smith, T.Q.; Mitroff, S.R. Stroboscopic Training Enhances Anticipatory Timing. *Int. J. Exerc. Sci.* **2012**, *5*, 344–353. [PubMed]
82. Deveau, J.; Ozer, D.J.; Seitz, A.R. Improved vision and on-field performance in baseball through perceptual learning. *Curr. Biol.* **2014**, *24*, R146–R147. [CrossRef]
83. Romeas, T.; Guldner, A.; Faubert, J. 3D-Multiple Object Tracking training task improves passing decision-making accuracy in soccer players. *Psychol. Sport Exerc.* **2016**, *22*, 1–9. [CrossRef]

Publisher's Note: MDPI stays neutral with regard to jurisdictional claims in published maps and institutional affiliations.

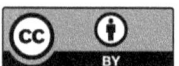

© 2020 by the authors. Licensee MDPI, Basel, Switzerland. This article is an open access article distributed under the terms and conditions of the Creative Commons Attribution (CC BY) license (http://creativecommons.org/licenses/by/4.0/).

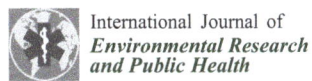

Article

Analysis of Performance Parameters of the Smash in Male and Female Professional Padel

Bernardino J. Sánchez-Alcaraz [1], Daniel T. Perez-Puche [1], Francisco Pradas [2], Jesús Ramón-Llín [3], Alejandro Sánchez-Pay [1,*] and Diego Muñoz [4]

1. Department of Physical Activity and Sport, Faculty of Sport Sciences, University of Murcia, C/Argentina, s/n, 30700 Murcia, Spain; bjavier.sanchez@um.es (B.J.S.-A.); danieltomas.perezp@um.es (D.T.P.-P.)
2. Department of Musical, Plastic and Corporal Expression, Faculty of Human Sciences and Education, University of Zaragoza, 50009 Zaragoza, Spain; franprad@unizar.es
3. Department of Musical, Plastic and Corporal Expression, University of Valencia, 46003 Valencia, Spain; jesus.ramon@uv.es
4. Department of Musical, Plastic and Corporal Expression, Faculty of Sport Sciences, University of Extremadura, 06006 Extremadura, Spain; diegomun@unex.es
* Correspondence: aspay@um.es; Tel.: +34-868-88-92-97

Received: 22 July 2020; Accepted: 24 September 2020; Published: 25 September 2020

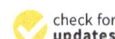

Abstract: The aim of this study was to analyze the distribution and effectiveness of the different types of smash in professional padel according to the area and direction of the strokes and the gender. Through systematic observation, 1.015 smashes from eight finals (four men's and four women's) of the professional matches were analyzed. The smashes were categorized into four types of smash: tray, flat, topspin and off the wall. The results showed both men's and women's that the tray is the most used smash by padel players, presenting a percentage of point continuity of almost 90%. The flat and topspin smashes are the strokes that achieve the highest percentage of winning points (near 60%), although this efficiency decreases significantly when the players move away from the net area ($p < 0.05$), especially in the flat smash. Men perform a higher percentage of winning smashes than women, mainly in the flat smash ($p = 0.02$). Furthermore, with regards to direction, flat and off the wall smashes are predominantly down the line strokes and women perform significantly more cross court topspin smashes than men ($p = 0.005$). The results shown could be used to design tasks and exercises by padel coaches at professional players.

Keywords: racket sports; technique; performance analysis; tactics

1. Introduction

Padel is a racket sport that was born in Mexico approximately 50 years ago [1] and has experienced enormous growth in the last decade both in the number of players and in the facilities for practicing it [2,3]. Currently it is practiced in more than 40 countries and it has an international tournament circuit in which the best padel players in the world participate [4]. This greater professionalization of padel has also produced an increase in scientific publications [5], especially those related to the performance analysis of the sport [6,7]. In this respect, most research has focused on three fundamental aspects: temporal parameters [8–11], players' movements and distance covered on the court [12–15] and game actions [16,17]. The results of these investigations have an enormous transfer and practical application in the design of training sessions adapted to the characteristics of the competition [18,19].

These studies, carried out on professional players, have determined that there are two basic tactical positions in padel: the offensive position, where the players play close to the net and the defensive position, where the players play near the baseline of the court [20]. Previous studies indicate the importance of occupying and maintaining positions close to the net to increase the likelihood of success [17,21]. Some research show that more than 80% of winning points are won from the offensive position and the winning players perform more attack strokes per point and per game [22]. Thus, the most commonly used strokes by players in the offensive position are volleys, followed by trays and smashes [12,17,23,24]. Moreover, 80% of the points in padel are finished with less than three attack shots, which reveal the offensive nature of such hits [22].

There is a continuous dichotomy during the development of the point, where players who are at the net try to keep this advantageous position, while the backcourt players try to recover it [21,25]. Players in the defensive position also perform different types of technical actions such as the lob or passing shot, varying both the height and direction of the strokes, with the aim of displacing the attacking pair so that they hit from more forced positions [7,26]. Therefore, the lobs will cause attacking players to hit the ball going above their heads. Over-head strokes (smash and tray) are the most successful shots during a match along with cross court lobs [12,27]. They are played from the middle and the net area, to maintain a positional advantage and increase the chances of winning a point [16,28]. The success of the smash as a winner depends, amongst other factors, on the area, direction, velocity and accuracy with which is executed [22,29]. The smash has become a very important and decisive shot. No previous studies have focused on this topic, even less observe the differences between males and females, which could affect the design of training sessions, depending on the gender. Due to the anthropometric and strength differences between male and female padel players, our hypotheses is that a male should use a more flat smash than a female to win the point, and the tray should be more used by women. Finally, for male and female players it could be possible that they have different behavior in the stroke direction.

Following the review conducted, there is research related to a performance analysis in padel, but mainly in male players. Research focused only on a female padel player is scarce [7]. In relation to match analysis, rally length or shots per rally are higher in female than male matches [17]. In addition, in the professional category, females perform 4% more smashes than males [17]. It seems therefore that the male and female matches develop differently and knowing the characteristics of one of the most decisive strokes in padel it would help to understand the differences between winning and losing according to gender. Thus, because of the importance of the smash as a decisive stroke in the point, the objective of this study will be to analyze the distribution and effectiveness of the different types of smash in professional padel depending on the area and direction of the shot and the gender of the players.

2. Materials and Methods

2.1. Sample and Variables

It is a descriptive and observational study of quantitative methodology. The sample included 1.015 smashes corresponding to eight finals (four men's and four women's matches) of the official circuit World Padel Tour 2019 held in Barcelona, Valladolid, Madrid, Santander and Murcia (Spain). The analyzed smashes were made by 20 professional padel players: 10 men (age = 32.35 ± 6.28 years old) and 10 women (age = 29.62 ± 5.91 years old) and the study was conducted in accordance with the Declaration of Helsinki of 2013. The following variables were analyzed:

- Type of smash: The different types of smash were classified into four shots, following the classification proposed by other authors in padel research [16,22]:

    1. Tray: Offensive stroke, without a bounce, which is made over the head and on the dominant side of the player. In this shot, before hitting the ball, the player opens the face of the racket pointing upwards and hits with a slice effect. The impact point on the ball is lower than in the other smashes.

2. Flat smash: Offensive stroke, without a bounce, which is made over the head and on the dominant side of the player. In the execution of this shot, the player hits the ball with a lot of power at the highest possible point, with a flat stroke (no effect), so that after bouncing on the opposite side, the ball could go out of court or return to the other side after rebounding against the wall.
3. Topspin smash: Offensive stroke, without a bounce, made over the head and hitting the ball from the non-dominant side (behind the player's head). In the execution of this shot the player hits the ball with a lot of power, with a topspin effect, accelerating the shot by arching the back so that, after bouncing the ball on the wall of the opposite side, it goes out over one of the sides walls of the court.
4. Off the wall smash: Offensive stroke, with a bounce, which is made above the head and on the dominant side of the player. This shot is made when the player, after receiving a lob, lets the ball bounce on his/her side and waits for the bounce on his/her back wall to make a smash. Depending on the player's aim, this shot can be done with a flat or slice effect.

- Shot effectiveness: The classification proposed by Courel-Ibáñez and Sánchez-Alcaraz (2017) was used to determinate smash effectiveness, distinguishing between the winner (the attacking player wins the point by making a smash), error (the attacking player fails the smash and loses the point) or continuity (the point continues after the smash).
- Hitting zone: The court was divided into six zones, depending on the court side (right or left) and the distance to the net (net, middle and baseline) when the player hit the ball (Figure 1). Baseline zone, from wall to the serve line (3 m); middle zone, from the serve line to 1/3 court area (3.5 m); net zone, from 1/3 court area to net (3.5 m).
- Shot direction: Two possible trajectories were distinguished: down the line and cross court (Figure 1).

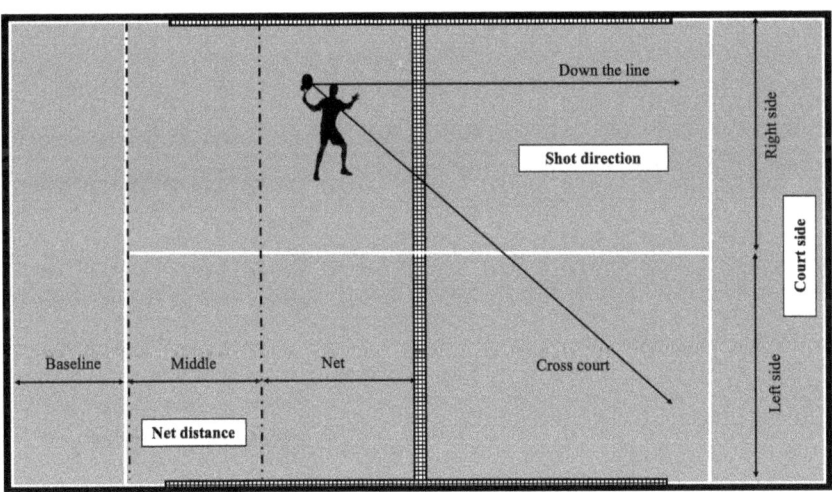

Figure 1. Hitting zones (net distance and court side) and shot direction.

2.2. Procedure

Data were collected through systematic observation, carried out by two observers who have a degree in Sports Science and are specialized in padel. Observers were specifically trained in the use of the observational instrument during two weeks. The training focused on the clear identification of the variables (type of smash, shot effectiveness, hitting zone and shot direction) and the use of the observational instrument software. At the end of the training process, each observer analyzed the same two sets in order to calculate the inter-observer reliability through the Multirater Kappa Free [30], obtaining values above 0.80. To ensure the consistency of the data, intra-observer reliability was evaluated at the end of the observation process, obtaining minimum values of 0.89. The kappa values obtained revealed a very high degree of agreement (>0.80) [31]. All the analyzed matches were retransmitted in streaming and later hosted on the World Padel Tour website (https://www.worldpadeltour.com/) [32], from where they were downloaded for the observation, collection and analysis of the data. LINCE specialized software was used for this process of recording and data collection [33].

2.3. Data Analysis

Firstly, a descriptive analysis of the data was carried out and the mean (M), standard deviation (SD), frequency (n) and percentage (%) were calculated on the whole sample. A comparison was made of the statistics of distribution and efficiency of the smashes according to gender and the playing side of the court using Pearson's Chi-Square test. Column proportions were compared using Z tests on the effectiveness of the smash according to the area and gender of the players. A significance level of $p < 0.05$ was established, which was adjusted according to Bonferroni in the Z tests. The associations among the categories of the variables were performed with corrected standardized residuals (CSR). The effect size was calculated using Crammer's V [34]. All data was analyzed with the IBM SPSS 25.0 statistical package for Macintosh (IBM Corp: Armonk, NY, USA).

3. Results

Figure 2 shows the results of the distribution percentages of the different smashes analyzed according to the type of smash, direction of hitting and court area comparing by gender. According to smash frequency, significant differences were found between genders ($\chi^2 = 26.423$; gl = 3; $p < 0.001$; $V = 0.161$). The female player performed significantly more tray strokes than male (CSR = 4.3. Otherwise, the male player made more flat (CSR = 3.7) and top-spin smashes (CSR = 3.0) than female players. Depending on the area of the court, most of the smashes were made in the middle area of the court for both genders. In relation to the direction of the smash, male players performed significantly more down the line strokes than female ($\chi^2 = 4.281$; gl = 1; $p = 0.039$; CSR = 2.1; $V = 0.065$).

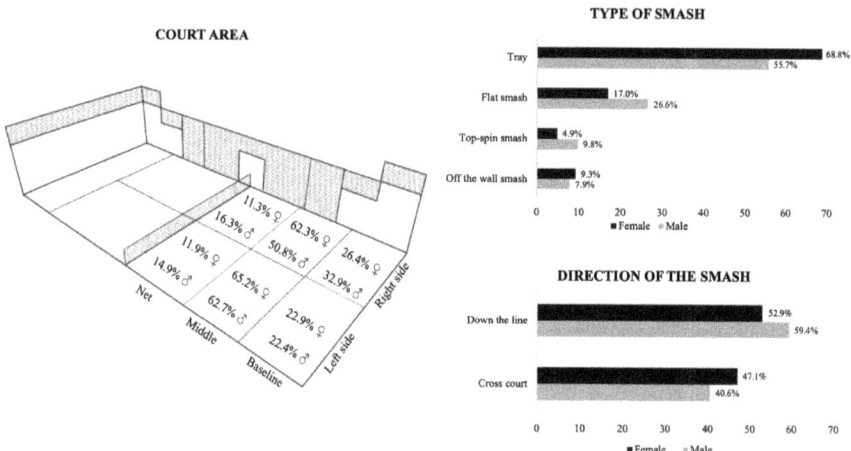

Figure 2. Percentages of distribution of all the smashes according to the area of the court (diagram on the left), type of smash (black bars) and direction of the smash (grey bars) by gender.

Depending on the hitting side, there was a trend towards a higher percentage of smashes in the middle zone in both genders. On the left side of the court, the smashes made in the different areas of the court were similar between male and female ($\chi^2 = 2.371$; gl = 2; $p > 0.05$; $V = 0.065$). By contrary, in the right side of the court male and female players played different ($\chi^2 = 9.497$; gl = 2; $p < 0.05$; $V = 0.145$). Male players made more smashes in the net (CSR = 1.8) and in the baseline (CSR = 1.5), and females played more smashes in middle area (CSR = 2.4).

Figure 3 shows the percentage of winning points depending on the type of smash and the area of the court by gender. In general lines, male and female players make more winning smashes in the net area than the others. Moreover, male players made more flat and top-spin smashes than females regardless of the hitting area. On the contrary, the female players made more winner shots with the tray stroke only at the net area.

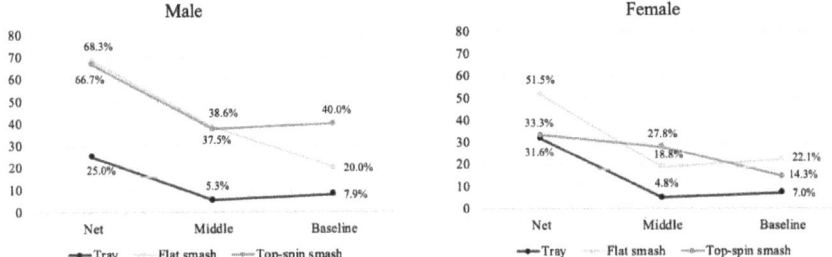

Figure 3. Percentage of winning points depending on the type of smash and the area of the court by gender.

The division by the type of smash (Table 1) showed differences in the distribution of hitting efficiency according to the gender of the players in the flat smash ($\chi^2 = 7.833$; gl = 2; $p < 0.05$; $V = 0.187$). The men performed a significantly higher percentage of winning flat smashes (CSR = 2.7) and less percentage of continuity of this stroke than the women (CSR = −2.8). No significant differences were found according to gender for the tray ($\chi^2 = 3.332$; gl = 2; $p > 0.05$), topspin ($\chi^2 = 2.376$; gl = 2; $p > 0.05$) and off the wall smashes ($\chi^2 = 1.333$; gl = 2 $p > 0.05$). Furthermore, the flat smash and topspin smash were the two smashes that produced more winners, while the tray and off the wall smashes were the smashes recording a higher percentage of continuity. The smash with the highest percentage of errors was the off the wall smash.

Table 1. Efficacy of the stroke depending on the type of smash and the gender of the players.

Type of Smash	Efficiency	Gender				Sig.
		Male		Female		
		N	%	N	%	
Tray	Continuity	261	89.7	295	87.0	
	Winner	21	7.2	23	6.8	0.189
	Error	9	3.1	21	6.2	
Flat	Continuity	61	43.9a	53	63.1b	
	Winner	72	51.8a	28	33.3b	0.020 *
	Error	6	4.3	3	3.6	
Topspin	Continuity	29	56.9	15	62.5	
	Winner	21	41.2	7	29.2	0.305
	Error	1	2.0	2	8.3	
Off the wall	Continuity	31	75.6	32	69.6	
	Winner	7	17.1	7	15.2	0.514
	Error	3	7.3	7	15.2	

Note: N = Number; % = Percentage; * = $p < 0.05$; a, b = indicate significant differences in the Z tests for comparison of column proportions from $p < 0.05$ adjusted according to Bonferroni.

Table 2 shows the differences in the percentages of distribution of the smash direction regarding players' gender and type of smash. Players' gender significantly determined the direction of the topspin smash ($\chi^2 = 7.203$; gl = 1; $p < 0.01$; CSR = 2.7; V = 0.31). Thus, while men equally distributed the direction of their topspin smashes, women performed more than 80% of their topspin smashes cross court. No significant differences were found between men and women in the direction of the flat smash ($\chi^2 = 2.635$; gl = 1; $p > 0.05$), tray ($\chi^2 = 0.260$; gl = 1; $p > 0.05$) and off the wall smash ($\chi^2 = 0.152$; gl = 1; $p > 0.05$). In general, both men and women hit a higher percentage of down the line flat and off the wall smashes, while the tray was directed equally down the line and cross court.

Table 2. Hitting direction depending on type of smash and players' gender.

Type of Smash	Direction	Male N	Male %	Female N	Female %	Sig.
Tray	Down the line	151	51.89	169	49.85	0.610
	Cross court	140	48.11	170	50.15	
Flat	Down the line	108	77.70	57	67.86	0.105
	Cross court	31	22.30	27	32.14	
Topspin	Down the line	25	49.02	4	16.67	0.007 *
	Cross court	26	50.98	20	83.33	
Off the wall	Down the line	26	63.41	31	67.39	0.697
	Cross court	15	36.59	15	32.61	

Note: N = Number; % = Percentage; * = $p < 0.05$

4. Discussion

Smash stroke is the game actions that produce the highest percentage of winner shots in padel [12,27] and has a great influence in match outcome. For that, the aim of this study was to analyze the distribution and effectiveness of the different types of smashes in professional padel according to court area, smash direction and players' gender. The results obtained showed that the tray stroke is the most widely used smash type, mainly for female players (Figure 2). In addition, this hit means, in almost 90% of cases, the continuity of the point, which would indicate an important technical domain for the players, since there are hardly any errors [26], although it is also easier for the opponents to defend [17]. On the other hand, the distribution of the smashes by court area showed that approximately 60% of the smashes were made in the middle area. These data confirm that the defending players seek to make high and deep lobs forcing the attacking players to hit the ball in situations far from the net, reducing the possibilities of achieving a winner [16,22]. In addition, on the right-side male players performed a greater number of smashes at the net and baseline areas than female. In the baseline area these differences could be due to anthropometric and strength differences that would allow the male players to make effective smashes further from the net. Regarding the smash effectiveness according to the hitting area (Figure 3), data showed that there is a direct relationship between the distance to the net in the hit and its effectiveness (mainly from the net area with the others). Thus, as the players hit closer to the net, the number of winners increased significantly, especially when using topspin and flat smashes. This could be explained by a favorable position for the attackers (decreasing the possibility of an error), and a shorter reaction time for the defenders. In this sense, coaches should include a high percentage of tray strokes in the training session (with the aim of keeping opponents away from the net), as well as working shots close to the net as a means of finishing the point.

Previous studies in professional padel have shown that players who are in defensive positions predominantly use the lob stroke to recover the net [7,26,35]. However, the attacking players try to maintain the offensive position [22], due to the greater probabilities of winning the point when they are in situations close to the net [16,17,22]. Therefore, in order to maintain the attacking position, it seems that players try to hit most of the balls sent by the defenders without bouncing, thus decreasing the frequency of the off the wall smash, using safer smashes like trays. However, the greater continuity of the hits for a good defense after the smash makes it necessary for the attacking players to look for other types of tactical actions that allow them to provoke successful situations in the point. Thus, it seems that varying the directions of the shots has been one of the fundamental tactical principles to achieve success in racket sports [25,36]. The results of this study showed that both men and women vary the directions of the down the line and cross court smashes in a balanced way, which would produce more movement on the part of the opponents swinging from one side of the court to the other, which may imply that they hit in more unfavorable situations making more mistakes [12,13].

Gender differences showed that men made a significantly higher percentage of winners than women (10% more topspin smashes and almost 20% more flat smashes). These results could be due to the anthropometric and strength differences between elite men and women players [37,38]. The results of these studies show that men padel players are taller, with greater muscle percentage and higher levels of vertical jump and grip strength than the women players, which would allow them to use the powerful smash successfully in positions further from the net. Regarding the hitting directions, it was observed that the women performed a significantly higher percentage of cross court flat and topspin smashes than the men. These differences may have a tactical explanation. While the men finish off a powerful smash down the line aiming to bring the ball to their field after the bounce on the back wall, the women do the cross court smashes with the aim of getting the ball to go over the side wall of the court (3 m high) [20]. In this way, the down the line smash, if not done with a lot of power, can cause the ball to bounce off the back wall at the opposite end with less force, offering a very favorable position for the return by the defending players [29]. With the results, coaches should work mostly on the flat stroke for the men and women, although women have a lower chance of winning than men.

In line with our hypothesis, males and females use one type of spike more than another, and with different performance (mainly in flat and top-spine strokes). The results of this study have important practical applications for the training of padel players, facilitating the design of tasks and exercises, as well as preparing them for competition taking into account the differences between the men's and women's categories. Moreover, knowledge of the effectiveness of the different types of smash depending on the court area in which the player is located will allow the training of perceptual and decisional mechanisms during the game by the player and the application of feedback about the behaviors by the coach [39,40]. However, this study has certain limitations that need to be taken into account when interpreting the results. For example, the use of some contextual variables such as the score (winning, drawing or losing) or the importance of the point (key moment) can influence decision-making in moments of pressure (choking) affecting performance [41]. In addition, other variables that influence smash effectiveness such as the position of the opponents or the speed of the smash have not been evaluated [29].

5. Conclusions

The tray was the most commonly used smash by padel players. Female players used more tray and less flat and topspin smashes than male players. Tray represents a percentage of point continuity of almost 90%. The flat and topspin smashes were the shots that achieved the highest percentage of winners, although this efficiency decreased significantly when the players moved away from the net area, especially in the flat smash. Regarding gender, men performed a significantly higher percentage of winning smashes than women. In addition, with regard to direction, flat smashes and off the wall smashes were predominantly down the line strokes and women performed significantly more cross court topspin smashes than men.

Author Contributions: Conceptualization, B.J.S.-A. and D.M.; methodology, B.J.S.-A., F.P., J.R.-L., A.S.-P. and D.M.; software, B.J.S.-A., D.T.P.-P.; validation, B.J.S.-A., D.T.P.-P., J.R.-L. and D.M.; formal analysis, B.J.S.-A. and A.S.P; investigation, B.J.S.-A., D.T.P.-P., J.R.-L., A.S.-P. and D.M.; resources, B.J.S.-A., J.R.-L., A.S.-P. and D.M.; data curation, B.J.S.-A., J.R.-L., A.S.-P. and D.M.; writing—Original draft preparation, B.J.S.-A., D.T.P.-P., and D.M.; writing—Review and editing, B.J.S.-A., F.P., J.R.-L., A.S.-P. and D.M.; visualization, B.J.S.-A., D.T.P.-P., F.P., J.R.-L., A.S.-P. and D.M.; supervision, B.J.S.-A., F.P., J.R.-L., A.S.-P. and D.M. All authors have read and agreed to the published version of the manuscript. Please turn to the CRediT taxonomy for the term explanation. Authorship must be limited to those who have contributed substantially to the work reported.

Funding: This research received no external funding.

Conflicts of Interest: The authors declare no conflict of interest.

References

1. Sánchez-Alcaraz, B.J. History of padel [Historia del pádel]. *Mater. Para. La Hist. Del. Deport.* **2013**, *11*, 57–60.
2. Courel-Ibáñez, J.; Sánchez-Alcaraz, B.J.; García, S.; Echegaray, M. Evolution of padel in spain according to practitioners' gender and age [Evolución del pádel en España en función del género y edad de los practicantes]. *Cult. Cienc. Y Deport.* **2017**, *12*, 39–46. [CrossRef]
3. Muñoz, D.; Sánchez-Alcaraz, B.J.; Courel-Ibáñez, J.; Romero, E.; Grijota, F.J.; Diaz, J. Study about profile and distribution of padel courts in the Autonomous Community of Extremadura. *E-Balonmano Com Rev. Cienc. Del. Deport.* **2016**, *12*, 223–230.
4. International Padel Federation. List of IPF Associated Countries. 2020. Available online: https://www.padelfip.com/es/federations/ (accessed on 1 July 2020).
5. Sánchez-Alcaraz, B.J.; Cañas, J.; Courel-Ibáñez, J. Analysis of scientific research in padel. *Agon Int. J. Sport Sci.* **2015**, *5*, 44–54.
6. Sánchez-Alcaraz, B.J.; Courel-Ibáñez, J.; Cañas, J. Temporal structure, court movements and game actions in padel: A systematic review [Estructura temporal, movimientos en pista y acciones de juego en pádel: Revisión sistemática]. *Retosnuevas Tend. En. Deport. Educ. Fís. Y Recreación* **2018**, *33*, 221–225.
7. Escudero-Tena, A.; Fernández-Cortes, J.; García-Rubio, J.; Ibáñez, S.J. Use and efficacy of the lob to achieve the offensive position in women's professional padel. Analysis of the 2018 wpt finals. *Int. J. Environ. Res. Public Health* **2020**, *17*, 4061. [CrossRef]
8. Courel-Ibáñez, J.; Sánchez-Alcaraz, B.J. Effect of situational variables on points in elite padel players [Efecto de las variables situacionales sobre los puntos en jugadores de pádel de élite]. *Apunt. Educ. Fis Y Deport.* **2017**, *127*, 68–74. [CrossRef]
9. Courel-Ibáñez, J.; Sánchez-Alcaraz, B.J.; Cañas, J. Game performance and length of rally in professional padel players. *J. Hum. Kinet.* **2017**, *55*, 161–169. [CrossRef]
10. Pradas, F.; Cachón, J.; Otín, D.; Quintas, A.; Arraco, S.I.; Castellar, C. Anthropometric, physiological and temporal analysis in elite female paddle players. *Retosnuevas Tend. En. Deport. Educ. Fís. Y Recreación* **2014**, *25*, 107–122.
11. Muñoz, D.; García, A.; Grijota, F.J.; Díaz, J.; Sánchez, I.B.; Muñoz, J. Influence of set duration on time variables in paddle tennis matches [Influencia de la duración del set sobre variables temporales de juego en pádel]. *Apunt. Educ. Fis.Y Deport.* **2016**, *123*, 69–75. [CrossRef]
12. Priego, J.I.; Olaso, J.; Llana, S.; Pérez, P.; Gonález, J.C.; Sanchís, M. Padel: A quantitative study of the shots and movements in the high-performance. *J. Hum. Sport Exerc.* **2013**, *8*, 925–931. [CrossRef]
13. Ramón-Llin, J.; Guzmán, J.F.; Martinez-Gallego, R.; Vučković, G.; James, N. Time-motion analysis of Pádel players in two matches of the 2011 pro tour. In *Performance Analysis of Sport IX*; Peter, D., O'Donoghue, P.G., Eds.; Routledge: London, UK, 2014.
14. Amieba, C.; Salinero Martín, J. General aspects of paddle tennis competition and its physiological demands [Aspectos generales de la competición del pádel y sus demandas fisiológicas]. *Agon Int. J. Sport Sci.* **2013**, *3*, 60–67.
15. Ramón-Llin, J.; Guzmán, J.; Llana, S.; Vuckovic, G.; Muñoz, D.; Sánchez-Alcaraz, B.J. Analysis of distance covered in padel based on level of play and number of points per match [Análisis de la distancia recorrida en pádel en función del nivel de juego y el número de puntos por partido]. *Retos Nuevas Tend. En. Educ. Fis Deport. Y Recreacion* **2020**, *39*, 205–209.

16. Courel-Ibáñez, J.; Sánchez-Alcaraz, B.J.; Muñoz, D. Exploring game dynamics in padel: Implications for assessment and training. *J. Strength Cond. Res.* **2019**, *33*, 1971–1977. [CrossRef] [PubMed]
17. Torres-Luque, G.; Ramirez, A.; Cabello-Manrique, D.; Nikolaidis, P.T.; Alvero-Cruz, J.R. Match analysis of elite players during paddle tennis competition. *Int. J. Perform. Anal. Sport* **2015**, *15*, 1135–1144. [CrossRef]
18. O'Donoghue, P. *Research Methods for Sports Performance Analysis*; Routledge: New York, NY, USA, 2010.
19. Hughes, M.D.; Barnett, T. What is performance analysis? In *Basics of Performance Analysis Cardiff*; Hughes, M.D., Ed.; Centre for Performance Analysis, UWIC Cardiff: Wales, UK, 2007.
20. Sánchez-Alcaraz, B.J. Padel tactic in initiation stage [Táctica del padel en la etapa de iniciación]. *Trances Rev. Transm. Del. Conoc. Educ. Y La Salud* **2013**, *5*, 109–116.
21. Courel-Ibáñez, J.; Sánchez-Alcaraz, B.J.; Cañas, J. Effectiveness at the net as a predictor of final match outcome in professional padel players. *Int. J. Perform. Anal. Sport* **2015**, *15*, 632–640. [CrossRef]
22. Sánchez-Alcaraz, B.J.; Courel-Ibáñez, J.; Muñoz, D.; Infantes, P.; Sáez de Zuramán, F.; Sánchez-Pay, A. Analysis of the attack actions in professional padel. *Apunt. Educ. Fís. Y Deport.* **2020**, in press.
23. García-Benítez, S.; Pérez-Bilbao, T.; Echegaray, M.; Felipe, J.L. The influence of gender on temporal structure and match activity patterns of professional padel tournaments. *Cult. Cienc. Y Deport.* **2016**, *33*, 241–247. [CrossRef]
24. Ramón-Llin, J.; Guzmán, J.F.; Llana, S.; James, N.; Vučković, G. Analysis of padel rally characteristics for three competitive levels. *Kinesiol. Slov.* **2017**, *23*, 39–49.
25. Ramón-Llin, J.; Guzmán, J.F.; Llana, S.; Martínez-Gallego, R.; James, N.; Vučković, G. The effect of the return of serve on the server pair's movement parameters and rally outcome in padel using cluster analysis. *Front. Psychol.* **2019**, *10*, 1–8. [CrossRef] [PubMed]
26. Muñoz, D.; Courel-Ibáñez, J.; Sánchez-Alcaraz, B.J.; Díaz, J.; Grijota, F.J.; Munoz, J. Analysis of the use and effectiveness of lobs to recover the net in the context of padel [Análisis del uso y eficacia del globo para recuperar la red en función del contexto de juego en pádel]. *Retosnuevas Tend. En. Deport. Educ. Fís. Y Recreación* **2017**, *31*, 19–22.
27. Carrasco, L.; Romero, S.; Sañudo, B.; de Hoyo, M. Game analysis and energy requirements of paddle tennis competition. *Sci. Sport* **2011**, *26*, 338–344. [CrossRef]
28. Lupo, C.; Condello, G.; Courel-Ibáñez, J.; Gallo, C.; Conte, D.; Tessitore, A. Effect of gender and match outcome on professional padel competition. *Ricyde Rev. Int. Cienc. Del. Deport.* **2018**, *51*, 29–41. [CrossRef]
29. Rivilla-García, J.; Muñoz, A.; Lorenzo, J.; van den Tillaar, R.; Navandar, A. Influence of opposition on overhead smash velocity in padel players. *Kinesiology* **2019**, *51*, 206–212. [CrossRef]
30. Randolph, J.J. *Free-Marginal Multirater Kappa: An. Alternative to Fleiss' Fixed-Marginal Multirater Kappa*; Joensuu University Learning and Instruction Symposium Joensuu: Helsinki, Finland, 2005.
31. Altman, D.G. *Practical Statistics for Medical Research*; Chapman and Hall: London, UK, 1991.
32. World Padel Tour. World Padel Tour Youtube Chanel. 2020. Available online: https://www.youtube.com/user/WorldPadelTourAJPP (accessed on 1 February 2020).
33. Gabin, B.; Camerino, O.; Anguera, M.T.; Castañer, M. Lince: Multiplatform sport analysis software. *Procedia Soc. Behav. Sci.* **2012**, *46*, 4692–4694. [CrossRef]
34. Cohen, J. *Statistical Power Analysis for the Behavioural Science*, 2nd ed.; Lawrence Erlbaum: Hillsdale, MI, USA, 1988.
35. Muñoz, D.; Sánchez-Alcaraz, B.J.; Courel-Ibáñez, J.; Diaz, J.; Julian, A.; Munoz, J. Differences in winning the net zone in padel between professional and advance players. *J. Sport Health Res.* **2017**, *9*, 223–231.
36. Loffing, F.; Sölter, F.; Hagemann, N.; Strauss, B. On-court position and handedness in visual anticipation of stroke direction in tennis. *Psychol. Sport Exerc.* **2016**, *27*, 195–204. [CrossRef]
37. Castillo-Rodríguez, A.; Hernández-Mendo, A.; Alvero-Cruz, J.R. Morphology of the elite paddle player—Comparison with other racket sports. *Int. J. Morphol.* **2014**, *32*, 177–182. [CrossRef]
38. Sánchez-Muñoz, C.; Muros, J.J.; Cañas, J.; Courel-Ibáñez, J.; Sánchez-Alcaraz, B.J.; Zabala, M. Anthropometric and physical fitness profiles of world-class male padel players. *Int. J. Environ. Res. Public Health* **2020**, *17*, 508. [CrossRef]
39. Del Villar, F.; González, L.G.; Iglesias, D.; Moreno, M.P.; Cervelló, E.M. Expert-novice differences in cognitive and execution skills during tennis competition. *Percept. Mot. Ski.* **2007**, *104*, 355–365. [CrossRef] [PubMed]

40. Nielsen, T.M.; McPherson, S.L. Response selection and execution skills of professionals and novices during singles tennis competition. *Percept. Mot. Ski.* **2001**, *93*, 541–555. [CrossRef]
41. Mesagno, C.; Geukes, K.; Larkin, P. Choking Under Pressure: A Review of Current Debates, Literature, and Interventions. In *Contemporary Advances in Sport Psychology: A Review*; Mellalieu, S., Hanton, S., Eds.; Routledge: New York, NY, USA, 2015.

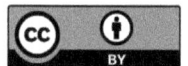

© 2020 by the authors. Licensee MDPI, Basel, Switzerland. This article is an open access article distributed under the terms and conditions of the Creative Commons Attribution (CC BY) license (http://creativecommons.org/licenses/by/4.0/).

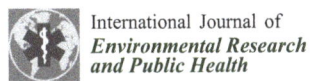

Article

Effects of *Tetraselmis chuii* Microalgae Supplementation on Ergospirometric, Haematological and Biochemical Parameters in Amateur Soccer Players

Víctor Toro [1], Jesús Siquier-Coll [1,*], Ignacio Bartolomé [1], María C. Robles-Gil [2], Javier Rodrigo [1] and Marcos Maynar-Mariño [1]

1. Department of Physiology, School of Sport Sciences, University of Extremadura, University Avenue, s/n CP: 10003 Cáceres, Spain; vtororom@alumnos.unex.es (V.T.); ignbs.1991@gmail.com (I.B.); rodbelly@hotmail.com (J.R.); mmaynar@unex.es (M.M.-M.)
2. Department of Didactics of Musical, Plastic and Corporal Expression, School of Teacher Training, University of Extremadura, University Avenue, s/n CP: 10003 Cáceres, Spain; mcroblesgil@unex.es
* Correspondence: jsiquier@alumnos.unex.es; Tel.: +34-927-257-460 (ext. 57833)

Received: 10 August 2020; Accepted: 18 September 2020; Published: 21 September 2020

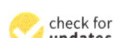

Abstract: This study aimed to analyse the effects of *Tetraselmis chuii* (TC) microalgae supplementation during thirty days on ergospirometric, haematological and biochemical parameters in amateur soccer players. Thirty-two amateur soccer players divided into a control group (CG; $n = 16$; 22.36 ± 1.36 years; 68.36 ± 3.53 kg) and a supplemented group (SG; $n = 16$; 22.23 ± 2.19 years; 69.30 ± 5.56 kg) participated in the double-blind study. SG ingested 25 mg of the TC per day, while CG ingested 200 mg per day of lactose powder. Supplementation was carried out for thirty days. The participants performed a maximal treadmill test until exhaustion. The ergospirometric values at different ventilatory thresholds and haematological values were obtained after the test. Heart rate decreased after supplementation with TC ($p < 0.05$). Oxygen pulse, relative and absolute maximum oxygen consumption increased in SG (pre vs. post; 19.04 ± 2.53 vs. 22.08 ± 2.25; 53.56 ± 3.26 vs. 56.74 ± 3.43; 3.72 ± 0.35 vs. 3.99 ± 0.25; $p < 0.05$). Haemoglobin and mean corpuscular haemoglobin increased in SG (pre vs. post; 15.12 ± 0.87 vs. 16.58 ± 0.74 $p < 0.01$; 28.03 ± 1.57 vs. 30.82 ± 1.21; $p < 0.05$). On the other hand, haematocrit and mean platelet volume decreased in SG ($p < 0.05$). TC supplementation elicited improvements in ergospirometric and haematological values in amateur soccer players. TC supplementation could be valuable for improving performance in amateur athletes.

Keywords: microalgae; soccer; ergogenic; ventilatory threshold

1. Introduction

Microalgae are photosynthetic eukaryotic microorganisms that live in the sea and were one of the first forms of life on Earth [1]. The number of microalgae species is estimated to range from 45,000 to more than 100,000 [2], and they have been used as a food source for humans for over a thousand years [3].

Microalgae can be considered a promising food due to their nutritional characteristics [4], and their industrial cultivation has increased in recent decades [5]. They have been used in the production of functional foods [6], animal feeds, biofuels [7] and cosmetics [8].

The effects of microalgae supplementation on humans have been studied previously [9,10], and marine bioactive peptides from microalgae have shown therapeutic potential in the treatment or prevention of disease [11]. The different effects of microalgae supplementation are anti-inflammatory [12], antioxidant [13], hypotensive [14] and hypolipidemic [15], among others. Supplementation with some microalgae such as spirulina and chlorella has been well studied [16,17]; however, the effect of supplementation with *Tetraselmis chuii* (TC) is unknown.

TC is green microalgae discovered in the 1950s, and is a unicellular, mobile, 4 to 15 μm size microseaweed, corresponding to the class Prasinophyceae [18]. It is present in the diet of mussels, oysters, clams, scallops and corals [19], representing a species of marine microalgae that is easy to grow and safe to eat [20]. Proportional to its size, TC has a high concentration of amino acids, essential fatty acids, vitamins and minerals (Table 1) [21,22].

Table 1. Composition of TC from Fitoplacton Marino S.L.

Component	Quantity	Component	Quantity
Proteins (mg/pill)	75.2 ± 2.51	Calcium (mg/g)	33.8 ± 0.26
Carbohydrates (mg/pill)	63.2 ± 2.67	Phosphorus (mg/g)	6.27 ± 1.87
Lipids (mg/pill)	13.4 ± 1.04	Magnesium (mg/g)	5.06 ± 0.09
Saturated fatty acids (mg/pill)	4.06 ± 0.41	Potassium (mg/g)	10.40 ± 0.56
Monounsaturated fatty acids (mg/pill)	7.05 ± 0.86	Sodium (mg/g)	14.33 ± 4.16
Polyunsaturated fatty acids (mg/pill)	6.26 ± 0.77	Chloride (mg/g)	17.77 ± 0.25
Leucine (mg/pill)	1.15 ± 0.08	Copper (mg/g)	0.006 ± 0.0
Arginine (mg/pill)	1.00 ± 0.06	Iron (mg/g)	2.01 ± 0.01
Glutamic acid (mg/pill)	1.75 ± 0.08	Manganese (mg/g)	5.06 ± 0.09
Aspartic acid (mg/pill)	1.39 ± 0.06	Iodine (mg/kg)	5.03 ± 5.78

The administration of sports supplements in soccer has become a standard procedure, often promoted by team physicians, coaches and even the parents of young players [23]. However, supplementation with microalgae is not common in sport, although their intake has been gradually introduced into sport due to the bioactive peptides they contain [24]. *Spirulina platensis* positively modifies bone marrow production and the cellular immune response, and may be effective as an adjuvant treatment in anaemia or immunodeficiency [25]. Similarly, other studies observed increases in maximum oxygen consumption (VO_{2max}) after supplementation with other microalgae, such as spirulina or chlorella [26,27]. Nevertheless, the literature about TC supplementation is scarce, and it would be interesting to know the impact of supplementation in humans due to its aforementioned properties. Therefore, this research aimed to evaluate the effects of TC microalgae supplementation during thirty days on ergospirometric parameters in amateur soccer players. In addition, the possible positive or negative effects on haematological and biochemical parameters were investigated.

2. Materials and Methods

2.1. Subjects

Thirty-two male players from a third division Spanish club participated in the study. The subjects were randomised into two groups: control group (CG; n = 16; 22.36 ± 1.36 years; 68.36 ± 3.53 kg; 1.74 ± 0.44 m) and supplemented group (SG; n = 16; 22.23 ± 2.19 years; 69.30 ± 5.56 kg; 1.73 ± 0.35 m). All participants were informed about the purpose of the study and signed a consent form before enrolling. The protocol was reviewed and approved by the Biomedical Ethics Committee of the University of Extremadura (Cáceres, Spain) following the guidelines of the Helsinki declaration of ethics, updated at the World Medical Assembly in Fortaleza (2013), for research involving human subjects (registration code: 99/2016). A code was assigned to each participant for the collection and treatment of the samples in order to maintain their anonymity. To be considered a healthy male and included in the study, participants had to comply with the inclusion criteria: not have haematological problems, not have altered values in the last blood analysis, not have anaemia problems, have four years of minimum training experience, be a nonsmoker, not have taken any supplementation, medication or over-the-counter medication, drug or alcohol in the previous two weeks and not to change their nutritional habits during the study.

At the beginning of the study, the participants completed a physical activity questionnaire (IPAQ) [28] and had a medical examination to detect any abnormalities. The participants performed 2.9 ± 0.55 metabolic equivalent of task (MET)-hour/day and no case abnormalities were reported.

2.2. Study Design

This research had a double-blind design. SG ingested a 25 mg capsule per day of powdered TC (TetraSOD®, El Puerto de Santa María, Andalucía, Spain) whereas CG ingested a 200 mg placebo tablet containing lactose powder. The nutritional value per day of the placebo pill was 22.6 kcal, 0.4 g water, 5.8 g carbohydrate, 0.1 g protein and 0.09 g lipids. Participants ingested the capsules for thirty days. Both capsules had identical designs to avoid interpretation among subjects. Participants were recommended to ingest all capsules at 10:00 a.m. for homogeneity of results. Table 1 shows the composition of TC [29].

The measurements were taken on the day previous to the beginning of the supplementation and after thirty days of supplementation. Participants did not intake TC on the day of the assessments. The assessments were performed after two days of inactivity to avoid the influence of training fatigue.

2.3. Blood Extraction and Determination of Haematological and Biochemical Parameters

Participants arrived between 8:00–9:00 a.m. for the extraction of 10 mL of venous blood from the antecubital vein. All extractions were carried out in fasting conditions. The blood sample was collected in a polypropylene tube. A 200 µL sample was taken from each blood tube and precipitated in a ladle and placed in the coulter (Coulter Electronics LTD, Model 6706319; Northwell Drive, Luton, UK) to obtain haematological data. For biochemical parameters, the blood was collected in 5 mL tubes containing ethylenediaminetetraacetic acid (EDTA) as anticoagulants and were centrifuged at 2500 rpm for 10 min. The plasma was separated and the biochemical parameters were determined by spectrophotometric techniques (Coulter Electronics LTD, Model CPA; Northwell Drive, Luton, UK).

2.4. Anthropometry

The anthropometric characteristics were measured in the morning at the same time after an overnight fast, always by the same researcher. A Seca© 769 (Seca, Hamburg, Germany) scale, with an accuracy of ±100 g; a Seca© 220 (Seca, Hamburg, Germany) measuring rod, accurate to ±1 mm; a Holtain© 610ND (Holtain, Crymych, UK) skinfold compass, accurate to ±0.2 mm; a Holtain© 604 (Holtain, Crymych, UK) bone diameter compass, accurate to ±1 mm; and a Seca© 201 (Seca, Hamburg, Germany) brand tape measure, accurate to ±1 mm, were used for the anthropometric assessments. The equations of the Spanish Group of Kinanthropometry [30] were used to calculate the muscle, fat and bone percentage. The anthropometric measurements obtained were height, weight, skinfolds (abdominal, suprailiac, subscapular, tricipital, thigh and leg), bone diameters (bistyloid, humeral biepicondyle and femoral biepicondyle) and muscle perimeters (relaxed arm and leg).

2.5. Nutritional Evaluation

All participants completed a nutritional survey in the first and last week of the study to guarantee that they were following a similar diet. The survey consisted of a 4-day daily nutritional record, of three preassigned week days, and one weekend day. The participants individually indicated the type, frequency and quantity (in grams) of each food consumed each day, and the nutritional composition of their diets was evaluated using different food composition tables [31].

2.6. Maximum Incremental Test and Threshold Determination

Subjects performed an incremental ergospirometric test on a treadmill (Ergofit Trac Alpin 4000, Germany). The test started with a warm-up at 8 km/h for 10 min and was increased by 1 km/h every two minutes until voluntary exhaustion. The tests were carried out in the laboratory with ambient conditions of 23 ± 2 °C (45–55% relative humidity). Physiological ergospirometric parameters were monitored with a gas analyser (Metamax model no. 762014-102, Cortex, Germany), and heart rate (HR) was monitored with a pulsometer (Polar® "Vantage M", Kempele, Finland) with sensor band (Polar® H10, Kempele, Finland). All tests were performed from 11:30 a.m. onwards in the same order to avoid the effects of circadian cycles.

After recording the test data, the ventilatory thresholds were determined according to the three-phase model [32]. The data were obtained at the aerobic threshold (VT1), the anaerobic threshold (VT2), maximum values of the incremental test and after three minutes of recovery.

2.7. Statistical Analysis

Statistical analyses were performed with SPSS 20.0 for Windows (SPSS Inc., Chicago, IL, USA). The normality of the distribution of variables was analysed using the Shapiro–Wilk test and the homogeneity of the variances with the Levene test. A paired samples t-test was used to compare the differences between pre- and post-supplementation and an independent samples t-test was used to compare the differences between CG and SG. A $p < 0.05$ was considered statistically significant. Results are expressed as means ± standard deviation.

3. Results

The results obtained are presented below, before supplementation (pre) and after supplementation (post). Table 2 shows the anthropometric values in both groups. No significant changes were observed between groups.

Table 2. Anthropometric values.

	CG (n = 16)			SG (n = 16)		
	Pre	Post	p Value	Pre	Post	p Value
Total weight (kg)	69.55 ± 4.70	69.10 ± 5.80	0.623	69.74 ± 5.89	69.05 ± 5.80	0.576
Σ6 skinfolds	68.00 ± 18.21	68.12 ± 17.95	0.891	68.38 ± 18.67	67.54 ± 18.05	0.401
Muscle percentage	48.39 ± 1.70	48.45 ± 2.67	0.678	48.48 ± 1.65	49.24 ± 2.28	0.245
Bone percentage	17.15 ± 0.83	17.17 ± 1.70	0.891	17.10 ± 0.87	17.15 ± 0.72	0.813
Fat percentage	10.41 ± 1.60	10.37 ± 1.70	0.451	10.30 ± 1.79	9.80 ± 1.39	0.378

CG: control group; SG: supplemented group; Σ: summation.

Table 3 shows the intake of macronutrients in both groups. There was no significant difference in total macronutrient intake.

Table 3. Nutritional assessment in the first and the last weeks of the study.

	CG (n = 16)			SG (n = 16)		
	Pre	Post	p Value	Pre	Post	p Value
Total intake (kcal/days)	2304.31 ± 321.21	2266.25 ± 307.27	0.556	2368.63 ± 347.41	2286.47 ± 339.74	0.347
Carbohydrates (g/days)	281.35 ± 35.24	277.43 ± 31.43	0.469	285.41 ± 28.31	279.51 ± 30.02	0.338
Proteins (g/days)	128.28 ± 25.62	130.84 ± 22.35	0.629	127.47 ± 26.67	130.32 ± 25.72	0.478
Lipids (g/days)	88.24 ± 21.24	85.45 ± 22.37	0.437	85.39 ± 26.81	82.25 ± 22.45	0.405

g: grams; kcal: kilocalories.

Table 4 shows the ergospirometric data of VT1 in both groups. There was a significant decrease in HR in the SG after TC supplementation ($p < 0.05$). There were no significant differences in the other parameters.

Table 4. Ergospirometric values corresponding to VT1.

	CG (n = 16)			SG (n = 16)		
	Pre	Post	p Value	Pre	Post	p Value
Speed (km/h)	10.55 ± 0.69	10.62 ± 1.12	0.567	10.71 ± 0.73	10.70 ± 1.09	0.897
HR (bpm)	155.95 ± 10.1	155.50 ± 11.55	0.821	156.50 ± 9.10	152.10 ± 9.51 *	0.041
Absolute VO_2 (L/min)	2.46 ± 0.22	2.47 ± 0.20	0.789	2.47 ± 0.30	2.48 ± 0.27	0.702
Relative VO_2 (mL/min/kg)	35.40 ± 2.50	35.80 ± 3.01	0.643	35.51 ± 2.87	36.59 ± 3.11	0.418
VCO_2 (L/min)	2.20 ± 0.25	2.22 ± 0.31	0.609	2.23 ± 0.26	2.21 ± 0.30	0.587
RER (VCO_2/VO_2)	0.90 ± 0.02	0.90 ± 0.01	0.803	0.90 ± 0.02	0.90 ± 0.03	0.789
O_2 pulse (mL/beat)	15.90 ± 2.09	15.99 ± 1.10	0.495	15.93 ± 2.10	16.05 ± 1.04	0.521
VE (L/min)	68.30 ± 11.05	68.52 ± 11.01	0.613	68.29 ± 11.38	69.50 ± 11.09	0.406
VE/VO_2	25.50 ± 2.36	25.55 ± 2.22	0.872	25.64 ± 2.76	25.77 ± 2.29	0.621
VE/VCO_2	28.59 ± 2.64	28.60 ± 2.13	0.883	28.60 ± 2.74	28.61 ± 2.04	0.813

CG: control group; SG: supplemented group; HR: heart rate; VO_2: oxygen consumption; VCO_2: carbon dioxide consumption; RER: respiratory exchange ratio; O_2: oxygen; VE: expired volume; p value: differences pre vs. post; *: $p < 0.05$ differences pre vs. post in SG.

Table 5 shows the results obtained for both groups at VT2. A significant decrease can be observed in HR in SG after TC supplementation compared to CG and baseline values ($p < 0.01$). There were no significant differences in the remaining parameters.

Table 5. Ergospirometric values at VT2.

	CG (n = 16)			SG (n = 16)		
	Pre	Post	p Value	Pre	Post	p Value
Speed (km/h)	15.45 ± 1.32	15.10 ± 1.12	0.701	15.50 ± 1.02	15.87 ± 1.34	0.831
HR (bpm)	184.23 ± 6.80	183.95 ± 7.75	0.696	186.57 ± 7.00	177.92 ± 7.75 ^	0.008
Absolute VO_2 (L/min)	3.33 ± 0.41	3.34 ± 0.24	0.845	3.34 ± 0.43	3.37 ± 0.36	0.439
Relative VO_2 (mL/min/kg)	47.60 ± 3.65	47.98 ± 3.56	0.793	47.71 ± 3.97	48.36 ± 3.26	0.278
VCO_2 (L/min)	3.40 ± 0.42	3.39 ± 0.30	0.868	3.41 ± 0.41	3.40 ± 0.27	0.512
RER (VCO_2/VO_2)	1.02 ± 0.01	1.01 ± 0.01	0.771	1.02 ± 0.02	1.01 ± 0.01	0.814
O_2 pulse (mL/beat)	18.49 ± 1.20	18.51 ± 1.28	0.882	18.52 ± 1.80	18.60 ± 1.26	0.708
VE (L/min)	108.34 ± 9.43	107.10 ± 9.90	0.791	108.14 ± 9.48	106.50 ± 10.00	0.451
VE/VO_2	29.80 ± 2.41	29.73 ± 2.48	0.702	29.83 ± 2.47	29.69 ± 2.58	0.512
VE/VCO_2	29.27 ± 2.29	29.45 ± 2.45	0.845	29.24 ± 2.23	29.49 ± 2.55	0.689

CG: control group; SG: supplemented group; HR: heart rate; VO_2: oxygen consumption; VCO_2: carbon dioxide consumption; RER: respiratory exchange ratio; O_2: oxygen; VE: expired volume; p value: differences pre vs. post; ^: $p < 0.05$ differences post CG vs. post SG.

Table 6 shows the maximum values obtained in the incremental test. Decreases in HRmax were observed after TC supplementation in SG compared to baseline ($p < 0.05$) and CG ($p < 0.05$). In SG, there were significant increases in oxygen pulse, and maximum absolute and relative oxygen consumption (VO_2) values ($p < 0.05$).

Table 6. Maximum values of the incremental test in both groups.

	CG (n = 16)			SG (n = 16)		
	Pre	Post	p Value	Pre	Post	p Value
Speed (km/h)	19.60 ± 0.89	19.58 ± 0.92	0.834	19.64 ± 0.93	19.82 ± 0.90	0.603
HR_{max} (bpm)	198.50 ± 5.18	198.38 ± 4.63	0.781	198.43 ± 6.28	194.42 ± 4.52 ^	0.046
Absolute VO_{2max} (L/min)	3.76 ± 0.39	3.74 ± 0.31	0.491	3.72 ± 0.35	3.99 ± 0.25 ^	0.031
Relative VO_{2max} (mL/min/kg)	54.49 ± 3.25	53.55 ± 3.40	0.309	53.56 ± 3.26	56.74 ± 3.43 ^	0.043
VCO_2 (L/min)	4.34 ± 0.40	4.35 ± 0.39	0.843	4.35 ± 0.59	4.32 ± 0.41	0.418
RER (VCO_2/VO_2)	1.17 ± 0.04	1.16 ± 0.03	0.619	1.17 ± 0.05	1.16 ± 0.04	0.626
O_2 pulse (mL/beat)	19.06 ± 2.40	19.08 ± 2.41	0.792	19.04 ± 2.53	22.08 ± 2.25 ^	0.045
VE (L/min)	144.00 ± 17.21	144.01 ± 18.98	0.925	142.14 ± 18.2	146.50 ± 19.35	0.221
VE/VO_2	36.50 ± 4.11	37.00 ± 4.09	0.213	36.63 ± 4.57	37.52 ± 4.02	0.426
VE/VCO_2	31.61 ± 2.23	31.98 ± 2.32	0.678	31.68 ± 2.73	32.49 ± 2.85	0.406

CG: control group; SG: supplemented group; HRmax: maximum heart rate; VO_{2max}: maximum oxygen consumption; VCO_2: carbon dioxide consumption; RER: respiratory exchange ratio; O_2: oxygen; VE: expired volume; p value: differences pre vs. post; ^: $p < 0.05$ differences post CG vs. post SG.

Table 7 shows the ergospirometric values obtained after 3 min of recovery at the end of the maximum incremental test. Significant decreases in HR in SG were found after TC supplementation compared to CG and baseline values ($p < 0.05$). There were no significant differences in the other parameters. Figure 1 shows the key findings.

Table 7. Ergospirometric results obtained after three minutes of recovery.

	CG (n = 16)			SG (n = 16)		
	Pre	Post	p Value	Pre	Post	p Value
HR (bpm)	131.23 ± 12.12	130.90 ± 12.20	0.705	131.10 ± 10.51	125.50 ± 10.29 ^	0.039
VO$_2$ (L/min)	0.95 ± 0.38	0.94 ± 0.19	0.645	0.96 ± 0.28	0.95 ± 0.36	0.715
Relative VO$_2$/kg (mL/min/kg)	13.29 ± 2.45	13.01 ± 2.15	0.479	13.57 ± 3.05	14.08 ± 2.05	0.255
Absolute VCO$_2$ (L/min)	1.20 ± 0.37	1.19 ± 0.25	0.631	1.22 ± 0.38	1.20 ± 0.20	0.521
RER (VCO$_2$/VO$_2$)	1.28 ± 0.10	1.29 ± 0.09	0.699	1.29 ± 0.11	1.28 ± 0.07	0.589
O$_2$ pulse (mL/beat)	7.32 ± 1.32	7.11 ± 1.01	0.306	7.38 ± 2.35	7.17 ± 0.94	0.201
VE (L/min)	46.90 ± 14.51	45.11 ± 12.36	0.218	46.14 ± 15.57	45.07 ± 13.40	0.349
VE/VO$_2$	45.40 ± 5.97	45.32 ± 5.68	0.521	45.58 ± 6.88	44.86 ± 5.08	0.180
VE/VCO$_2$	35.28 ± 3.70	35.26 ± 3.57	0.844	35.34 ± 3.83	35.31 ± 3.47	0.719

CG: control group; SG: supplemented group; HR: heart rate; VO$_2$: oxygen consumption; VCO$_2$: carbon dioxide consumption; RER: respiratory exchange ratio; O$_2$: oxygen; VE: expired volume; p value: differences pre vs. post; ^: $p < 0.05$ differences post CG vs. post SG.

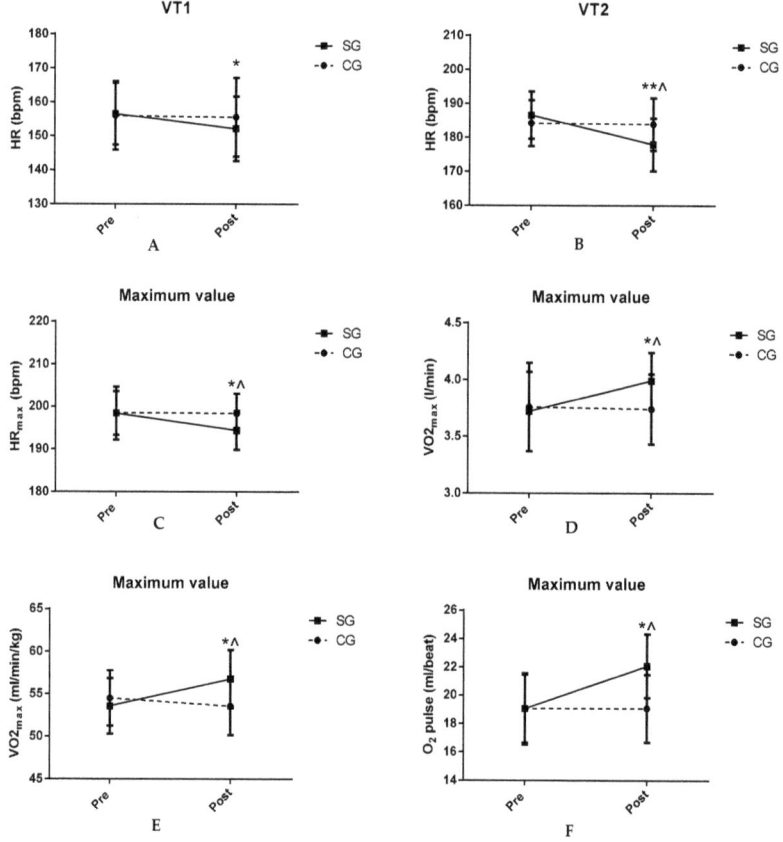

Figure 1. Cont.

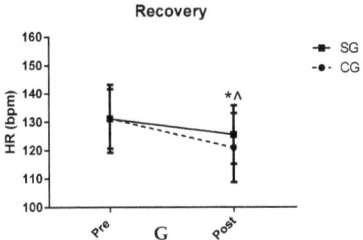

Figure 1. Results of the incremental test: (**A**) ergospirometric values corresponding to VT1; (**B**) ergospirometric values corresponding to VT2; (**C–F**) maximum values of the incremental test; (**G**) results obtained after three minutes of recovery. CG: control group; SG: supplemented group; HR: heart rate; VO_2: oxygen consumption; * $p < 0.05$ differences pre vs. post in SG; ** $p < 0.01$ differences pre vs. post in SG; ^ $p < 0.05$ differences post CG vs. post SG.

Table 8 shows the biochemical parameters studied in both groups. There were increases in glucose ($p < 0.01$), uric acid ($p < 0.05$) and creatinine ($p < 0.01$) values after TC supplementation in SG. In addition, the previous parameters after TC supplementation were higher in SG compared to CG.

Table 8. Biochemical values of both groups.

	CG (n = 16)			SG (n = 16)		
	Pre	Post	p Value	Pre	Post	p Value
Glucose (mg/dL)	84.02 ± 8.29	85.10 ± 6.30	0.417	83.01 ± 10.31	91.01 ± 5.40 ^	0.007
Cholesterol (mg/dL)	113.11 ± 20.81	110.78 ± 25.15	0.327	112.27 ± 22.73	107.78 ± 24.40	0.219
Triglycerides (mg/dL)	51.44 ± 26.20	49.60 ± 20.30	0.415	50.79 ± 35.39	43.59 ± 19.07	0.105
Uric acid (mg/dL)	5.74 ± 0.72	5.75 ± 0.73	0.735	5.76 ± 0.76	6.04 ± 0.77 ^	0.035
HDL (mg/dL)	52.02 ± 6.50	53.60 ± 7.61	0.621	51.14 ± 6.35	55.54 ± 7.50	0.195
LDL (mg/dL)	50.37 ± 20.21	49.12 ± 20.11	0.569	50.97 ± 20.62	43.58 ± 20.91	0.077
GOT (U/L)	36.23 ± 13.76	36.11 ± 12.93	0.877	36.79 ± 14.91	36.06 ± 11.96	0.421
GPT (U/L)	27.45 ± 14.12	26.88 ± 12.31	0.521	27.32 ± 15.12	25.88 ± 10.38	0.451
GGT (U/L)	21.40 ± 18.06	22.02 ± 17.21	0.610	21.53 ± 19.07	22.25 ± 17.46	0.653
Creatinine (mg/dL)	0.96 ± 0.11	0.97 ± 0.10	0.690	0.96 ± 0.10	1.07 ± 0.12 ^	0.043

CG: control group; SG: supplemented group; HDL: high density lipoprotein; LDL: low density lipoprotein; GOT: glutamic-oxaloacetic transaminase; GPT: glutamic-pyruvic transaminase; GGT: gamma-glutamyl transferase; p value: differences pre vs. post; ^: $p < 0.05$ differences post CG vs. post SG.

Table 9 shows the values obtained for the different haematological parameters studied in both groups. There were increases in haemoglobin ($p < 0.01$) and mean corpuscular haemoglobin (MCH) ($p < 0.05$) values after TC supplementation in SG compared to CG and baseline values. Haematocrit values and MPV decreased in SG after TC supplementation ($p < 0.05$).

Table 9. Haemogram of both groups in the different evaluations.

	CG (n = 16)			SG (n = 16)		
	Pre	Post	p Value	Pre	Post	p Value
Red blood cells (millions)	5.40 ± 0.31	5.39 ± 0.35	0.734	5.43 ± 0.34	5.42 ± 0.39	0.569
Haemoglobin (gr %)	15.25 ± 0.80	15.24 ± 0.84	0.459	15.12 ± 0.87	16.58 ± 0.74 **^	0.008
Haematocrit (%)	48.29 ± 2.72	48.45 ± 2.15	0.743	48.03 ± 2.15	46.68 ± 2.05 *^	0.045
MCV (fL)	88.00 ± 2.55	87.84 ± 3.08	0.585	88.10 ± 2.75	87.49 ± 4.05	0.418
MCH (Pg)	28.31 ± 1.60	29.26 ± 1.69	0.476	28.03 ± 1.57	30.82 ± 1.21 *	0.042
Platelets (thousands)	223.67 ± 70.05	225.39 ± 65.56	0.702	222.72 ± 90.05	241.31 ± 46.99	0.216
MPV (fL)	9.00 ± 1.42	9.01 ± 1.20	0.833	9.02 ± 1.13	8.04 ± 1.05 *^	0.041
Leukocytes (thousands)	6.57 ± 1.17	6.53 ± 1.73	0.704	6.55 ± 1.67	6.51 ± 1.73	0.491
Lymphocytes ($10^3/\mu L$)	1.90 ± 0.60	1.89 ± 0.33	0.755	1.89 ± 0.61	1.88 ± 0.42	0.306
Neutrophils ($10^3/\mu L$)	3.78 ± 1.10	3.75 ± 1.12	0.649	3.77 ± 1.24	3.76 ± 1.09	0.703
Monocytes ($10^3/\mu L$)	0.40 ± 0.12	0.41 ± 0.20	0.805	0.39 ± 0.15	0.41 ± 0.24	0.498
Basophils ($10^3/\mu L$)	0.05 ± 0.02	0.06 ± 0.05	0.876	0.05 ± 0.03	0.06 ± 0.06	0.614
Eosinophil ($10^3/\mu L$)	0.28 ± 0.18	0.27 ± 0.19	0.859	0.28 ± 0.19	0.26 ± 0.20	0.592
ESR (mm)	6.59 ± 2.80	6.41 ± 2.90	0.621	6.53 ± 3.61	6.43 ± 2.73	0.217

CG: control group; SG: supplemented group; MCV: medium corpuscular volume; MCH: mean corpuscular haemoglobin; MPV: mean platelet volume; ESR: erythrocyte sedimentation rate; p value: differences pre vs. post; ^ $p < 0.05$ differences post CG vs. post SG.

4. Discussion

The aim of the present study was to analyse the effect of TC (TetraSOD® El Puerto de Santa Maria, Andalucía, Spain) supplementation on ergospirometric, haematological and biochemical parameters in amateur soccer players. To our knowledge, this is the first study to evaluate the impact of TC supplementation in athletes. TC supplementation during thirty days produced decreases in HR and increased absolute VO_{2max}, relative VO_{2max}, oxygen pulse, haemoglobin and mean corpuscular haemoglobin (MCH) ($p < 0.05$) In addition, glucose, uric acid and creatinine were higher in SG. No changes were observed in CG, which could indicate that the changes in SG could be due to TC supplementation. It should be noted that there were no differences in nutritional intake. All biochemical parameters were maintained in normal ranges. No negative effects on the body were observed.

TetraSOD® is a unique commercial product composed of 100% lyophilised TC that is currently marketed for food and nutraceutical applications. In 2017, the European Union gave approval to the company to market its lyophilised TC for use in dietary supplements such as TetraSOD®, at levels of up to 250 mg/day [20].

The decrease of HR in SG could be positively related to arterial stiffness [33,34]. Previous studies have investigated the effects of the supplementation of other green microalgae, the microalgae chlorella, on arterial stiffness. Otsuki et al. (2013) analysed the effect of 200 mg chlorella supplementation in fourteen men over twelve weeks in a double-blind trial [35]. They concluded that chlorella supplementation could decrease arterial stiffness due to the nutrients it contains. Another study analysed the supplementation of 200 mg of chlorella in thirty-two subjects, with the authors concluding that multicomponent supplementation derived from chlorella decreased arterial stiffness [36]. Thus, it could be assumed that differences in HR may be due to changes in arterial stiffness; when artery walls lose their elastic properties and become stiff, they elicit a rise in systolic blood pressure and the heart's workload [37].

Some components present in TC may positively affect arterial stiffness; minerals such as potassium could decrease it [38], as well as unsaturated fatty acids through their anti-inflammatory function [39]. According to the results obtained, TC could reduce arterial stiffness due to the nutrients it contains and, therefore, decrease HR. The decrease in HR is related to the increase in O_2 pulse [40]. This could indicate a better metabolic economy of effort by the body.

Concerning ergospirometric values, SG recorded an increase in absolute and relative VO_{2max} ($p < 0.05$). Other research has analysed the effect of supplementation with other microalgae in different groups. For example, Hernández-Lepe et al. (2018) evaluated an exercise programme with and without spirulina, and a nonexercise programme with and without spirulina, in sedentary overweight and obese people [26]. They observed that supplementation of 4.5 g/day for six weeks with spirulina increased the relative VO_{2max} in the groups that consumed the microalgae without the exercise programme. Additionally, they reported a decrease in resting HR and an increase in the maximum lactate steady state. Another crossover and double-blind study reported a rise in relative VO_{2max} after twice-daily supplementation with chlorella (200 mg) for four weeks in ten young people [41]. In a double-blind trial by Zempo-Miyaki et al. (2017), a multicomponent supplement derived from chlorella (200 mg) for four weeks in thirty-four healthy men increased relative $VO_{2\ max}$ in an incremental maximal test on a cycle ergometer [27].

Curiously, the maximal speed in the test before and after the supplementation in SG was similar, whereas there was an increase in absolute and relative VO_{2max}. The rise in VO_2 could be due to an increase in O_2 pulse and haemoglobin. The calcium content of TC could generate an increase in oxygen transport by the haemoglobin. Calcium performs several vital functions in red blood cells that affect oxygen transport and coagulation, and increase the cell half-life [42,43]. Increases in intracellular calcium appear to promote the ability of red blood cells to supply oxygen [43].

TC contains carotenoids and polyphenols [20] that have antioxidant properties [44]. Several investigations observed that spirulina supplementation increases some enzymatic antioxidant systems [45,46]. The antioxidant properties of TC could explain the performance increase observed in this study.

Haemoglobin and MCH concentrations increased after TC supplementation in SG ($p < 0.01$ in haemoglobin; $p < 0.05$ in MCH). Microalgae have been used in animals as supplements to improve iron deficiencies [47]. Nasirian et al. (2017) investigated the effects of *Spirulina platensis* (15 and 30 mg/kg body weight) for five weeks on haematological parameters in diabetic rats [48]. They observed that *Spirulina platensis* supplementation of 30 mg/kg body weight improved total red blood cells, haemoglobin, MCH, mean cell volume and whole white blood cells. The authors hypothesised that *Spirulina platensis* could stimulate erythropoietin formation. In humans, Selmi et al. (2011) analysed the effect of 500 mg spirulina supplementation for twelve weeks in forty older volunteers [49]. They reported an increase in MCH in subjects of both sexes, whereas MCV and MCH concentration increased in males. They concluded that more studies are needed to confirm the results in humans. It should be noted that the participants in the previous studies were animals and older people, a different population to those of the present study.

The increases in haemoglobin concentration in SG despite a drop in haematocrit are discordant. This phenomenon could be related to the presence of some haematopoietic factor in the algae. The chlorides present in the microalgae could explain this increase [9], as cobalt chloride is an erythropoietic factor [50]. Another mineral, such as iron, could explain this increase in haemoglobin. The effects of iron on erythropoiesis and haemoglobin levels have been previously reported [51]. Finally, the bioactive peptides present in the microalgae could play a significant role as they have immunomodulation, antihypertensive or anticancer properties [52]. We believe that during the TC digestion process some bioactive peptide with haematopoietic properties can be obtained. In addition, we believe that the high levels of sodium and chloride present in TC could increase fluid retention and generate hypervolaemia, thereby decreasing haematocrit [53,54]. Further research is needed to explain the results obtained. We think that it is a finding of interest for sports performance.

This study has many limitations as it is a preliminary study of algae, which at this moment has not been previously investigated. First, the intensity and volume of training during the study could influence the results. The team's coach confirmed that the number of training hours and days did not change during the study in both groups. However, the intensity could have been modified. Second, the number of participants in this study was small and micronutrients intake was not considered. Third, there are no studies on these microalgae to compare results, so studies on other algae have been used. Fourth, the state of hydration could not be evaluated to verify the increase in plasma volume.

Current results need to be confirmed with larger sample sizes, and different populations and concentrations of TC to analyse the potential effects of various doses, and establish a dose–response relationship. It would be interesting for future studies to investigate the antioxidant properties of TC as well as the effect on elite athletes, and analyse the intake of micronutrients.

5. Conclusions

The data obtained in this investigation suggest that the daily supplementation of 25 mg of TC (TetraSOD®) during thirty days could modify the ergospirometric and haematological parameters analysed in amateur soccer players. The absence of abnormal values in biochemical parameters would indicate that the TC microalgae would not have negative effects on our body. Although these are preliminary results, we suggest that TC could be an ergogenic alternative for athletes. The intake of TC significantly improved the values of the hemogram, which would probably be the cause of the ergospirometric changes. The reasons for ergospirometric and haematological changes after TC administration are not well understood, and further research is needed to elucidate this topic.

Author Contributions: Conceptualisation, V.T. and M.M.-M.; methodology, M.M.-M. and M.C.R.-G.; formal analysis, J.S.-C. and I.B.; investigation, M.M.-M. and J.R.; data curation, J.R.; writing—original draft preparation, V.T. and M.M.-M.; writing—review and editing, J.S.-C., I.B. and M.C.R.-G.; visualisation, J.R.; supervision, M.M.-M. All authors have read and agreed to the published version of the manuscript.

Funding: This research received no external funding.

Acknowledgments: We want to thank the Fitoplancton Marino S.L. company for providing us with the microalgae *Tetraselmis chuii* for this study.

Conflicts of Interest: The authors declare a possible conflict of interest in that the Fitoplancton Marino S.L. company provided us with the microalgae *Tetraselmis chuii* used for this study. However, Fitoplancton Marino S.L did not participate in the design of the study, collection of data, interpretation of results or writing of the manuscript.

References

1. Falkowski, P.G.; Katz, M.E.; Knoll, A.H.; Quigg, A.; Raven, J.A.; Schofield, O.; Taylor, F.J.R. The evolution of modern eukaryotic phytoplankton. *Sciencie* **2004**, *305*, 354–360. [CrossRef]
2. Guiry, M.D. How many species of algae are there? *J. Phycol.* **2012**, *48*, 1057–1063. [CrossRef] [PubMed]
3. Milledge, J.J. Commercial application of microalgae other than as biofuels: A brief review. *Rev. Environ. Sci. Bio/Technol.* **2011**, *10*, 31–41. [CrossRef]
4. Benedetti, M.; Vecchi, V.; Barera, S.; Dall'Osto, L. Biomass from microalgae: The potential of domestication towards sustainable biofactories. *Microb. Cell Fact.* **2018**, *17*, 1–18. [CrossRef]
5. Plaza, M.; Herrero, M.; Cifuentes, A.; Ibáñez, E. Innovative Natural Functional Ingredients from Microalgae. *J. Agric. Food Chem.* **2009**, *57*, 7159–7170. [CrossRef]
6. Caporgno, M.P.; Mathys, A. Trends in Microalgae Incorporation into Innovative Food Products with Potential Health Benefits. *Front. Nutr.* **2018**, *5*, 58. [CrossRef] [PubMed]
7. Lum, K.K.; Kim, J.; Lei, X.G. Dual potential of microalgae as a sustainable biofuel feedstock and animal feed. *J. Anim. Sci. Biotechnol.* **2013**, *4*, 53. [CrossRef]
8. Wang, H.-M.D.; Chen, C.-C.; Huynh, P.; Chang, J.-S. Exploring the potential of using algae in cosmetics. *Bioresour. Technol.* **2015**, *184*, 355–362. [CrossRef]
9. Levine, I.; Fleurence, J. *Microalgae in Health and Disease Prevention*; Academic Press: San Diego, CA, USA, 2018; ISBN 978-0-12-811405-6.
10. Kay, R.A.; Barton, L.L. Microalgae as food and supplement. *Crit. Rev. Food Sci. Nutr.* **1991**, *30*, 555–573. [CrossRef]
11. Kim, S.-K.; Kang, K.-H. Medicinal effects of peptides from marine microalgae. In *Advances in Food and Nutrition Research*; Elsevier: San Diego, CA, USA, 2011; Volume 64, pp. 313–323. ISBN 1043-4526.
12. Barbalace, M.C.; Malaguti, M.; Giusti, L.; Lucacchini, A.; Hrelia, S.; Angeloni, C. Anti-Inflammatory Activities of Marine Algae in Neurodegenerative Diseases. *Int. J. Mol. Sci.* **2019**, *20*, 3061. [CrossRef]
13. Ismail, M.; Hossain, M.; Tanu, A.R.; Shekhar, H.U. Effect of spirulina intervention on oxidative stress, antioxidant status, and lipid profile in chronic obstructive pulmonary disease patients. *Biomed Res. Int.* **2015**, *2015*, 486120. [CrossRef] [PubMed]
14. Fallah, A.A.; Sarmast, E.; Dehkordi, S.H.; Engardeh, J.; Mahmoodnia, L.; Khaledifar, A.; Jafari, T. Effect of Chlorella supplementation on cardiovascular risk factors: A meta-analysis of randomized controlled trials. *Clin. Nutr.* **2018**, *37*, 1892–1901. [CrossRef]
15. Torres-Duran, P.V.; Ferreira-Hermosillo, A.; Juarez-Oropeza, M.A. Antihyperlipemic and antihypertensive effects of Spirulina maxima in an open sample of Mexican population: A preliminary report. *Lipids Health Dis.* **2007**, *6*, 33. [CrossRef] [PubMed]
16. Sathasivam, R.; Radhakrishnan, R.; Hashem, A.; Abd Allah, E.F. Microalgae metabolites: A rich source for food and medicine. *Saudi J. Biol. Sci.* **2019**, *26*, 709–722. [CrossRef]
17. Karkos, P.D.; Leong, S.C.; Karkos, C.D.; Sivaji, N.; Assimakopoulos, D.A. Spirulina in clinical practice: Evidence-based human applications. *Evid.-Based Complement. Altern. Med.* **2011**, *2011*, 531053. [CrossRef] [PubMed]
18. Butcher, R.W. An introductory account of the smaller algae of British coastal waters Part I. Introduction and Chlorophyceae. In *Fishery Investigations*; HMSO: Iver, UK, 1959; Volume 4, pp. 1–74.
19. Kumaran, P.; Saifuddin, N.; Janarthanan, S. Potential of microalgae Tetraselmis Chuii as feedstock for biodiesel application. *Int. Rev. Mech. Eng.* **2014**, *8*, 283–288.

20. Mantecón, L.; Moyano, R.; Cameán, A.M.; Jos, A. Safety assessment of a lyophilized biomass of Tetraselmis chuii (TetraSOD®) in a 90 day feeding study. *Food Chem. Toxicol.* **2019**, *133*, 110810. [CrossRef]
21. de Jesús Bonilla-Ahumada, F.; Khandual, S.; Lugo-Cervantes, E.C. Microencapsulation of algal biomass (Tetraselmis chuii) by spray-drying using different encapsulation materials for better preservation of beta-carotene and antioxidant compounds. *Algal Res.* **2018**, *36*, 229–238. [CrossRef]
22. Tibbetts, S.M.; Milley, J.E.; Lall, S.P. Chemical composition and nutritional properties of freshwater and marine microalgal biomass cultured in photobioreactors. *J. Appl. Phycol.* **2015**, *27*, 1109–1119. [CrossRef]
23. Hespel, P.; Maughan, R.J.; Greenhaff, P.L. Dietary supplements for football. *J. Sports Sci.* **2006**, *24*, 749–761. [CrossRef]
24. Gammone, M.A.; Gemello, E.; Riccioni, G.; D'Orazio, N. Marine bioactives and potential application in sports. *Mar. Drugs* **2014**, *12*, 2357–2382. [CrossRef] [PubMed]
25. Simsek, N.; Karadeniz, A.; Karaca, T. Effects of the Spirulina platensis and Panax ginseng oral supplementation on peripheral. *Rev. Méd. Vét* **2007**, *158*, 483–488.
26. Hernández-Lepe, M.; López-Díaz, J.; Juárez-Oropeza, M.; Hernández-Torres, R.; Wall-Medrano, A.; Ramos-Jiménez, A. Effect of arthrospira (Spirulina) maxima supplementation and a systematic physical exercise program on the body composition and cardiorespiratory fitness of overweight or obese subjects: A double-blind, randomized, and crossover controlled trial. *Mar. Drugs* **2018**, *16*, 364. [CrossRef] [PubMed]
27. Zempo-Miyaki, A.; Maeda, S.; Otsuki, T. Effect of Chlorella-derived multicomponent supplementation on maximal oxygen uptake and serum vitamin B2 concentration in young men. *J. Clin. Biochem. Nutr.* **2017**, 17–36.
28. Hagströmer, M.; Oja, P.; Sjöström, M. The International Physical Activity Questionnaire (IPAQ): A study of concurrent and construct validity. *Public Health Nutr.* **2006**, *9*, 755–762. [CrossRef]
29. Barat, M.; Ferrús, M.A.; Font, G.; Hardisson, A.; Herrera, A.; Lorente, F.; Marcos, A.; Martín, M.R.; Martínez, M.R.; Martínez, A.; et al. Report of the Scientific Committee of the Spanish Agency for Food Safety and Nutrition on a request for initial assessment for marketing of the marine microalgae Tetraselmis chuii under Regulation (EC) No 258/97 on novel foods and novel food ingredients. *Rev. Com. Científico AESAN* **2013**, *18*, 11–28.
30. Porta, J.; Galiano, D.; Tejedo, A.; González, J.M. Valoración de la composición corporal. Utopías y realidades. In *Manual de Cineantropometría.*; Esparza Ros, F., Ed.; FEMEDE: Madrid, Spain, 1993; pp. 113–170.
31. Moreiras, O.; Carbajal, A.; Cabrera, L.; Cuadrado, C. *Tablas de Composición de Alimentos: Guía de Prácticas*; Pirámide: Madrid, Spain, 2016; ISBN 9788436836233.
32. Skinner, J.S.; Mclellan, T.H. The transition from aerobic to anaerobic metabolism. *Res. Q. Exerc. Sport* **1980**, *51*, 234–248. [CrossRef]
33. Chu, C.-Y.; Lin, T.-H.; Hsu, P.-C.; Lee, W.-H.; Lee, H.-H.; Chiu, C.-A.; Su, H.-M.; Lee, C.-S.; Yen, H.-W.; Voon, W.-C. Heart rate significantly influences the relationship between atrial fibrillation and arterial stiffness. *Int. J. Med. Sci.* **2013**, *10*, 1295. [CrossRef]
34. Fei, D.-Y.; Arena, R.; Arrowood, J.A.; Kraft, K.A. Relationship between arterial stiffness and heart rate recovery in apparently healthy adults. *Vasc. Health Risk Manag.* **2005**, *1*, 85. [CrossRef]
35. Otsuki, T.; Shimizu, K.; Iemitsu, M.; Kono, I. Multicomponent supplement containing Chlorella decreases arterial stiffness in healthy young men. *J. Clin. Biochem. Nutr.* **2013**, *53*, 166–169. [CrossRef]
36. Otsuki, T.; Shimizu, K.; Maeda, S. Changes in arterial stiffness and nitric oxide production with Chlorella-derived multicomponent supplementation in middle-aged and older individuals. *J. Clin. Biochem. Nutr.* **2015**, *57*, 228–232. [CrossRef] [PubMed]
37. Logan, J.G.; Kim, S.-S. Resting heart rate and aortic stiffness in normotensive adults. *Korean Circ. J.* **2016**, *46*, 834–840. [CrossRef] [PubMed]
38. Sun, Y.; Byon, C.H.; Yang, Y.; Bradley, W.E.; Dell'Italia, L.J.; Sanders, P.W.; Agarwal, A.; Wu, H.; Chen, Y. Dietary potassium regulates vascular calcification and arterial stiffness. *JCI Insight* **2017**, *2*. [CrossRef] [PubMed]
39. Monahan, K.D.; Feehan, R.P.; Blaha, C.; McLaughlin, D.J. Effect of omega-3 polyunsaturated fatty acid supplementation on central arterial stiffness and arterial wave reflections in young and older healthy adults. *Physiol. Rep.* **2015**, *3*, e12438. [CrossRef] [PubMed]
40. Lavie, C.J.; Milani, R.V.; Mehra, M.R. Peak exercise oxygen pulse and prognosis in chronic heart failure. *Am. J. Cardiol.* **2004**, *93*, 588–593. [CrossRef]
41. Umemoto, S.; Otsuki, T. Chlorella-derived multicomponent supplementation increases aerobic endurance capacity in young individuals. *J. Clin. Biochem. Nutr.* **2014**, *55*, 143–146. [CrossRef]

42. Steffen, P.; Jung, A.; Nguyen, D.B.; Müller, T.; Bernhardt, I.; Kaestner, L.; Wagner, C. Stimulation of human red blood cells leads to Ca2+-mediated intercellular adhesion. *Cell Calcium* **2011**, *50*, 54–61. [CrossRef]
43. Bogdanova, A.; Makhro, A.; Wang, J.; Lipp, P.; Kaestner, L. Calcium in red blood cells—a perilous balance. *Int. J. Mol. Sci.* **2013**, *14*, 9848–9872. [CrossRef]
44. Haoujar, I.; Cacciola, F.; Abrini, J.; Mangraviti, D.; Giuffrida, D.; Oulad El Majdoub, Y.; Kounnoun, A.; Miceli, N.; Fernanda Taviano, M.; Mondello, L. The Contribution of Carotenoids, Phenolic Compounds, and Flavonoids to the Antioxidative Properties of Marine Microalgae Isolated from Mediterranean Morocco. *Molecules* **2019**, *24*, 4037. [CrossRef]
45. Kalafati, M.; Jamurtas, A.Z.; Nikolaidis, M.G.; Paschalis, V.; Theodorou, A.A.; Sakellariou, G.K.; Koutedakis, Y.; Kouretas, D. Ergogenic and antioxidant effects of spirulina supplementation in humans. *Med Sci Sport. Exerc* **2010**, *42*, 142–151. [CrossRef]
46. Lu, H.-K.; Hsieh, C.-C.; Hsu, J.-J.; Yang, Y.-K.; Chou, H.-N. Preventive effects of Spirulina platensis on skeletal muscle damage under exercise-induced oxidative stress. *Eur. J. Appl. Physiol.* **2006**, *98*, 220. [CrossRef] [PubMed]
47. Gao, F.; Guo, W.; Zeng, M.; Feng, Y.; Feng, G. Effect of microalgae as iron supplements on iron-deficiency anemia in rats. *Food Funct.* **2019**, *10*, 723–732. [CrossRef] [PubMed]
48. Nasirian, F.; Mesbahzadeh, B.; Maleki, S.A.; Mogharnasi, M.; Kor, N.M. The effects of oral supplementation of spirulina platensis microalgae on hematological parameters in streptozotocin-induced diabetic rats. *Am. J. Transl. Res.* **2017**, *9*, 5238.
49. Selmi, C.; Leung, P.S.C.; Fischer, L.; German, B.; Yang, C.-Y.; Kenny, T.P.; Cysewski, G.R.; Gershwin, M.E. The effects of Spirulina on anemia and immune function in senior citizens. *Cell. Mol. Immunol.* **2011**, *8*, 248. [CrossRef] [PubMed]
50. Lippi, G.; Franchini, M.; Guidi, G.C. Cobalt chloride administration in athletes: A new perspective in blood doping? *Br. J. Sports Med.* **2005**, *39*, 872–873. [CrossRef] [PubMed]
51. Rishi, G.; Subramaniam, V.N. The relationship between systemic iron homeostasis and erythropoiesis. *Biosci. Rep.* **2017**, *37*, 1–17. [CrossRef]
52. Fan, X.; Bai, L.; Zhu, L.; Yang, L.; Zhang, X. Marine algae-derived bioactive peptides for human nutrition and health. *J. Agric. Food Chem.* **2014**, *62*, 9211–9222. [CrossRef]
53. Savoie, F.A.; Asselin, A.; Goulet, E.D.B. Comparison of sodium chloride tablets–induced, sodium chloride solution–induced, and glycerol-induced hyperhydration on fluid balance responses in healthy men. *J. Strength Cond. Res.* **2016**, *30*, 2880–2891. [CrossRef]
54. Mora-Rodriguez, R.; Hamouti, N. Salt and fluid loading: Effects on blood volume and exercise performance. In *Acute Topics in Sport Nutrition*; Karger Publishers: Basel, Switzerland, 2012; Volume 59, pp. 113–119.

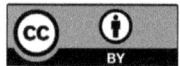

© 2020 by the authors. Licensee MDPI, Basel, Switzerland. This article is an open access article distributed under the terms and conditions of the Creative Commons Attribution (CC BY) license (http://creativecommons.org/licenses/by/4.0/).

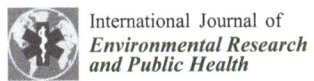

Article

The Effect of Wearing a Customized Mouthguard on Body Alignment and Balance Performance in Professional Basketball Players

Hae Joo Nam [1], Joon-Hee Lee [2,*], Dae-Seok Hong [1] and Hyun Chul Jung [2]

1. Department of Health Rehabilitation, O-san University, 45 Cheonghak-ro, Osan-si, Gyeonggi-do 18119, Korea; tjlove@osan.ac.kr (H.J.N.); spoho@osan.ac.kr (D.-S.H.)
2. Department of Coaching, College of Physical Education, Kyung Hee University (Global Campus), 1732 Deokyoungdaero, Giheung-gu, Yongin-si, Gyeonggi-do 17014, Korea; jhc@khu.ac.kr
* Correspondence: borracho@khu.ac.kr; Tel.: +82-31-201-2758

Received: 6 August 2020; Accepted: 31 August 2020; Published: 3 September 2020

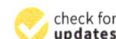

Abstract: The present study examined the influence of a customized mouthguard on body alignment and balance performance in professional basketball players. Twenty-three professional male basketball players, aged 25.8 ± 8.6 years old, were voluntarily assigned to participate in three treatments, including no treatment (no mouthguard), acute treatment (wearing a mouthguard), and repeated treatments (8 weeks follow-up). Body alignment status, such as spinal and pelvic posture and balance performance, were measured at each time point using a 3D Formetric III (Germany) and a postural control device (Posturomed 202, Germany), respectively. A repeated MANOVA analysis with a Bonferroni post hoc test was applied, and the adjusted p-value was set at 0.02. No significant treatment effect was observed in body alignment ($p = 0.302$). However, univariate analysis showed a significant difference in pelvic torsion, where it was decreased after acute and repeated mouthguard treatments compared to no treatment ($p < 0.001$). Kyphotic angle also increased significantly following 8 weeks of treatment compared to no treatment ($p < 0.001$) and acute treatment ($p < 0.002$). There was a significant treatment effect on balance performance ($p < 0.001$). Both static and dynamic balance performance improved following 8 weeks of treatment ($p < 0.001$). Our study revealed that a customized mouthguard provides a benefit to balance performance. Notably, repeated treatment impacts on balance performance more than acute treatment. Although our findings did not show a significant effect on body alignment, some positive results, such as pelvic torsion and kyphotic angle, may provide substantial information for developing future longitudinal studies with large sample sizes.

Keywords: body alignment; static balance; dynamic balance; basketball; mouthguard

1. Introduction

Sports athletes commonly undergo highly intensive training to gain specialized physical strength and develop skills and specific movement patterns needed for competitions. However, unilateral training or incorrect movements can induce the muscular imbalance between the left and right sides of the body, which may interfere with well-balanced bodily development [1]. It is also known that asymmetric loads during repeated training can increase the risk of spinal deformation and structural scoliosis due to the unilateral mechanical action of force [2]. It has been reported that the prevalence of sports-related spinal deformity, such as functional scoliosis, was 33.5% in a sample of 571 athletes [3]. Such spinal deformity can alter the characteristics of spinal muscles, including muscle spindle activity [4], which interferes with the interactions between various body components [5].

Consequently, this causes instability when maintaining a standing posture, while also affecting balance performance [6].

Muscular imbalance throughout the asymmetrical movements negatively influence body alignment [7]. In particular, the misaligned spinal column can cause back pain and negatively impact on athletic performance in professional athletes [8,9]. For instance, basketball training involves numerous movements, such as rapid acceleration and deceleration, as well as continued jumping movements. Athletes also require higher physiological demand (77–95% HRmax) with intermittent movements to rapidly transit from defense to offense motions [10]. They often experience muscular injuries, including ankle and lumber sprains, when eccentric load is applied on the legs during pivoting and jumping. Sudden deceleration while changing direction, bad landing after jumping, and failed direction control have been also reported as major causes of injury [11]. The athlete's lumbar pain is mainly characterized by "postural back pain", which leads to an asymmetrical position by repeating excessive training for a long period of time, and the deformed body alignment causes dislocation when the load is concentrated in the local region of the spine. Thus, it makes it difficult to maintain normal spinal curvature. The deformed body alignment can affect the core muscles' strength and a decrease in the range of motion reduces the extensor strength [12]. In addition, when the hip joint is displaced, there is a difference in the height of the left and right sides of the pelvis, and the lengths of both legs are changed; thus, the balance of the pelvis is collapsed and makes it difficult to maintain the midline of the spine [13].

To safely protect physical functions from undesirable movement patterns, it is important to maintain proper positional state and posture in each part of the body. In particular, proper position and posture of the head and neck may play an important role in postural maintenance and function, where muscles in the head and neck area form a balance with each other to help perform movements by maintaining the posture of the spine connected to the area and controlling the mandibular movement. A previous case study reported that a female professional basketball player who suffered the temporomandibular joint dysfunction (TMJ) improved her postural control after six months of wearing an occlusal splint during training and competitions [14]. In the same way, Mannheimer and Rosenthal [15] reported that the position of the cervical spine changes temporomandibular joint (TMJ) disorder and changes the direction of the head and consequently changes the position of the mandible. Therefore, the position of the appropriate mandibular joint can improve the exercise ability when the movement occurs, and the muscle strength can be changed according to the position of the jaw [16]. Recently, there have been reports of improvements in performance by changing the position of the jaw joints after wearing a mouthguard [17–19]. However, a lack of studies may limit our understanding of the effectiveness of wearing a mouthguard on body alignment and balance performance in professional athletes. Therefore, the present study examined the acute and repeated effects of wearing a customized mouthguard on body alignment and balance performance in professional basketball players. We hypothesized that maintaining a stable occlusion state of the temporomandibular joint (TMJ) through wearing a mouthguard will change the body alignment and improve both static and dynamic balance performance in professional basketball players.

2. Materials and Methods

2.1. Participants

Twenty-six professional male basketball players who are currently affiliated with the Korean Basketball League voluntarily participated in the study. Participants received an oral explanation of the purpose of the study, the study procedure, the potential risks and benefits, and completed a written consent approved by Institutional Review Board of the university (KHUIRB-019). During the study period, three players were unable to complete the experiment due to personal reasons or orthopedic injury; thus, twenty-three players completed the study. The participants' average age, career length, height, and body mass were 25.8 ± 8.6 years old, 16.3 ± 5.4 years, 187.5 ± 5.2 cm, and 83.4 ± 8.26 kg, respectively.

2.2. Study Procedure

Prior to the experiment, all participants were instructed to visit a designated dentist to undergo an oral examination, temporomandibular disorder test, and diagnostic model test. Subsequently, mouthguards were custom made for players who were determined to have no problem wearing a mouthguard. Participants were familiarized with all the measurements, including body alignment and balance performance tests, at least one week prior to the experiment. A total of three measurements, including body alignment and balance performance tests, were performed with no treatment (without wearing a mouthguard), acute treatments (wearing a mouthguard) and repeated treatments (8 weeks follow-up). There was a seven-day wash-out period between treatments. Participant underwent the measurements without a mouthguard for no treatment and with a mouthguard for acute and repeated treatments. Basketball players were encouraged to wear the mouthguard for at least 3 h a day during strength and conditioning training as well as technical training for the 8-week follow-up period.

2.3. Mouthguard

The customized mouthguard was produced by fabricating a plaster model based on an impression taken with irreversible hydrocolloid impression material on the maxillomandibular dentition of the subjects. Subsequently, Drufomat 2 (Dreve-Dentamid GmbH., Unna., Germany) was used with an ethylene vinyl acetatecopolymer sheet to produce the mouthguard by a traditional laminate method involving thermos compression molding in accordance with the recommendation given by the Korean Academy of Sports Dentistry (Figure 1).

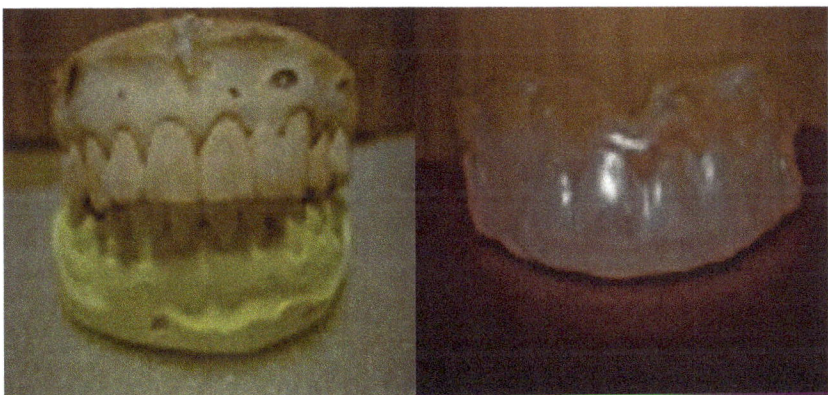

Figure 1. An example of a customized mouthguard.

2.4. Measurement of Body Alignment

For spinal and pelvic posture, Formetric III3D (Formetric, Diers International GmbH, Schlangenbad, Germany) developed by the Institut fur Experimenteller Biomechanik (University of Münster, Germany) was used, and a videorastereogaphy method was used, where a halogen light source is projected on the back surface of the subject and the image is processed by a raster method. Image acquisition time was approximately 6 s, where the position of four anatomical landmarks—vertebra prominence (VP; C7), sacrom point (SP), left lumbar dimple (DL), and right lumbar dimple (DR)—was automatically established and the values were determined based on anatomical calculations (error: ±0.05 mm). Measurement postures are shown in Figure 2 and the variables used during the measurements are shown in Table 1.

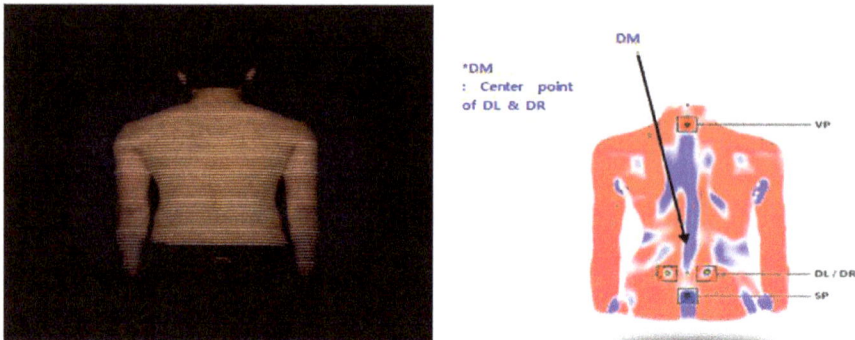

Figure 2. Posture for Formetric III testing and anatomical points (2006).

Table 1. Body alignment variables.

Variables	Definition	Unit
Torsion Trunk	Left and right rotation of trunk	[°]
Trunk Imbalance	From the VP to vertical line and angle of connect line from VP to DM	[°]
Trunk Inclination	Anterior and posterior inclination of trunk in the side position	[°]
Pelvic Tilt	Length of both pelvic tilts	[mm]
Pelvic Torsion	Contrary anterior and posterior torsion of both pelvic sides	[°]
Pelvic Rotation	Left and right rotation of both pelvic sides	[°]
Kyphotic Angle	Maximum kyphotic angle in the thoracic vertebrae part	[°]
Lordotic Angle	Maximum lordotic angle in the lumbar vertebrae part	[°]
Lateral Deviation	Lateral deviation length to connection line of VP and DM	[mm]
Surface Rotation	Surface rotation angle to connection line of VP and DM	[°]

2.5. Measurement of Balance Performance

The study measured static balance ability, where the posture was maintained with the body remaining stationary and the center of gravity was maintained on the supporting base without moving. Dynamic balance ability was measured where the posture was maintained while the body was moving. A postural control device (Posturomed 202, Haider Bioswing, Pullenreuth, Germany) was used to measure the left and right postural sway when standing one-legged on the left and right leg. Two measurements, 10 s each, were taken for each posture, with a 1-min rest interval between measurements. The maximum value was recorded.

2.6. Statistical Analysis

All data analysis was performed with SPSS for Windows (version 23.0, SPSS Inc., Chicago, IL, USA) and the mean (M) and standard deviation (SD) of all measured values were calculated. A repeated multivariate analysis of variance (MANOVA) analysis with a Bonferroni post hoc test was applied to examine the treatment effects (baseline, acute, and repeated treatment). The adjusted significance level of all statistical values was set at 0.02.

3. Results

3.1. Changes in Body Alignment

The results of body alignment are presented in Table 2. A total of 10 variables were examined to estimate the spinal and pelvic posture. No significant treatment effect was observed in body alignment

(F = 6.476, p = 0.302). However, univariate analysis showed a significant difference in pelvic torsion (p = 0.001) where both acute (p = 0.015) and repeated treatment (p = 0.006) of wearing a mouthguard reduced the pelvic torsion compared to no treatment. A significant difference in kyphotic angle was observed between different treatments (p < 0.001). The kyphotic angle improved significantly following 8 weeks of wearing mouthguard compared to the baseline (p = 0.002) and acute treatment (p = 0.001). However, other variables, including trunk torsion, trunk inclination, trunk imbalance, pelvic tilt, pelvic rotation, lordotic angle, surface rotation max, and lateral deviation max, were not different between different treatments.

Table 2. Changes in body alignment condition (mean ± SD).

Variables	NT	AT	RT	F-Value	p-Value
Trunk torsion [°]	2.0 ± 6.81	1.6 ± 4.11	3.0 ± 4.43	0.782	0.451
Trunk inclination [°]	2.4 ± 2.92	1.8 ± 2.38	1.5 ± 1.83	2.928	0.075
Trunk imbalance [°]	−0.3 ± 1.17	−0.3 ± 0.77	0.04 ± 0.67	2.628	0.098
Pelvic tilt [mm]	−0.7 ± 7.96	0.1 ± 6.62	0.3 ± 4.33	0.423	0.580
Pelvic torsion [°]	4.3 ± 2.93a	2.9 ± 2.38b	2.1 ± 2.01b	9.569	<0.001
Pelvis rotation [°]	−1.8 ± 4.36	−0.5 ± 2.96	−0.3 ± 2.09	3.094	0.063
Kyphotic angle [°]	37.3 ± 6.37a	38.6 ± 6.36a	41.9 ± 5.99b	13.197	<0.001
Lordotic angle [°]	31.7 ± 8.84	33.4 ± 8.56	34.3 ± 9.12	3.223	0.072
Surface rotation max [°]	0.2 ± 7.60	−2.0 ± 5.00	−1.0 ± 4.07	1.979	0.169
Lateral deviation max [mm]	2.4 ± 9.22	1.9 ± 7.52	2.8 ± 6.30	0.314	0.675

Note. Different letters indicate a significant difference between treatments. NT, no treatment; AT, acute treatment; RT, repeated treatment.

3.2. Changes in Balance Performance

With respect to the measurement results of balance performance, a significant treatment effect was observed across time (F = 3.942, p < 0.001). Univariate analysis revealed that almost all categories of static and dynamic balance variables improved significantly after wearing an acute and repeated mouthguard compared to no treatment (p < 0.01). Particularly, athletes became more stable following 8 weeks of repeated treatment. The results from analysis of changes in static and dynamic balance are shown in Table 3.

Table 3. Changes in static and dynamic balance performance (mean ± SD).

	Variables	NT	AT	RT	F-Value	p-Value
Static	RF X axis	1368.4 ± 812.93a	592.2 ± 477.59b	327.0 ± 211.19c	33.817	<0.001
	RF Y axis	425.1 ± 339.77a	190.3 ± 168.24b	327.0 ± 211.19a	7.665	0.004
	Sum of RF X + Y axis	1502.4 ± 887.03a	660.3 ± 525.93b	374.8 ± 224.90c	33.044	<0.001
	LF X axis	1619.9 ± 1137.99a	504.0 ± 355.42b	258.4 ± 191.59c	31.606	<0.001
	LF Y axis	390.3 ± 305.74a	155.7 ± 94.36b	99.3 ± 52.53c	20.193	<0.001
	Sum of LF X + Y axis	1738.8 ± 1179.47a	563.2 ± 370.38b	300.2 ± 199.55c	33.046	<0.001
Dynamic	RF X axis	1164.6 ± 508.36a	660.0 ± 285.47b	327.0 ± 211.19c	42.657	<0.001
	RF Y axis	446.8 ± 172.96a	363.8 ± 163.83a	272.0 ± 122.69b	16.306	<0.001
	Sum of RF X + Y axis	1400.2 ± 549.12a	847.0 ± 352.71b	595.6 ± 208.65c	40.962	<0.001
	LF X axis	1280.0 ± 680.85a	669.6 ± 363.73b	412.0 ± 214.88c	34.069	<0.001
	LF Y axis	409.5 ± 180.06a	306.0 ± 128.76a	261.8 ± 106.02b	10.670	0.001
	Sum of LF X + Y axis	1449.3 ± 710.18a	819.6 ± 398.35b	562.8 ± 251.46c	32.918	<0.001

Note. RF, right foot; LF, left foot; NT, no treatment; AT, acute treatment; RT, repeated treatment. Different letters indicate a significant difference between treatments.

4. Discussion

Changes in the body alignment caused by repeated unilateral movements have been recognized as one of the major factors for inducing chronic inflammation, pain, deformation of the vertebrae, and inhibiting the growth of young athletes [20,21]. This study investigated the influence of a customized mouthguard on body alignment and balance performance in professional basketball players. Our findings showed that wearing a customized mouthguard provides a positive effect on balance performance, but no significant effect was observed in body alignment. Notably, repeated treatment over an 8-week period provides a greater impact on balance performance than acute treatment.

Although no significant impact on body alignment was observed in the present study, univariate analyses showed a significant effect on pelvic torsion and kyphotic angle, where it was improved following acute or repeated treatments. Pelvic torsion angle is a factor used to identify pelvic deviation, which refers to the antero-posterior displacement of the left and right pelvis, and as the angle deviates from the normal range of 0°, there is a high probability of abnormal changes. In the present study, the pelvic torsion angle decreased significantly after wearing the mouthguard, which represents the improvement of pelvic balance. It is well understood that the TMJ and nearby muscles share a functional relationship. Abnormalities in TMJ function caused by various factors have been known to weaken the head and neck muscles [22], as well as abdominal and leg muscles. Maintaining safe teeth conditions and jaw repositioning by wearing a customized mouthguard have been shown to improve athletic performance, such as maximal aerobic power, vertical jump, and sprint performance [23].

Kyphotic angle is a variable that reflects the spinal curvature related to the antero-posterior aspect, and is indicative of how much the back is curved towards the front. Relative to the fully curved state, 47°–50° represents the normal range. In the present study, the subjects showed curvature values in the range of 37°–42°, which showed a difference of about 10° as compared to the normal range. Wojtys et al. found an association between the accumulated training time and the increase in thoracic kyphosis and lumbar lordosis [24]. They reported that repeated movements or overload training could cause organic adaptations with potential muscular imbalances and could determine postural changes, which are specific to the practiced modality. These biomechanical compensations may influence the growth processes and lead to the development of various postural patterns [25]. Although the characteristics of each sport may have a major impact on athletes' postural patterns, excessive exercise load and repetitive motion, such as running and jumping, could cause a limited range of motion and muscle stiffness that could also affect the postural imbalance.

Over the past several years, many studies have been conducted to figure out the determinant factors that can affect the body posture, and the evaluations of respiration and head and neck position have been introduced as determinant factors [26,27]. Recently, studies have reported the role of trigeminal afferences and dental occlusion in proprioception and visual and postural stabilization [28,29]. Sakaguchi et al. [29] examined the association between mandibular position and posture changes, suggesting that occlusal contact may vary during standing and walking if there is a difference in leg length or hip joint or other postural deformations. Another study also reported that body posture could be changed by different dental occlusion positions [30].

Balance or postural stability is a necessary component in both daily activities and sport [31]. Postural stability can be defined as the ability of an individual to remain centered on the ground, which includes feedback from the sensory system that determines continuous neuromuscular changes [32]. Balance ability is associated with the improvement of performance and the reduction of injury factors [33,34]. Contrary to changes in spinal alignment, postural balance ability showed significantly large differences in all categories of static and dynamic balance. Basketball athletes require a high level of balance ability, and the inherent sense of acceptance from the hip is important because of the complexity of the basketball technique. However, various movements, such as deceleration and acceleration, switching direction, and box-out, can develop the unbalanced conditions [35]. Additionally, basketball techniques, including a one-leg jump shoot, foot twist motions, pivot motion, airborne rebounds, and dribbling, include potential risks for developing unbalanced conditions [36]. Therefore, the improvement of balance ability is believed to be of significant help in predicting and maintaining instantaneous movements for basketball players during competitions.

Mouthguards are typical safety devices recommended for use by athletes in various sports to decrease the risk of oral–facial injuries. Basketball players are more likely to hit an opponent in repeated movements such as deceleration, acceleration, jumping, and turning. For this reason, some basketball players use a variety of mouthguards during the season or during training to prevent tooth injuries and protect the maxilla from possible extreme collisions [37]. Recently, as research progresses on the connection between TMJ, the surrounding muscles, and posture, the mouthguard is used as protective equipment, a TMJ occlusion correction treatment device, and equipment to improve performance [14]. Previous studies reported that among various physical fitness factors, wearing a mouthguard can promote functional improvement [38,39]. Previous studies also reported that wearing a mouthguard or mandibular orthopedic repositioning appliance (MORA) had the effect of strengthening head and neck muscles and enhancing leg strength and power performance [40]. Moreover, wearing a mouthguard resulted in a positive change and improvement in the center of posture and balance ability [41], while Yoshinobu et al. reported that just by stabilizing occlusion, balance was maintained quickly, which would allow for an improved sense of balance and postural stability and maintain safe stationary posture after movement [42]. In this study, the repeated treatment of wearing a mouthguard resulted in better static and dynamic balance performance than acute treatment. However, some studies reported that wearing a mouthguard did not improve balance performance in trained men and women [39] and collegiate male athletes [43]. These inconsistent results between the studies may be associated with different subject groups, test equipment, and treatment periods.

Although this study provides substantial information about the implication of mouthguards for body alignment and balance performance among professional basketball players, there are some limitations that need to be considered when interpreting the data. The duration that each athlete wore the mouthguard was not recorded in the present study. Thus, it is difficult to evaluate the dose–response effects. However, basketball players were encouraged to wear the mouthguard by coaches and researchers during strength conditioning and technical training to meet the minimum requirement hours (3 h). This study was a crossover study, but participants were not randomly allocated to the different treatments due to the game schedules, which may have created bias in the results. In future studies, randomized allocation needs to be applied to confirm the effectiveness of mouthguards on body alignment and balance performance in basketball players.

5. Conclusions

The present study suggests that wearing a mouthguard improves balance performance. In particular, the repeated treatment of wearing a mouthguard over an 8-week period had a more positive impact on changes in balance performance than acute treatment. Although our findings did not show a significant effect on body alignment, some positive results, such as for pelvic torsion and kyphotic angle, may provide substantial information for developing future longitudinal studies with large sample sizes.

Author Contributions: Conceptualization, H.J.N. and J.-H.L.; Methodology, H.J.N. and J.-H.L.; Formal analysis, H.J.N. and J.-H.L.; Investigation, H.J.N., D.-S.H., and J.-H.L.; Data curation, H.J.N., D.-S.H., and J.-H.L.; Writing—original draft preparation, H.J.N. and J.-H.L.; Writing—Review and editing, H.C.J.; Supervision, J.-H.L.; Funding acquisition, J.-H.L. All authors have read and agreed to the published version of the manuscript.

Funding: This work was supported by a grant from Kyung Hee University in 2019, grant number KHU-20191041.

Acknowledgments: The authors wish to thank the professional basketball players who participated in this study.

Conflicts of Interest: The authors declare no conflict of interest.

References

1. Jeon, K.; Kim, S. Effect of unilateral exercise on spinal and pelvic deformities, and isokinetic trunk muscle strength. *J. Phys. Ther. Sci.* **2016**, *28*, 844–849. [CrossRef] [PubMed]
2. Yoo, J.C.; Suh, S.W.; Jung, B.J.; Hur, C.Y.; Chae, I.J.; Kang, C.S.; Wang, J.H.; Moon, W.N.; Cheon, E.M. Asymmetric Exercise and Scoliosis-A Study on Volleyball Athletes. *Kor. J. Orthop. Assoc.* **2001**, *36*, 455–460. [CrossRef]

3. Omey, M.L.; Micheli, L.J.; Gerbino, P.G. Idiopathic scoliosis and spondylosis in the female athlete. *Clin. Orthop.* **2000**, *372*, 74–84. [CrossRef] [PubMed]
4. Sadat-Ali, M.; Al-Othman, A.; Bubshait, D.; Al-Dakheel, D. Does scoliosis causes low bone mass? A comparative study between siblings. *Eur. J. Spine.* **2008**, *17*, 944–947. [CrossRef] [PubMed]
5. Nault, M.L.; Allard, P.; Hinse, S.; Le Blanc, R.; Caron, O.; Labelle, H.; Sadeghi, H. Relations between standing stability and body posture parameters in adolescent idiopathic scoliosis. *Spine* **2002**, *27*, 1911–1917. [CrossRef] [PubMed]
6. Yagi, M.; Kaneko, S.; Yato, Y.; Asazuma, T. Standing balance and compensatory mechanisms in patients with adult spinal deformity. *Spine* **2017**, *42*, 584–591. [CrossRef]
7. Modi, H.; Srinivasalu, S.; Mehta, S.; Yang, J.H.; Song, H.R.; Suh, S.W. Muscle imbalance in volleyball players initiates scoliosis in immature spines: A screening analysis. *Asian Spine J.* **2008**, *2*, 38. [CrossRef]
8. Gravara, M.; Hadzik, A. Postural variables in girls practicing volleyball. *Biomed. Hum. Kinet.* **2009**, *1*, 67–71.
9. Hawrylak, A.; Skolimowski, T.; Barczyk, K.; Biec, E. Asymetry of trunk in athletes of different kind of sports. *Pol. J. Sports Med.* **2001**, *17*, 232–235.
10. Scanlan, A.T.; Fox, J.L.; Borges, N.R.; Tucker, P.S.; Dalbo, V.J. Temporal changes in physiological and performance responses across game-specific simulated basketball activity. *J. Sport Health Sci.* **2018**, *7*, 176–182. [CrossRef]
11. Drakos, M.C.; Domb, B.; Starkey, C.; Callahan, L.; Allen, A.A. Injury in the National Basketball Association: A 17-year overview. *Sports Health* **2010**, *2*, 284–290. [CrossRef] [PubMed]
12. Neumann, D.A. *Kinesiology of the Musculoskeletal System: Foundations for Physical Rehabilitation*, 1st ed.; St. Mosby: Michigan, MI, USA, 2002.
13. Morimoto, T.; Sonohata, M.; Kitajima, M.; Yoshihara, T.; Hirata, H.; Mawatari, M. Hip-Spine Syndrome: The Coronal Alignment of the Lumbar Spine and Pelvis in Patients with Ankylosed Hips. *Spine Surg. Relat. Res.* **2019**, *4*, 37–42. [CrossRef] [PubMed]
14. Baldini, A.; Beraldi, A.; Nota, A.; Danelon, F.; Ballanti, F.; Longoni, S. Gnathological postural treatment in a professional basketball player: A case report and an overview of the role of dental occlusion on performance. *Ann. Stomatol.* **2012**, *3*, 51.
15. Mannheimer, J.S.; Rosenthal, R.M. Acute and chronic postural abnormalities as related to craniofacial pain and temporomandibular disorders. *Dent. Clin. N. Am.* **1991**, *35*, 185–208. [PubMed]
16. Gelb, H.; Mehta, N.R.; Forgiane, A.G. The relationship between jaw posture and muscular strength in sports dentistry: A reappraisal. *J. Craniomandib. Pract.* **1996**, *14*, 320–325. [CrossRef] [PubMed]
17. Cetin, C.; Kececi, A.D.; Erdogan, A.; Baydar, M.L. Influence of custom-made mouth guards on strength, speed and anaerobic performance of teakwondo athletes. *Dent. Traumatol.* **2009**, *25*, 272–276. [CrossRef]
18. Queiroz, A.F.; de Brito, R.B.; Ramacciato, J.C.; Motta, R.H.; Florio, F.M. Influence of mouthguards on the physical performance of soccer players. *Dent. Traumatol.* **2013**, *26*, 450–454. [CrossRef]
19. Allen, C.R.; Dabbs, N.C.; Zachary, C.S.; Garmer, J.C. The acute effect of a commercial bite-aligning mouth-piece on strength and power in recreationally trained men. *J. Strength Cond. Res.* **2014**, *28*, 499–503. [CrossRef]
20. Gravara, M.; Hadzik, A. The body posture in young athletes compared to their peers. *Med. Sport.* **2009**, *25*, 115–124.
21. Grabara, M. Body posture of young female basketball players. *Biomed. Hum. Kinet.* **2012**, *4*, 76–81. [CrossRef]
22. Rocha, C.P.; Croci, C.S.; Caria, P.H. Is there relationship between temporomandibular disorders and head and cervical posture? A systematic review. *J. Oral Rehabil.* **2013**, *40*, 875–881. [CrossRef] [PubMed]
23. Martins, R.S.; Girouard, P.; Elliott, E.; Mekary, S. Physiological responses of a jaw-repositioning custom-made mouthguard on airway and their effects on athletic performance. *J. Strength Cond. Res.* **2020**, *34*, 422–429. [CrossRef] [PubMed]
24. Wojtys, E.; Ashton-Miller, J.; Huston, L.; Moga, P. The assocation between athletic training time and the sagittal curvature of the immature spine. *Am. J. Sports Med.* **2000**, *28*, 490–498. [CrossRef]
25. Boldori, L.; Da Solda, M.; Marelli, A. Anomalies of the trunk. An analysis of their prevalence in young athletes. *Minerva. Pediatr.* **1999**, *51*, 259–264. [PubMed]
26. Kantor, E.; Poupard, L.; Le Bozec, S.; Bouisset, S. Does body stability depend on postural chain mobility or stability area? *Neurosci. Lett.* **2001**, *308*, 128–132. [CrossRef]
27. Gangloff, P.; Louis, J.P.; Perrin, P.P. Dental occlusion modifies gaze postural stabilization in human subjects. *Neurosci. Lett.* **2000**, *293*, 203–206. [CrossRef]

28. Milani, R.S.; De Pierre, D.D.; Lapeyre, L.; Pourreyron, L. Relationship between dental occlusion and posture. *J. Craniomandib. Pract.* **2000**, *18*, 127–134. [CrossRef]
29. Sakaguchi, K.; Mehta, N.R.; Abdallah, E.F.; Forgione, A.G.; Hirayama, H.; Kawasaki, T.; Yokoyama, A. Examination of the relationship between mandibular position and body posture. *Cranio. Oct.* **2007**, *25*, 237–249. [CrossRef]
30. Blum, C.A. Chiropractic perspective of dental occlusion's affect on posture. *J. Chiroprac. Edu.* **2004**, *18*, 38.
31. Guskiewicz, K.M.; Ross, S.E.; Marshall, S.W. Postural stability and neuropsychological deficits after concussion in collegiate athletes. *J. Athl. Train.* **2001**, *36*, 263–273.
32. Huang, M.H.; Brown, S.H. Age differences in the control of postural stability during reaching tasks. *Gait Posture* **2013**, *38*, 837–842. [CrossRef] [PubMed]
33. Gribble, P.A.; Hertel, J.; Plisky, P. Using the Star Excursion Balance Test to assess dynamic postural-control deficits and outcomes in lower extremity injury: A literature and systematic review. *J. Athl. Train.* **2012**, *47*, 339–357. [CrossRef] [PubMed]
34. Hrysomallis, C. Balance ability and athletic performance. *Sports Med.* **2011**, *41*, 221–232. [CrossRef] [PubMed]
35. Scanian, A.; Dascombe, B.; Reabum, P. A comparison of the activity demands of elite and sub-elite Australian men's basketball competition. *J. Sports Sci.* **2011**, *29*, 1153–1160. [CrossRef]
36. Ben Abdelkrim, N.; El Fazaa, S.; El Ati, J. Time-motion analysis and physiological data of elite under-19-year-old basketball players during competition. *Br. J. Sports Med.* **2007**, *41*, 69–75. [CrossRef]
37. Ferrari, C.H.; de Medeiros, J.M.F. Dental trauma and level of information: Mouth-guard use in different contact sports. *Dent. Traumatol.* **2002**, *18*, 144–147. [CrossRef]
38. Duddy, F.A.; Weissman, J.; Lee, R.A.S.; Paranjpe, A.; Di Paolo, C. Influence of different types of mouth guards on strength and performance of collegiate athletes: A controlled-randomized trial. *Dent. Traumatol.* **2012**, *28*, 263–267. [CrossRef]
39. Dumm-Lewis, C.; Luk, H.Y.; Comstock, B.A.; Szivak, T.K.; Hooper, D.R.; Kupchak, B.R.; Watts, A.M.; Putney, B.J.; Volek, H.J.S.; Denegar, C.R.; et al. The effects of a customized over-counter mouth guard on neuromuscular force and power production in trained men and women. *J. Strength Cond. Res.* **2012**, *26*, 1085–1093. [CrossRef]
40. Morales, J.; Solana-Tramunt, M.; Miró, A.; García, M. Effects of jaw clenching while wearing a customized bite-aligning mouthpiece on strength in healthy young men. *J. Strength Cond. Res.* **2016**, *30*, 1102–1110.
41. Tardieu, C.; Dumitrescu, M.; Giraudeau, A.; Blanc, J.L.; Cheynet, F.; Borel, L. Dental occlusion and postural control in adults. *Neurosci. Lett.* **2009**, *450*, 221–224. [CrossRef]
42. Maeda, Y.; Emura, I.; Nakamura, K.; Nishida, K.; Nokubi, T. Study on the role of occlusal support for the body equilibrium function among elderly people -Examination with static and dynamic configuration-. *J. Jpn. Prosthodont. Soc.* **1995**, *39*, 900–905. [CrossRef]
43. Golem, D.L.; Arent, S.M. Effects of over-the-counter jaw-repositioning mouth guards on dynamic balance, flexibility, agility, strength, and power in college-aged male athletes. *J. Strength Cond. Res.* **2015**, *29*, 500–512. [CrossRef] [PubMed]

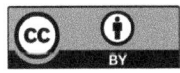

© 2020 by the authors. Licensee MDPI, Basel, Switzerland. This article is an open access article distributed under the terms and conditions of the Creative Commons Attribution (CC BY) license (http://creativecommons.org/licenses/by/4.0/).

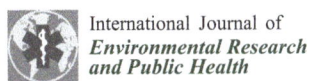

Article

Hormonal Changes in High-Level Aerobic Male Athletes during a Sports Season

Javier Alves [1], Víctor Toro [2], Gema Barrientos [1,*], Ignacio Bartolomé [2], Diego Muñoz [2] and Marcos Maynar [2]

1 Department of Sport Science, Faculty of Education, Pontifical University of Salamanca, C/Henry Collet, 52-70, CP: 37007 Salamanca, Spain; fjalvesva@upsa.es
2 Department of Physiology, Faculty of Sports Science Faculty, University of Extremadura, University Avenue, s/n CP: 10003 Cáceres, Spain; vtororom@alumnos.unex.es (V.T.); ignbs.1991@gmail.com (I.B.); diegomun@unex.es (D.M.); mmaynar@unex.es (M.M.)
* Correspondence: gbarrientosvi@upsa.es; Tel.: +34-923-125-027

Received: 25 July 2020; Accepted: 10 August 2020; Published: 12 August 2020

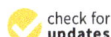

Abstract: The aim of this study was to determine the possible changes in plasma of several hormones such as Luteinizing Hormone, Testosterone, Cortisol and Insulin in endurance runners during the sports season. Twenty-one high-level male endurance runners (22 ± 3.2 years, 1.77 ± 0.05 m) participated in the study. Basal plasma hormones were measured at four moments during the season (initial, 3, 6 and 9 months), and were analyzed using ELISA (enzyme-linked immunosorbent assay). Testosterone and Luteinizing Hormone (LH) suffered very significant decreases ($p < 0.01$) at 3 months compared with the beginning and an increase ($p < 0.05$) at 6 and 9 months compared with 3 months. Insulin level was significantly lower ($p < 0.05$) at 3, 6 and 9 months compared with the initial test. Insulin and cortisol were associated inversely ($r = 0.363$; $\beta = -0.577$; $p = 0.017$) and positively ($r = 0.202$; $\beta = 0.310$; $p = 0.043$), respectively, with the amount of km per week performed by the runners. There was a significant association between km covered at a higher intensity than the anaerobic threshold and I ($r = 0.580$; $\beta = -0.442$; $p = 0.000$). Our findings indicate that testosterone, LH and insulin were more sensitive to changes in training volume and intensity than cortisol in high-level endurance runners. Basal testosterone and LH concentrations decrease in athletes who perform a high volume of aerobic km in situations of low energy availability.

Keywords: hormones; LH; testosterone; cortisol; insulin; athletes

1. Introduction

Endurance athletes modulate the volume and intensity of their constant training throughout the sports season in order to produce adaptations and achieve their best performance in previously established competitive periods [1]. This exercise causes stress in the organism that induces important changes in the endocrine system to recover the initial homeostasis [2].

Cortisol (C) is the main glucocorticoid of the organism, its secretion is produced in the adrenal glands and it is controlled through a negative feedback mechanism by the hypothalamus–pituitary–adrenal axis [3]. It is a hormone modulated by circadian rhythms, but factors such as mental stress, dehydration or food can alter its production [4]. In endurance activities, its blood values increase, as its catabolic function contributes to maintaining adequate energy levels through protein degradation, hydrolysis of triglycerides and even adding additional energy from carbohydrates through gluconeogenesis in the liver [5]. At the end of physical activity, the concentrations of this hormone begin to decrease, and it may take up to 48 h to recover its basal values after maximum effort [6].

Testosterone (T) is an anabolic hormone that participates in multiple physiological functions, intervenes in muscle protein synthesis, stimulates bone remodeling and erythropoiesis [7] and regulates the function of lactate transporter proteins thus promoting lactate oxidation as a fuel during exercise [8]. T is secreted by the Leydig cells in the testicles and its concentration in blood is controlled by the hypothalamic–pituitary–testicular (HPT) axis [9]. It has been reported that athletes who undergo long-term continuous training may have reduced levels of chronic basal T, status defined as "Exercise-Hipogonadal Male Condition" [10]. Previous studies have shown that its low levels would be caused by the negative relationship between C and T [11,12]. Hackney, Szczepanowska and Viru have hypothesized whether this inhibition would be caused by a dysfunction of the axis at the peripheral level, through direct inhibition of the Leydig cells in the testicles, or at the central level, reducing the release of Luteinizing Hormone (LH) in the pituitary that would affect the production of T at the testicular level [13].

LH is secreted in the anterior pituitary gland. LH is part of a pathway comprising the hypothalamus, pituitary gland, and gonads [14]. The release of LH is stimulated by gonadotropin-releasing hormone (GnRH) [15]. After acute physical exercise, LH usually decreases [16,17]. During the training phases, a reduction in LH secretion was found in runners [18].

The T/C ratio is a variable that relates to the anabolic/catabolic balance in athletes and is widely used for monitoring and evaluating the body's response to chronic exercise-induced stress [19]. Authors such as Meeusen et al. [20] think that the ratio cannot be used as a means of control since they reported studies where decreases of 30% of the ratio did not always worsen the athletes' performance.

Another important hormone involved during physical exercise is insulin (I), related to energy balance and blood glucose control [21]. Horton, Grunwald, Lavely and Donahoo reported a decrease in plasma I concentration during exercise, followed by an increase during the hours after exercise to favor glycogen repletion, a decrease in carbohydrate oxidation, and an increase in fat oxidation [22]. Aerobic endurance athletes have lower baseline values and higher insulin sensitivity than sedentary subjects to support fatty acid oxidation [23].

In summary, hormones have been defined as important mediators in the body's response and adaptations to exercise-induced stress. Their acute responses to different stimuli and their modifications over short periods have been extensively investigated [24,25]. However, few studies have shown hormonal changes in high-level endurance runners during a sports season, so the aim of this study was to determine the baseline values of T, C, LH and I and their changes throughout a sports season where training loads are modulated to obtain several peaks of performance.

2. Materials and Methods

2.1. Participants

The athletes were studied every three months at four moments during an athletic season. The measures were made during the first week of October, January, April and July. Athletes were informed of the purpose of the study and signed an informed consent form prior to enrolment. A code was assigned to each participant for the collection and treatment of the samples in order to maintain their anonymity. This research was carried out under the Helsinki Declaration ethical guidelines, updated at the World Medical Assembly in Fortaleza (Brazil) in 2013 for research with human subjects, and the Ethics Committee of the University of Extremadura approved the protocol (52/2012).

Twenty-one high-level aerobic male runners (22 ± 3.2 years, 1.77 ± 0.05 m) participated in the present survey, all of them were living in the area of Caceres (Spain), at a latitude of 39° 28' 35.36" N. Each athlete had at least five years of training experience, and all of them were participants in national and international tournaments (1500 and 5000 m race modalities). All subjects were required to have a stable body weight throughout the sports season (no weight changes >3%). Significant changes in fat mass and fat-free mass (FFM) are associated with circulating T concentrations due to their role in energy metabolism and adipogenesis [26]. The participants did not take regular medication, anti-inflammatory medications or nutritional supplementation during the two weeks prior to the measurements. None of the subjects had taken hormonal medication in the previous year or during the study since any high-level athlete is obliged to conform to drug testing in competition or out of competition.

2.2. Nutritional Evaluation

All participants were instructed to complete a 3-day diet record, including one weekend day and two weekdays, on the provided nutritional questionnaire; each participant weighed and indicated the amount in grams of each food consumed. The athletes' dietary intakes were obtained using a food composition table [27].

2.3. Anthropometrics Measurements

Subjects reported to the laboratory after an overnight fast and had to abstain from hard training and/or competition for at least 72 h before testing. The participants' morphological characteristics were measured in the morning and always at the same time (09:00 a.m.). Body height was measured to the nearest 0.1 cm using a wall-mounted stadiometer (Seca©, Hamburg, Germany), and body weight was measured to the nearest 0.01 kg using calibrated electronic digital scales, (Seca©, Hamburg, Germany) in barefoot conditions. Fat mass and fat-free mass content was estimated from the sum of 6 skinfolds ($\Sigma 6$) (abdominal, suprailiac, tricipital and subscapularis, thigh and calf). Skinfold thicknesses were measured with a Harpenden caliper (Holtain Skinfold Caliper, Crosswell, UK) and converted to % of body fat using the equations of Jackson and Pollock [28]. All measurements were made by the same operator, accredited in kinanthropometric techniques (level 1), in accordance with the International Society for the Advancement of Kinanthropometry (ISAK) recommendations [29].

2.4. Exercise Test until Exhaustion

A running test on a treadmill (Powerjoc, UK) equipped with a gas analyzer (Metamax, Cortex Biophysik Gmbh, Germany) and a Polar pulsometer (Polar Vantage M, Norway) was used to evaluate the maximum oxygen uptake (VO_2 max). All the tests were performed between 10 and 12 a.m. Exercise test consisted of a 10 min warm-up at 10 km/h followed by incremental runs until voluntary exhaustion, starting at 10 km/h and increasing it by 1 km/h every 400 m, with a stable slope of 1%. During the incremental test, VO_2 max was determined according to the following criteria: the respiratory exchange ratio (RER) had to exceed 1; stabilization in oxygen uptake (VO_2) together with an increment in carbon dioxide (CO_2) elimination and in the ventilatory volume (VE), induced by the increases in the test velocity.

After recording the test data, the ventilatory thresholds were determined according to the three-phase model to monitor training [30]. The data were obtained at the aerobic threshold (VT_1) and the anaerobic threshold (VT_2) to determine training load intensity.

2.5. Training Characteristics

Figure 1 details the timeline of periodization and testing during the season. Athletes had a four-week adaptation before the initial measurement (October), where they performed 85.71 ± 13.62 km per week and a four-week transition period after the second competitive period. The first preparatory period began in October through December and the second one during March through May. Competitive periods were coincident with January and February when the athletes performed cross country competitions (10,000–12,000 m approximately), and the second competitive period was in June-July when they performed track and field competitions between 1500 and 5000 m. A GPS pack equipped with pulsometers (Polar Vantage M. Norway) was used to track the training loads during the season.

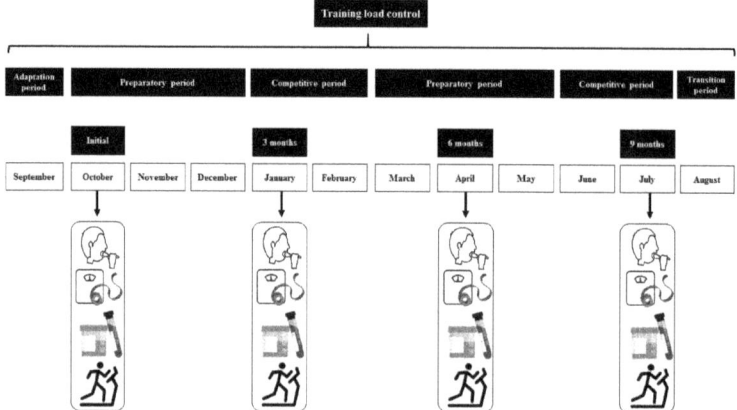

Figure 1. Periodization and testing during the season.

Table 1 summarizes training characteristics in the athletes. In addition, they performed two weekly sessions of resistance training during the whole athletics season. In general, the volume of the training was high (3 sets of 8–12 repetitions of whole-body exercises) while the intensity was low-moderate (30–70% of 1RM) depending on the period of the season.

Table 1. Training characteristics in the athletes during the season.

Training Load	Initial	3 Months	6 Months	9 Months
Total (km/week)	85.71 ± 13.62	105.9 ± 16.85	93.33 ± 14.34	74.76 ± 14.09
>VT$_2$ (km/week)	4.29 ± 0.68	12.71 ± 2.02	18.67 ± 2.86	16.45 ± 3.10
<VT$_2$ (km/week)	81.43 ± 12.94	93.24 ± 14.83	74.67 ± 11.47	58.31 ± 10.99

VT$_2$: anaerobic threshold; >VT$_2$: intensity above anaerobic threshold; <VT$_2$: intensity below anaerobic threshold.

2.6. Sample Collection

Always at nine o'clock in the morning, to limit the impact of circadian rhythms on hormonal concentrations, after weighing the participants, ten milliliters of antecubital venous blood was drawn from each participant. Venous blood samples were obtained using EDTA as anticoagulant. Blood was immediately centrifuged at 3000 rpm during 10 min (P-selecta, MEDITRONIC) using a plastic syringe with a stainless-steel needle. The blood sample was collected in a polypropylene tube. Then, the blood sample was centrifuged at 3000 rpm for 15 min at room temperature (23 ± 1 °C) to separate plasma from erythrocytes. Plasma was placed in sterile tubes and stored at −80 °C until use.

2.7. Analytical Determination

The hormone determination was carried out using the ELISA (enzyme-linked immunosorbent assay) with an ER-500 (Sinnowa, Germany), using the commercial tests for I, C, T and LH. All hormonal measurements were performed by the same technician and were made with duplicate determination. Between and within coefficients of variation for all assays were less than 10% for all biochemical analyses.

2.8. Statistical Analysis

The statistical analysis was carried out with IBM SPSS Statistic software version 21.0 (IBM Co., Armonk, NY, USA). The results are expressed as x ± s, where x is the mean values and s is the standard deviation. All variables used in the study were checked for normality of distribution before the analyses (Kolmogorov–Smirnov tests). The data were analyzed by repeated measurements analysis of variance (ANOVA) with the Bonferroni post hoc test for moment/period as the categorical variable.

Partial eta squared (η_p^2) was used as an effect size measure of ANOVA. Threshold values for assessing magnitudes of standardized effects were $\eta_p^2 \geq 0.01$, $\eta_p^2 \geq 0.06$ and $\eta_p^2 \geq 0.14$ for small, medium and large, respectively [31]. The equality of variances between the differences was assessed with Mauchly's test of sphericity. When sphericity was violated, Greenhouse–Geisser corrected p-values were used. Simple linear regression analysis was conducted to examine the associations between hormones and km trained per week. A $p \leq 0.05$ was considered statistically significant.

3. Results

Table 2 shows ergospirometric and body composition variables in the runners during the season. In our study, VO$_2$ max, VT$_2$, RER, heart rate maximum (HRM), fat mass, fat-free mass and Σ6 skinfolds did not show significant changes during the season. Weight suffered significant decreases ($p < 0.05$) at 6 and 9 months compared with initial values.

Table 2. Ergospirometric and body composition parameters in the athletes during the season.

Parameters	Initial	3 Months	6 Months	9 Months	η_p^2
VO$_2$ max (mL/min/kg)	68.12 ± 4.63	67.53 ± 9.54	68.55 ± 6.97	68.60 ± 7.36	0.05
VT$_2$ (% VO$_2$ max.)	91.02 ± 2.43	92.43 ± 3.59	91.02 ± 3.08	90.96 ± 2.07	0.06
RER	1.05 ± 0.03	1.05 ± 0.04	1.05 ± 0.05	1.04 ± 0.04	0.01
HR maximum	190.4 ± 9.48	193.1 ± 7.80	193.5 ± 9.06	193.8 ± 7.19	0.04
Weight (kg)	65.50 ± 7.30	65.45 ± 7.36	64.67 ± 7.03 *	64.80 ± 7.34 *	0.07
Fat mass (%)	8.18 ± 1.04	8.23 ± 1.04	8.19 ± 1.29	8.21 ± 1.07	0.04
Fat-free mass (kg)	60.15 ± 6.70	60.07 ± 6.75	59.38 ± 6.45	59.48 ± 6.73	0.02
Σ6 skinfold (mm)	45.65 ± 10.88	46.49 ± 10.69	44.92 ± 8.16	45.37 ± 9.11	0.03

VO$_2$ max: maximum oxygen uptake; VT$_2$: ventilatory anaerobic threshold; HR maximum: heart rate maximum; Σ6: sum of 6 skinfolds * $p < 0.05$ initial vs. 3/6/9 months; η_p^2: partial eta squared.

Nutritional intake of the athletes during the season is shown in Table 3. The athletes followed a diet using established energy and macronutrient guidelines for adequate athletic performance [32]. Energy availability (EA) is defined as the amount of energy intake (kcal day^{-1}) −exercise energy expenditure (kcal day^{-1})] /FFM. An appropriate energy balance equates to ≥45 calories per day per kg of FFM (kcal/kg/FFM/d) [33].

Table 3. Nutritional intake.

Parameters	Initial	3 Months	6 Months	9 Months
Energy (kcal/d)	2855.21 ± 511.32	2515.48 ± 427.18	2902.37 ± 522.62	3108.78 ± 770.12
EA (kcal/kg/FFM/d)	43.58 ± 4.32	41.87 ± 3.15	48.88 ± 5.63	52.26 ± 4.87
HC (g/kg/d)	5.26 ± 1.21	5.18 ± 1.14	6.25 ± 1.38	6.13 ± 1.50
Proteins (g/kg/d)	1.73 ± 0.79	1.69 ± 0.35	1.85 ± 0.53	1.89 ± 0.63
Lipids (g/kg/d)	1.78 ± 0.40	1.63 ± 0.28	1.58 ± 0.52	1.72 ± 0.74

HC: carbohydrates; FFM: fat-free mass; EA: energy availability.

Plasmatic concentrations of hormones are shown in Table 4.

Table 4. Hormonal changes during the season.

Parameters	Initial	3 Months	6 Months	9 Months	η_p^2
Insulin (μIU/mL)	10.25 ± 7.99	7.81 ± 6.15 **	7.62 ± 5.50 **	9.89 ± 5.32 *	0.51
LH (mIU/mL)	8.85 ± 4.10	6.30 ± 2.86 **	7.59 ± 2.32 #	7.95 ± 3.49 #	0.29
Testosterone (ng/mL)	6.59 ± 0.92	5.83 ± 1.10 **	6.72 ± 0.94 #	7.01 ± 1.50 #	0.32
Cortisol (ng/mL)	89.26 ± 21.85	91.41 ± 27.32	98.06 ± 31.28	103.9 ± 38.04	0.05
T/C	0.07 ± 0.01	0.06 ± 0.02	0.07 ± 0.02	0.07 ± 0.02	0.03

LH: luteinizing hormone; T: testosterone; C: cortisol; * $p < 0.05$ differences between initial vs. 3/6/9 months; ** $p < 0.01$ differences between initial vs. 3/6/9 months; # $p < 0.05$ differences between 3 months vs. 6/9 months; η_p^2: partial eta squared.

Analysis of the data revealed changes in plasmatic concentrations of total T, LH and I during the sports season. T and LH suffered very significant decreases ($p < 0.01$) at 3 months compared with the initial test, and an increase ($p < 0.05$) at 6 and 9 months compared with 3 months. I concentrations were significantly lower at 3, 6 ($p < 0.01$) and 9 ($p < 0.05$) months compared with the initial test (Figure 2). There were no statistical differences in plasmatic C concentration and T/C ratio during the athletic season.

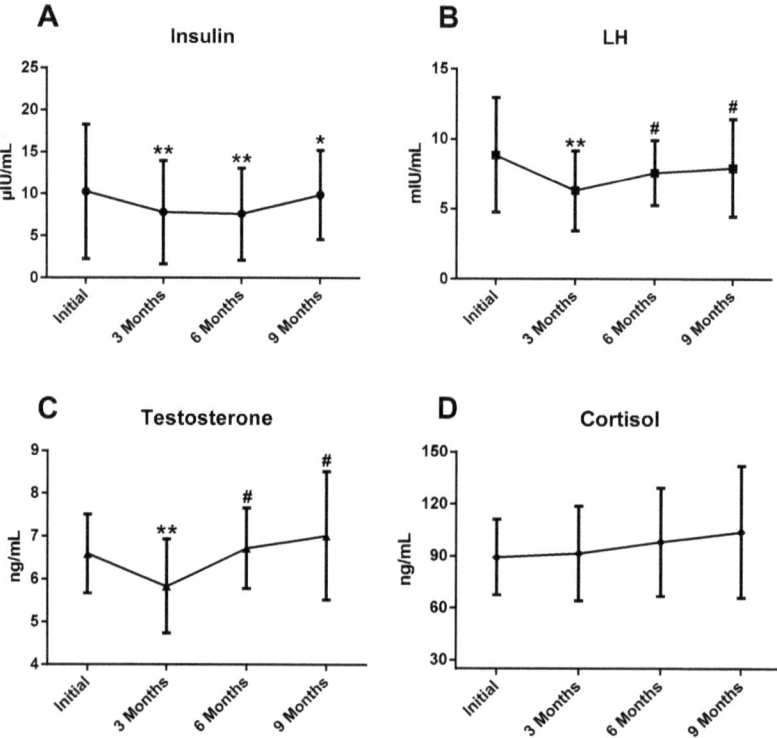

Figure 2. This figure shows the key findings. (**A**) Insulin changes during season; (**B**) LH changes during season; (**C**) testosterone changes during season; (**D**) cortisol changes during season; LH: luteinizing hormone; * $p < 0.05$ differences between initial vs. 3/6/9 months; ** $p < 0.01$ differences between initial vs. 3/6/9 months; # $p < 0.05$ differences between 3 months vs. 6/9 months.

Simple linear regressions between the plasmatic hormones and km trained are shown in Tables 5 and 6. Plasmatic concentrations of I and C were inversely (r = 0.363; β = −0.577; p = 0.017) and positively (r = 0.202; β = 0.310; p = 0.043) associated, respectively, with the amount of km trained per week.

Table 5. Simple linear regression between the plasmatic concentration of hormones and total km trained.

Hormones	β (95% CI)	SE	r	R²	p
Insulin	−0.577 (−0.984/0.030)	0.255	0.363	0.142	0.017
LH	−1.105 (−2.769/−0.440)	0.585	0.113	0.025	0.302
Testosterone	−2.145 (−5.247/−3.543)	1.109	0.131	0.028	0.213
Cortisol	0.310 (−0.124/0.544)	0.167	0.202	0.075	0.043

LH: luteinizing hormone; β: beta coefficient; SE: standard error; CI: confidence interval; R^2: coefficient of determination; r: Pearson's coefficient of correlation; p: p value.

Table 6. Simple linear regression between the plasmatic concentration of hormones and km trained with intensity higher than VT_2.

Hormones	β (95% CI)	SE	r	R^2	p
Insulin	−0.442 (−0.579/−0.306)	0.069	0.580	0.336	0.000
LH	−0.320 (−0.707/0.068)	0.195	0.178	0.032	0.104
Testosterone	0.276 (−0.812/1.364)	3.638	0.056	0.003	0.615
Cortisol	0.238 (−0.004/0.081)	2.150	0.193	0.037	0.079

LH: luteinizing hormone; β: beta coefficient; SE: standard error; CI: confidence interval; R^2: coefficient of determination; r: Pearson's coefficient of correlation; p: p value.

There was a significant association between km trained at a higher intensity than VT_2 and I (r = −0.580; β = −0.442; p = 0.000).

4. Discussion

The purpose of our longitudinal study was to observe the changes in plasma basal concentrations of LH, T, C and I in high-level endurance runners, as well as the possible changes that occur during a sports season in relation to the training performed.

VO_2 max and VT_2 did not show significant changes during the season in our athletes. High values of VO_2 max are required in endurance athletes, although it is not a determinant variable among homogeneous groups [34]. Body composition and running economy are other variables related to performance in endurance runners [35,36].

The findings of this research agree with those observed in other studies in which they found that training throughout a sports season produces adaptations in the endocrine system with the aim of improving the athletes' performance [2]. The basal concentrations of the different hormones in the study showed significant changes during the sports season although they remained within the normal reference values for humans [37,38].

C did not suffer significant changes during the season, since athletes were examined in the laboratory without having carried out intense exercise the previous days. Mäestu, Jürimäe and Jürimäe reported that C did not change when training volume was increased [39]. In our study, C showed a positive association with the volume of km performed per week. Purge, Jürimäe and Jürimäe also observed a significant relation between C and mean training volume in elite male rowers [40]. It is known that during long-term aerobic exercise hypercortisolemia occurs which contributes to maintaining adequate energy levels during training [9]. The C prevents the re-esterification of fatty acids released by the catecholamine-induced lipolysis [41]. The activation of catabolic processes is an essential tool for adaptation in high-stress conditions [42].

Cortisol is usually elevated in energy-deficient conditions. Increases in cortisol circulation have been observed in studies of severe caloric restriction or fasting [43]. As mentioned above, during endurance exercise C concentrations increase, and previous studies have reported an inhibitory effect of C on T synthesis [9,44] that could interfere with athletes' recovery and performance, since it participates in protein synthesis and erythropoiesis [45], and could even negatively affect their health due to low bone mineral density and infertility [10].

It has been reported that chronic endurance training may have negative effects on the basal concentration of T, which leads to chronic low levels of this hormone as a consequence of the accumulation of aerobic training over years [46]. In our research, athletes suffered a significant decrease in basal T levels at 3 months accompanied by a significant decrease in LH, a fact that would indicate that there is an alteration of the HPT axis at the central level, decreasing the secretion of GnRH from the hypothalamus that would affect the release of LH and, consequently, the Leydig cells would not be stimulated for T synthesis [47,48]. This could be caused by the fact that in this period the runners trained the highest volume of km per week of the entire season, which forced them to carry out longer training sessions with less recovery between sessions that would promote maintaining high concentrations of C during this phase. MacConnie [48] reported a decrease in LH pulse frequency in highly trained runners. Several studies have reported a negative relationship between T concentrations and high volumes of aerobic training, where the HPT axis is altered in runners who performed more than 100 km/week as occurred with our athletes [49,50]. Flynn et al., observed a decrease in T after the training volume had been increased by 88% for two weeks in swimmers [51].

However, in a recent review suggesting that running mileage alone is not enough to predict the low T concentrations [52], it was proposed that the alterations in the endocrine–reproductive hormonal system observed in endurance runners are related to the development of low energy availability (LEA) [33]. In healthy and active women, it has been established that an adequate energy intake is ≥45 kcal/kg FFM [53]; whether intake in men is similar is currently under debate [52]. In our study, runners reported an energy intake lower than 45 kcal/kg FFM initially and especially at 3 months, a period when the runners ran more km/week, and basal T and LH concentrations were the lowest of the season. De Souza [53] concluded that it is difficult to consume the energy required by athletes who perform chronic strenuous exercise, resulting in an energy deficit that causes alterations in the hypothalamic- pituitary- gonadal axis.

Another factor that could contribute to the decrease in basal T values is the variation in the annual circadian rhythms that this hormone suffers from as a consequence of exposure to the sun, thus, higher peak concentrations have been verified during the summer months, and lower levels during the winter as occurred in our research, since the third month of the study corresponded to the month of January in our region [54]. Low circulating vitamin D concentrations have been associated with a lower total T concentration [55]. Lombardi et al. [56] confirmed the importance of sun exposure and solar irradiance in the vitamin D and T concentrations in professional soccer players during two sports seasons, also, significant correlations between vitamin D and T were reported.

In the second part of the season, at 6 and 9 months, we observed an increase in the basal concentrations of T and LH. It seems that hormonal changes as a consequence of LEA are reversible when the subjects have adequate energy available [57], as occurred in the runners of our study when they performed less km/week and they had adequate energy intake. In addition, the target competitions to be carried out in these periods were shorter distances and higher intensities (maximum 16 min), where the athletes trained less km per week and with greater intensity (more weekly sessions >VT_2). Previous studies have reported that high-intensity training produces an increase in T [11,58], which could be a consequence of the large reduction in night time C concentrations that occur during these training sessions compared to aerobic training [59]. T could play an essential role in muscle metabolism during the tapering phase [39,60]. T seems to increase the ability of the muscle to refill its glycogen stores through increased activity of muscle glycogen synthetase [61].

This would be very important for adequate regeneration after prolonged exercise and during intensive training periods [62]. Other factors mentioned above are important, such as the annual variation suffered by this hormone; the measures taken at 6 and 9 months correspond to the months of April and July, respectively, where there are more hours of sun exposure and solar irradiance, during those periods which could have favored the increase in vitamin D concentrations and basal T concentrations [63].

As for the I, there was a decrease in its basal values with respect to the initial ones throughout the season, more visible in the periods of greater volume of km trained, also, remarkable negative associations were revealed with the number of km trained per week. Jürimäe, Purge and Jürimäe [64] reported an inverse correlation between I and training volume in elite rowers ($r = -0.399$, $p < 0.05$). Other study reported a significantly lowered maximal exercise-induced level of I [41]. Reduced insulin levels have been observed in energy-deficient athletes [43].

During prolonged training, the I level decreases because the catecholamine increase inhibits the I secretion [65]. This phenomenon could favor glucose homeostasis with increased glucose availability for the central nervous system [41]. It has been widely reported that training improves insulin sensitivity [66], which can be considered a positive adaptation produced in runners to enhance the use of fatty acids as fuel [23]. Previous studies with athletes have reported a decrease in the plasma

I concentration during exercise, followed by an increase during the hours after the end of exercise, in that time there is a decrease in the oxidation of carbohydrates and an increase in the oxidation of fats to favor the repletion of glycogen [22].

The small number of participants and the absence of control of I sensitivity are limitations of the present study. Basal vitamin D concentrations could not be analyzed during the season to observe its circannual rhythm and the possible relationship with the hours of sun and its irradiation. Using Dual-energy X-ray absorptiometry (DXA) or Bioelectrical Impedance Analysis (BIA) are methods that could provide more accurate data on the body composition of subjects (fat mass and fat-free mass) that would have allowed a better assessment of changes in muscle mass and its relationship with dietary intake and hormonal concentrations. Blood samples were not drawn for lactate collection during the treadmill running test.

5. Conclusions

Our findings indicate that basal concentrations of T, LH and I in endurance runners are modified throughout the sports season as a consequence of the different training loads, volume and intensity of km they perform per week and energy availability.

In summary, runners who train with a high volume of aerobic km achieve adaptations in the endocrine system, although performing this training with low energy availability causes decreases in basal LH and T concentrations.

Author Contributions: Conceptualization, M.M. methodology, M.M.; formal analysis, M.M., I.B., V.T. and G.B.; data curation, M.M. and V.T.; writing—original draft preparation, J.A., G.B. and D.M.; writing—review and editing, M.M., J.A. and G.B.; All authors have read and agreed to the published version of the manuscript.

Funding: This research did not receive any specific grant from funding agencies in the public, commercial, or not-for-profit sectors.

Acknowledgments: The authors gratefully acknowledge the collaboration of athletes.

Conflicts of Interest: The authors declare no conflict of interest.

References

1. Zinner, C.; Wahl, P.; Achtzehn, S.; Reed, J.L.; Mester, J. Acute hormonal responses before and after 2 weeks of HIT in well trained junior triathletes. *Int. J. Sports Med.* **2014**, *35*, 316–322. [CrossRef]
2. Hackney, A.C.; Lane, A.R. Exercise and the regulation of endocrine hormones. In *Molecular and Cellular Regulation of Adaptation to Exercise*; Bouchard, C., Ed.; Elsevier Academic Press: San Diego, CA, USA, 2015; Volume 135, pp. 293–311, ISBN 1877-1173.
3. Brownlee, K.K.; Moore, A.W.; Hackney, A.C. Relationship between circulating cortisol and testosterone: Influence of physical exercise. *J. Sports Sci. Med.* **2005**, *4*, 76.
4. Duclos, M.; Tabarin, A. Exercise, training, and the hypothalamo–pituitary–adrenal axis. In *Hormone Use and Abuse by Athletes*; Springer: Boston, MA, USA, 2011; pp. 9–15.
5. Viru, A.; Viru, M. Cortisol-essential adaptation hormone in exercise. *Int. J. Sports Med.* **2004**, *25*, 461–464. [CrossRef] [PubMed]
6. Anderson, T.; Lane, A.R.; Hackney, A.C. Cortisol and testosterone dynamics following exhaustive endurance exercise. *Eur. J. Appl. Physiol.* **2016**, *116*, 1503–1509. [CrossRef]
7. Zitzmann, M.; Nieschlag, E. Testosterone levels in healthy men and the relation to behavioural and physical characteristics: Facts and constructs. *Eur. J. Endocrinol.* **2001**, *144*, 183–197. [CrossRef]
8. Enoki, T.; Yoshida, Y.; Lally, J.; Hatta, H.; Bonen, A. Testosterone increases lactate transport, monocarboxylate transporter (MCT) 1 and MCT4 in rat skeletal muscle. *J. Physiol.* **2006**, *577*, 433–443. [CrossRef] [PubMed]
9. Daly, W.; Seegers, C.A.; Rubin, D.A.; Dobridge, J.D.; Hackney, A.C. Relationship between stress hormones and testosterone with prolonged endurance exercise. *Eur. J. Appl. Physiol.* **2005**, *93*, 375–380. [CrossRef] [PubMed]
10. Hackney, A.C. Effects of endurance exercise on the reproductive system of men: The "exercise-hypogonadal male condition". *J. Endocrinol. Investig.* **2008**, *31*, 932–938. [CrossRef]

11. Cumming, D.C.; Quigley, M.E.; Yen, S.S.C. Acute suppression of circulating testosterone levels by cortisol in men. *J. Clin. Endocrinol. Metab.* **1983**, *57*, 671–673. [CrossRef]
12. Vervoorn, C.; Quist, A.M.; Vermulst, L.J.M.; Erich, W.B.M.; De Vries, W.R.; Thijssen, J.H.H. The behaviour of the plasma free testosterone/cortisol ratio during a season of elite rowing training. *Int. J. Sports Med.* **1991**, *12*, 257–263. [CrossRef]
13. Hackney, A.C.; Szczepanowska, E.; Viru, A.M. Basal testicular testosterone production in endurance-trained men is suppressed. *Eur. J. Appl. Physiol.* **2003**, *89*, 198–201. [CrossRef]
14. Raju, G.A.R.; Chavan, R.; Deenadayal, M.; Gunasheela, D.; Gutgutia, R.; Haripriya, G.; Govindarajan, M.; Patel, N.H.; Patki, A.S. Luteinizing hormone and follicle stimulating hormone synergy: A review of role in controlled ovarian hyper-stimulation. *J. Hum. Reprod. Sci.* **2013**, *6*, 227. [CrossRef] [PubMed]
15. Millar, R.P.; Lu, Z.-L.; Pawson, A.J.; Flanagan, C.A.; Morgan, K.; Maudsley, S.R. Gonadotropin-releasing hormone receptors. *Endocr. Rev.* **2004**, *25*, 235–275. [CrossRef]
16. An, E.; Wilson, A. Exercise and gonadal function. *Hum. Reprod.* **1993**, *8*, 1747–1761.
17. Elias, A.N.; Wilson, A.F.; Pandian, M.R.; Chune, G.; Utsumi, A.; Kayaleh, R.; Stone, S.C. Corticotropin releasing hormone and gonadotropin secretion in physically active males after acute exercise. *Eur. J. Appl. Physiol. Occup. Physiol.* **1991**, *62*, 171–174. [CrossRef]
18. Lehmann, M.; Gastmann, U.; Petersen, K.G.; Bachl, N.; Seidel, A.; Khalaf, A.N.; Fischer, S.; Keul, J. Training-overtraining: Performance, and hormone levels, after a defined increase in training volume versus intensity in experienced middle-and long-distance runners. *Br. J. Sports Med.* **1992**, *26*, 233–242. [CrossRef] [PubMed]
19. De Luccia, T. Use of the testosterone/cortisol ratio variable in sports. *Open Sports Sci. J.* **2016**, *9*, 104–113. [CrossRef]
20. Meeusen, R.; Duclos, M.; Foster, C.; Fry, A.; Gleeson, M.; Nieman, D.; Raglin, J.; Rietjens, G.; Steinacker, J.; Urhausen, A. Prevention, diagnosis, and treatment of the overtraining syndrome: Joint consensus statement of the European College of Sport Science and the American College of Sports Medicine. *Med. Sci. Sports Exerc.* **2013**, *45*, 186. [CrossRef]
21. Comitato, R.; Saba, A.; Turrini, A.; Arganini, C.; Virgili, F. Sex hormones and macronutrient metabolism. *Crit. Rev. Food Sci. Nutr.* **2015**, *55*, 227–241. [CrossRef]
22. Horton, T.J.; Grunwald, G.K.; Lavely, J.; Donahoo, W.T. Glucose kinetics differ between women and men, during and after exercise. *J. Appl. Physiol.* **2006**, *100*, 1883–1894. [CrossRef]
23. Goodpaster, B.H.; He, J.; Watkins, S.; Kelley, D.E. Skeletal muscle lipid content and insulin resistance: Evidence for a paradox in endurance-trained athletes. *J. Clin. Endocrinol. Metab.* **2001**, *86*, 5755–5761. [CrossRef] [PubMed]
24. Popovic, B.; Popovic, D.; Macut, D.; Antic, I.B.; Isailovic, T.; Ognjanovic, S.; Bogavac, T.; Kovacevic, V.E.; Ilic, D.; Petrovic, M. Acute Response to Endurance Exercise Stress: Focus on Catabolic/Anabolic Interplay Between Cortisol, Testosterone, and Sex Hormone Binding Globulin in Professional Athletes. *J. Med. Biochem.* **2019**, *38*, 6–12. [PubMed]
25. Wahl, P.; Mathes, S.; Köhler, K.; Achtzehn, S.; Bloch, W.; Mester, J. Acute metabolic, hormonal, and psychological responses to different endurance training protocols. *Horm. Metab. Res.* **2013**, *45*, 827–833. [CrossRef] [PubMed]
26. Yassin, A.A.; Doros, G. Testosterone therapy in hypogonadal men results in sustained and clinically meaningful weight loss. *Clin. Obes.* **2013**, *3*, 73–83. [CrossRef] [PubMed]
27. Moreiras, O. *Tablas de Composición de Alimentos*, 16th ed.; Pirámide: Madrid, Spain, 2013.
28. Jackson, A.S.; Pollock, M.L. Practical Assessment of Body Composition. *Phys. Sportsmed.* **1985**, *13*, 76–90. [CrossRef]
29. Stewart, A.; Marfell-Jones, M.; Olds, T.; de Ridder, H. *International Standards for Anthropometric Assessment*; ISAK: Lower Hutt, New Zealand, 2011.
30. Skinner, J.S.; Mclellan, T.H.; McLellan, T.H. The Transition from Aerobic to Anaerobic Metabolism. *Res. Q. Exerc. Sport* **1980**, *51*, 234–248. [CrossRef]
31. Cohen, J. *Statistical Power Analysis for the Behavioral Sciences*; Routledge Academic: New York, NY, USA, 1988.

32. Rodriguez, N.R.; DiMarco, N.M.; Langley, S.; American Dietetic Association; Dietitians of Canada; American College of Sports Medicine: Nutrition and Athletic Performance. Position of the American Dietetic Association, Dietitians of Canada, and the American College of Sports Medicine: Nutrition and Athletic Performance. *J. Am. Diet. Assoc.* **2009**, *109*, 509–527. [CrossRef]
33. Dipla, K.; Kraemer, R.R.; Constantini, N.W.; Hackney, A.C. Relative energy deficiency in sports (RED-S): Elucidation of endocrine changes affecting the health of males and females. *Hormones* **2020**. [CrossRef]
34. Basset, F.A.; Chouinard, R.; Boulay, M.R. Training profile counts for time-to-exhaustion performance. *Can. J. Appl. Physiol.* **2003**, *28*, 654–666. [CrossRef]
35. Berg, K. Endurance training and performance in runners—Research limitations and unanswered questions. *Sports Med.* **2003**, *33*, 59–73. [CrossRef]
36. Rabadán, M.; Díaz, V.; Calderón, F.J.; Benito, P.J.; Peinado, A.B.; Maffulli, N. Physiological determinants of speciality of elite middle- and long-distance runners. *J. Sports Sci.* **2011**, *29*, 975–982. [CrossRef] [PubMed]
37. Hackney, A.; Sinning, W.E.; Bruot, B.C. Reproductive hormonal profiles of endurance-trained and untrained males. *Med. Sci. Sports Exerc.* **1988**, *20*, 60–65. [CrossRef] [PubMed]
38. Volek, J.S.; Ratamess, N.A.; Rubin, M.R.; Gomez, A.L.; French, D.N.; McGuigan, M.M.; Scheett, T.P.; Sharman, M.J.; Häkkinen, K.; Kraemer, W.J. The effects of creatine supplementation on muscular performance and body composition responses to short-term resistance training overreaching. *Eur. J. Appl. Physiol.* **2004**, *91*, 628–637. [CrossRef] [PubMed]
39. Mäestu, J.; Jürimäe, J.; Jürimäe, T. Hormonal reactions during heavy training stress and following tapering in highly trained male rowers. *Horm. Metab. Res.* **2003**, *35*, 109–113. [CrossRef]
40. Purge, P.; Jürimäe, J.; Jürimäe, T. Hormonal and psychological adaptation in elite male rowers during prolonged training. *J. Sports Sci.* **2006**, *24*, 1075–1082. [CrossRef]
41. Urhausen, A.; Gabriel, H.; Kindermann, W. Blood hormones as markers of training stress and overtraining. *Sports Med.* **1995**, *20*, 251–276. [CrossRef]
42. Petibois, C.; Cazorla, G.; Deleris, G. The biological and metabolic adaptations to 12 months training in elite rowers. *Int. J. Sports Med.* **2003**, *24*, 36–42. [CrossRef]
43. Elliott-Sale, K.J.; Tenforde, A.S.; Parziale, A.L.; Holtzman, B.; Ackerman, K.E. Endocrine effects of relative energy deficiency in sport. *Int. J. Sport Nutr. Exerc. Metab.* **2018**, *28*, 335–349. [CrossRef]
44. Lane, A.R.; Anderson, T.; Hackney, A.C. Relationship Between Cortisol and Free Testosterone in Response to Exhaustive Endurance Exercise. *Age* **2015**, *22*, 19–28.
45. Shahani, S.; Braga-Basaria, M.; Maggio, M.; Basaria, S. Androgens and erythropoiesis: Past and present. *J. Endocrinol. Investig.* **2009**, *32*, 704–716. [CrossRef]
46. Hackney, A.C.; Lane, A.R. Low testosterone in male endurance-trained distance runners: Impact of years in training. *Hormones* **2018**, *17*, 137–139. [CrossRef] [PubMed]
47. Krsmanovic, L.Z.; Hu, L.; Leung, P.-K.; Feng, H.; Catt, K.J. The hypothalamic GnRH pulse generator: Multiple regulatory mechanisms. *Trends Endocrinol. Metab.* **2009**, *20*, 402–408. [CrossRef] [PubMed]
48. MacConnie, S.E.; Barkan, A.; Lampman, R.M.; Schork, M.A.; Beitins, I.Z. Decreased hypothalamic gonadotropin-releasing hormone secretion in male marathon runners. *N. Engl. J. Med.* **1986**, *315*, 411–417. [CrossRef] [PubMed]
49. Hooper, D.R.; Kraemer, W.J.; Saenz, C.; Schill, K.E.; Focht, B.C.; Volek, J.S.; Maresh, C.M. The presence of symptoms of testosterone deficiency in the exercise-hypogonadal male condition and the role of nutrition. *Eur. J. Appl. Physiol.* **2017**, *117*, 1349–1357. [CrossRef]
50. De Souza, M.J.; Arce, J.C.; Pescatello, L.S.; Scherzer, H.S.; Luciano, A.A. Gonadal hormones and semen quality in male runners. *Int. J. Sports Med.* **1994**, *15*, 383–391. [CrossRef]
51. Flynn, M.G.; Pizza, F.X.; Brolinson, P.G. Hormonal responses to excessive training: Influence of cross training. *Int. J. Sports Med.* **1997**, *18*, 191–196. [CrossRef]
52. Hackney, A.C. Hypogonadism in Exercising Males: Dysfunction or Adaptive-Regulatory Adjustment? *Front. Endocrinol. (Lausanne)* **2020**, *11*, 1–16. [CrossRef]
53. De Souza, M.J.; Koltun, K.J.; Williams, N.I. The Role of Energy Availability in Reproductive Function in the Female Athlete Triad and Extension of its Effects to Men: An Initial Working Model of a Similar Syndrome in Male Athletes. *Sports Med.* **2019**, *49*, 125–137. [CrossRef]

54. Bellastella, G.; Pane, E.; Iorio, S.; De Bellis, A.; Sinisi, A.A. Seasonal variations of plasma gonadotropin, prolactin, and testosterone levels in primary and secondary hypogonadism: Evidence for an independent testicular role. *J. Endocrinol. Investig.* **2013**, *36*, 339–342.
55. Chen, C.; Zhai, H.; Cheng, J.; Weng, P.; Chen, Y.; Li, Q.; Wang, C.; Xia, F.; Wang, N.; Lu, Y. Causal Link between Vitamin D and Total Testosterone in Men: A Mendelian Randomization Analysis. *J. Clin. Endocrinol. Metab.* **2019**, *104*, 3148–3156. [CrossRef]
56. Lombardi, G.; Vitale, J.A.; Logoluso, S.; Logoluso, G.; Cocco, N.; Cocco, G.; Cocco, A.; Banfi, G. Circannual rhythm of plasmatic vitamin D levels and the association with markers of psychophysical stress in a cohort of Italian professional soccer players. *Chronobiol. Int.* **2017**, *34*, 471–479. [CrossRef] [PubMed]
57. Wong, H.K.; Hoermann, R.; Grossmann, M. Reversible male hypogonadotropic hypogonadism due to energy deficit. *Clin. Endocrinol. (Oxf.)* **2019**, *91*, 3–9. [CrossRef] [PubMed]
58. Cumming, D.C.; Wheeler, G.D.; McColl, E.M. The effects of exercise on reproductive function in men. *Sports Med.* **1989**, *7*, 1–17. [CrossRef] [PubMed]
59. Hackney, A.C.; Viru, A. Twenty-four-hour cortisol response to multiple daily exercise sessions of moderate and high intensity. *Clin. Physiol.* **1999**, *19*, 178–182. [CrossRef] [PubMed]
60. Flynn, M.G.; Pizza, F.X.; Boone, J.B.; Andres, F.F.; Michaud, T.A.; Rodriguez-Zayas, J.R. Indices of training stress during competitive running and swimming seasons. *Int. J. Sports Med.* **1994**, *15*, 21–26. [CrossRef]
61. Gillespie, C.A.; Edgerton, V.R. The role of testosterone in exercise-induced glycogen supercompensation. *Horm. Metab. Res.* **1970**, *2*, 364–366. [CrossRef]
62. Kuoppasalmi, K.; Adlercreutz, H. Interaction between catabolic and anabolic steroid hormones in muscular exercise. *Exerc. Endocrinol.* **1985**, 65–98. [CrossRef]
63. Smith, R.P.; Coward, R.M.; Kovac, J.R.; Lipshultz, L.I. The evidence for seasonal variations of testosterone in men. *Maturitas* **2013**, *74*, 208–212. [CrossRef]
64. Jürimäe, J.; Purge, P.; Jürimäe, T. Adiponectin and stress hormone responses to maximal sculling after volume-extended training season in elite rowers. *Metabolism* **2006**, *55*, 13–19. [CrossRef]
65. Hartley, L.H.; Mason, J.W.; Hogan, R.P.; Jones, L.G.; Kotchen, T.A.; Mougey, E.H.; Wherry, F.E.; Pennington, L.L.; Ricketts, P.T. Multiple hormonal responses to prolonged exercise in relation to physical training. *J. Appl. Physiol.* **1972**, *33*, 607–610. [CrossRef]
66. Borghouts, L.B.; Keizer, H.A. Exercise and insulin sensitivity: A review. *Int. J. Sports Med.* **2000**, *21*, 1–12. [CrossRef] [PubMed]

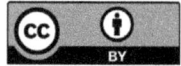

© 2020 by the authors. Licensee MDPI, Basel, Switzerland. This article is an open access article distributed under the terms and conditions of the Creative Commons Attribution (CC BY) license (http://creativecommons.org/licenses/by/4.0/).

MDPI
St. Alban-Anlage 66
4052 Basel
Switzerland
Tel. +41 61 683 77 34
Fax +41 61 302 89 18
www.mdpi.com

International Journal of Environmental Research and Public Health Editorial Office
E-mail: ijerph@mdpi.com
www.mdpi.com/journal/ijerph

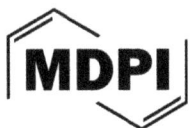

www.ingramcontent.com/pod-product-compliance
Lightning Source LLC
LaVergne TN
LVHW070510100526
838202LV00014B/1829